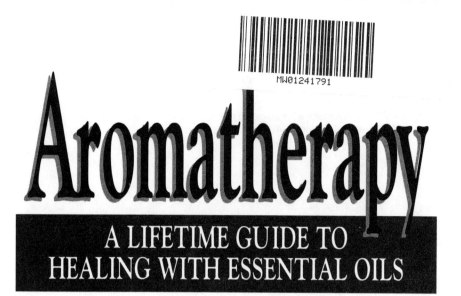

Aromatherapy

A LIFETIME GUIDE TO HEALING WITH ESSENTIAL OILS

VALERIE GENNARI COOKSLEY

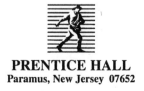

PRENTICE HALL
Paramus, New Jersey 07652

Library of Congress Cataloging-in-Publication Data

Cooksley, Valerie.
    Aromatherapy : a lifetime guide to healing with essential oils/
Valerie Cooksley.
        p.   cm.
    Includes bibliographical references and index.
    ISBN 0-13-349424-1 (cloth).—ISBN 0-13-349432-2 (pbk.)
    1.Aromatherapy—Popular works.   I.Title.
RM666.A68C66   1996   95-53852
615′.321—dc20   CIP

Printed in the United States of America

10 9 8 7 6 5 4   (C)   10 9 8   (P)

ISBN 0-13-349424-1 (C)   ISBN 0-13-349432-2 (P)

This book is reference work based on research by the author. The opinions expressed herein
are not necessarily those of or endorsed by the publisher. The directions stated in this book are
in no way to be considered as a substitute for consultation with a duly licensed doctor.

ATTENTION: CORPORATIONS AND SCHOOLS
Prentice Hall books are available at quantity discounts with bulk purchase for
educational, business, or sales promotional use. For information, please write to: Prentice
Hall Career & Personal Development Special Sales, 240 Frisch Court, Paramus, New
Jersey 07652. Please supply: title of book, ISBN number, quantity, how the book will be
used, date needed.

PRENTICE HALL
Career & Personal Development
Paramus, NJ 07652
A Simon & Schuster Company

On the World Wide Web at http://www.phdirect.com

Prentice-Hall International (UK) Limited, *London*
Prentice-Hall of Australia Pty. Limited, *Sydney*
Prentice-Hall Canada Inc., *Toronto*
Prentice-Hall Hispanoamericana, S.A., *Mexico*
Prentice-Hall of India Private Limited, *New Delhi*
Prentice-Hall of Japan, Inc., *Tokyo*
Simon & Schuster Asia Pte. Ltd., *Singapore*
Editora Prentice-Hall do Brasil, Ltda., *Rio de Janeiro*

This book is dedicated to my parents, my family, and to those special people who have touched my life with their positive influence and support, and to the Creator, whose gifts of nature leave me awed and humbled.

Acknowledgment

It is with heartfelt appreciation that I thank the following people for their contributions to this book and to my profession:

Marguerite Scace, who lovingly encouraged me to make nursing a career and who now rests in the arms of the Great Physician.

Martha Petit, who introduced me as a young girl to the healing powers of nature through her simple wisdom and generous teachings. Martha, I will never forget our walks through the woods. You are an angel whose presence will forever touch me.

Beth Tait, whose strength and connection to the earth continue to inspire me.

Dr. Peter Grimm for his commitment to healing and patient education, and to Dr. Bruce Milliman for his brilliant insights into natural medicine. You've both shown me the positive virtues of physician as facilitator.

Kate Billings and Jane Gilchrist who, by example, have empowered me and supported my belief that *it can be done.*

Dr. Kurt Schnaubelt, whose scientific approach to aromatherapy helped create the foundation on which I could build.

Dr. Karen Erickson, who painstakingly reviewed the book for herbal and medical accuracy, and shared her wealth of knowledge in the naturopathic and midwifery fields.

This book would never have been written without the support and dedication of the following:

Doug Corcoran, my editor, who had this vision and asked me to share in it.

Sharon Faiola-Petersen, who helped me take those first steps through her creative writing and enthusiasm. Your talents gave form to this vision.

The Pacific Institute of Aromatherapy, Essex Laboratories, Inc., Aroma Vera, Energy Essentials, Natus Corporation, Noevir U.S.A., Inc., Joseph B. Stephenson Foundation, Inc., American Cancer Society Washington Division, Inc., and Wellness Productions Inc., who have all contributed time and valuable information.

The skilled and dedicated people at Prentice Hall Publishing who had a creative hand in the production of this book.

Last, but certainly not least, I wish to warmly thank my dear family: my husband Bill for his belief in me and steadfast support, and my three sons, Jeremy, Kristopher, and Ryan, who have patiently endured many months of mediocre meals and a pre-occupied Mom while I buried myself in this project. And to my sister Christine, whose words of encouragement were immensely needed and continue to be appreciated.

Introduction

Today, more and more of us are seeking simple, safe, and natural alternatives—everything from healthcare and cosmetics to even the materials we build our homes with.

Aromatherapy: A Lifetime Guide to Healing with Essential Oils is a down-to-earth, hands-on guide to preventative self-care and healing through aromatherapy. My hope is that you will find it so practical and easy to use, it will be found in your kitchen, bathroom, and/or bedroom, stained and scented with essential oils and worn and tattered from frequent and enthusiastic use. This book features easy-to-follow "recipes" for the reader who wants to know how to use aromatherapy in the simplest, most straightforward manner. The greater part of the book focuses on common ailments with corresponding recipes for essential oil blends and recommended lifestyle changes. I have included case histories and personal stories of how aromatherapy has impacted my health and lifestyle as well as those of many others.

This book is designed for anyone interested in using natural alternatives to complement conventional medicine: the young mother who desires natural care for her family, the avid athlete who needs relief from aching muscles, the environmentally conscious person who avoids harmful chemicals, or the stressed-out executive who needs to unwind.

I have made an effort in this book to dispel many of the misconceptions about aromatherapy. Essential oils are not magical or mystical things.

You do not need to wear love beads or Birkenstocks to enjoy them, nor do you need a graduate degree in biochemistry to use them correctly. They are as real and down-to-earth as the herbs in your kitchen pantry and the flowers growing in your garden.

As with all herbal medicine, aromatherapy assists the body in balancing itself in order for healing to take place, and for a state of wellness to be maintained. An increasing number of people are now actively participating in their own healthcare, no longer surrendering to others their own personal responsibility for overall wellness. Nearly half of the "acute" conditions in the United States are now being treated without direct physician intervention.

Do not, however, misunderstand the message of this book. While aromatherapy can be used as a primary tool for healing, it should not be viewed as a replacement for medical/surgical treatment or diagnosis. Rather, it is a *complementary* therapy which can assist your body during the healing process. It embraces holistic healing through lifestyle enhancement, natural prevention, and botanical medicine. The key to success in healing everyday common ailments is found in prevention and early treatment. Be patient with the more chronic ailments, those which have existed for a long time, as they usually take longer to remedy. And please do not try to treat a serious condition on your own, but consult a physician.

Aromatherapy has survived the ages and now is experiencing a reawakening for good reason. What better way to improve our health, appearance, and the environment around us, than through the sensual, "scentual" natural pleasures of aromatherapy. Humankind has come around full circle, returning to nature, to find health and wellness.

Contents

PART ONE

Introduction to Aromatherapy
1

Chapter 1
3
WHAT YOU NEED TO KNOW

PART TWO

A Self-Help Guide to Natural Healing with Essential Oils and Successful Recipes for over 100 Health Challenges
21

Chapter 2   25
AROMATHERAPY TREATMENTS
FOR THE DIGESTIVE SYSTEM

Chapter 3   60
AROMATHERAPY TREATMENTS FOR EYE, EAR, NOSE, AND THROAT PROBLEMS

Chapter 4   92
AROMATHERAPY TREATMENTS FOR THE RESPIRATORY SYSTEM

Chapter 8   197
AROMATHERAPY TREATMENTS FOR CHILDREN

PART THREE

Enjoying The Aromatic Lifestyle: Three of the Most Common Methods Made Simple
289

Chapter 11   291
THE AROMATIC BATH—YOUR PERSONAL SPA

Chapter 12   306
ALL-OVER BODY TREATMENTS AND SPECIAL CARE FOR SMALL AREAS

Chapter 13   320
BREATHE EASY—THE IN'S AND OUT'S OF INHALATION

PART FOUR
The Pure Essentials
337

Chapter 14   339
ESSENTIAL OIL REFERENCE GUIDE

Chapter 15   367
BLENDING HOW-TO'S AND HELPFUL HINTS

Index   385

"The Lord hath created medicines out of the earth;
and he that is wise will not abhor them."

Ecclesiaticus 38:4

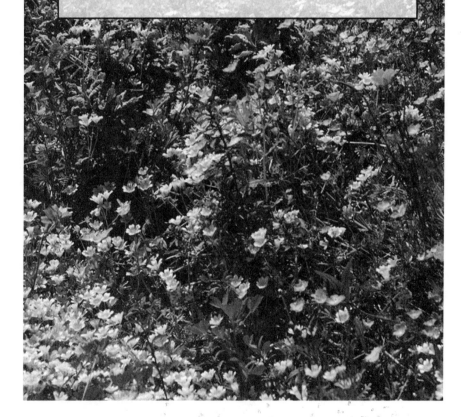

PART ONE

Introduction
to Aromatherapy

CHAPTER 1

What You Need to Know

However eager you may be to dive right into chapters covering your areas of special interest or personal needs, you first need to go over some of the "essentials" so you will be able to better utilize the information in this book. Most of what I will be sharing with you concerns common ailments and their treatment with aromatherapy applications.

This chapter deals with the fundamentals of aromatherapy. I have attempted to demystify this natural herbal healing art, as well as to simplify its medicinal applications for safe and confident use of essential oils in promoting a lifestyle of health and wellness. If you want more in-depth information, you can refer to the later parts of this book for essential oil characteristics, methods of application, and blending instructions. Others of you may wish to refer directly to that ailment chapter that is of particular personal interest.

For a definition many people can relate to, aromatherapy simply means the "study of scent." I invite you into a whole new fragrant world that awaits you, blending ancient knowledge and art with scientific knowledge to support natural healing for a lifetime.

Aromatherapy is more thoroughly defined as the *skilled* and *controlled* use of essential oils for physical and emotional health and well-being. Science is now confirming what has been known for centuries: essential oils have healing properties on both physical and emotional lev-

3

els. Absorbed through the skin and via the olfactory-brain connection through inhalation, they have been considered among the most therapeutic and rejuvenating of all botanical extracts throughout the ages.

What Are Essential Oils and How Are They Produced?

Only nature can produce whole essential oils. They are tiny droplets contained in glands, glandular hairs, sacs, or veins of different plant parts: leaves, stems, bark, flowers, roots, and fruits. They are the "essence" of that particular plant form. They are responsible for giving the botanical its unique scent and "fingerprint." When you brush against your rosemary bush in the garden, or sniff a rose growing in the hedgerow, you experience the essential oils being released into the air. Essential oils are volatile, which means they turn from a liquid to a gas very readily at room temperature or higher. They aren't oily at all, but rather a water-like fluid. Rupture of the essential oil glands, or simply heat exposure, will help release these natural, memory-evoking, volatile scents. This is one of the reasons why we experience more fragrances in the summer than in the winter. Obviously there are fewer plants blooming in winter, but also because the weather is so much colder, and the air denser, molecules are moving at a slower rate and the essential oils are less likely to evaporate. This makes it more difficult for us to pick up their scent.

Volatile comes from the Latin root "volare," which means "to fly."

At the Geneva Conference, Essential oils were defined as: "the exclusive product of the extraction of the volatile aromatic principles contained in the substances of which they bear the name." Essential oils are highly concentrated forms of the plant part in which they were derived; however, the oils can also change composition and location from one part of the plant to another. Take the Orange Tree, for example. Neroli oil is obtained from the blossoms, orange oil from the citrus fruit itself, and petitgrain essential oil from the leaves of the tree.

To give you an idea of how potent these oils are, consider this: one drop of essential oil equals about thirty cups of herbal tea in terms of concentration. When you make a cup of chamomile tea by pouring boiling water over the dried herb, and letting it steep, you are extracting miniscule amounts of the essential oil present in that herbal tea along with water-sol-

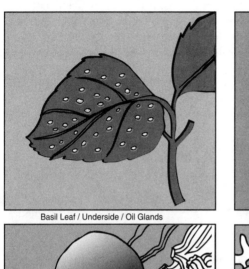

Basil Leaf / Underside / Oil Glands   Lemon Balm / Bulging Oil Gland

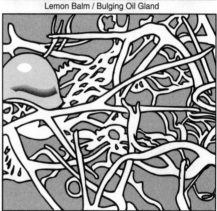

Oil Gland of Thyme   Lavender Bud Oil Gland

Essential Oil Glands of Plants

Plants contain from .01 to 10% essential oil content. The average amount found in most aromatic plants is about 1 to 2%. It is interesting to note that the amount nature has provided in its original plant form strongly correlates to the amounts used in aromatherapy applications.

uble constituents. Sometimes these oils can be 75 to 100 times more concentrated than the fresh herb. This is one reason why they should be used with caution and knowledge of their potency.

Steam distillation is the most common process for obtaining the essential oils from the plant. The steam is forced into a vat of plant material, where it breaks open and ruptures these glands releasing the precious oil. Following a cold-water bath (cooling phase), the volatile oils are collected to be bottled. This is an economical and popular method used. However, it still may take hundreds, or even thousands of pounds of plant parts to distill a single pound of the essential oil. Therefore, some essential oils will vary greatly in their cost.

Steam Distillation Process

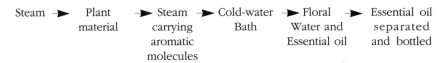

Steam → Plant material → Steam carrying aromatic molecules → Cold-water Bath → Floral Water and Essential oil → Essential oil separated and bottled

Essential oils can also be squeezed or cold-expressed from the fruit. This is how many citrus essential oils are obtained, since their oils are present in the rind of the fruit, and the heat from the steam method would alter their composition. This method is called *expression.*

Experiment: Squeeze a lemon or orange rind into a candle flame to see tiny fireworks. Because essential oils are flammable, you can see firsthand that they are present.

Expression Process

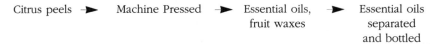

Citrus peels → Machine Pressed → Essential oils, fruit waxes → Essential oils separated and bottled

Another method employed is called *solvent extraction.* Technically, this process does not produce an essential oil. Rather the outcome is a highly scented concentrate used primarily in the perfume and food industry. Solvents are used to "pull out" the soluble plant molecules; therefore they are not complete. Resins, concretes, absolutes, and pomades are often

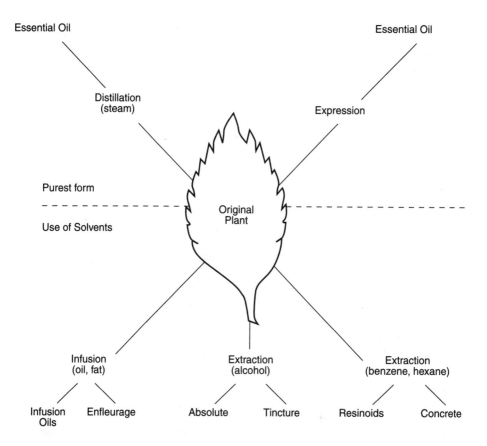

Various Extraction Methods

Note the only *true essential oils* are obtained from *distillation* and *expression* methods. These are the highest grade and purest essential oils produced and are the most desirable for aromatherapy application.

All other methods shown actually produce aromatic products, which contain various proportions of the essential oil along with the solvent. They may contain large amounts of solvent (tincture, enfluerage, infusion oils) or minute traces of the solvent (absolute, resinoids). These are primarily employed in the perfume industry (absolutes, concrete), herbal medicine (tinctures, infusion oils), and skincare (infusion oils).

the products of this type of extraction. *Enfluerage* is a form of solvent extraction whereby the plant, usually its floral parts, is layered onto fat in several layers. Over time and many layerings, the fat absorbs many of the scented molecules. Because some plants have inherently low essential oil content, and other methods would destroy these fragile essences, this method has its advantages. In what is one of the earliest forms of obtaining isolated essences by an ancient culture, the Egyptians used this method to make scented unguents and various cosmetics.

How to Know When It's the "Real Thing"

There are several variables that can affect the quality and quantity of a particular essential oil. The quality and intensity of essential oils vary due to the plant variety, time of harvest, soil condition, method of cultivation, and the process of extraction. All these factors play a significant role in the end result. It is important to know the origin of the oils and the reputation of the company providing them. Beware of synthetic versions made possible by recent advances in chemistry. When a very high quality essential oil is used, less of it is needed to obtain the desired effect. Also, it is important to note that essential oils obtained from cold pressing and distillation methods often produce the highest quality oils for aromatherapy use. When using a cheaper, perhaps adulterated oil, you naturally increase your risks considerably. This is why dealing with reputable producers and distributors is important. As a consumer, you can insist that manufacturers assure that their oils are pure and 100% natural.

Some aromatherapy companies are now offering their services of essential oil testing to guarantee purity. This procedure is called *gas chromatography* and involves very expensive, highly technical measurement and computation equipment.

A highly trained chemist will be able to decipher whether or not the test sample is genuine or adulterated and with what, as well as where and even what time of year the oil was produced. Chemists have been able to duplicate some of the major chemical constituents in the laboratory. Only a portion of the whole essential oil is synthetically produced in this way. Many, if not all, aromatherapists believe the "whole" or entire essential oil in its natural form should be used to insure its greatest therapeutic value. Otherwise, one increases the risk of toxicity.

Gas chromatography shows the "fingerprint" of an essential oil.

Essential oils should be purchased and stored in dark-colored glass bottles, such as amber. Because of the variables in production discussed earlier, you can expect to see a cost variation among different oils. For example, a shelf of 1/3-ounce bottles of different essential oils can range from $5.00 to $30.00. However, if you find a whole range of essential oils all the same price, that probably means they have been "stretched" or adulterated with cheaper synthetic scents to get them cheap enough to equal out. Ask the store owner the place of purchase and if they are 100% pure, authentic essential oils. Read labels carefully.

Bulgarian Rose oil takes approximately four thousand pounds of hand- picked flower petals to make 1 pound of oil, making it one of the most expensive oils that can be purchased. In comparison, Lavender, French fine, yields one pound of essential oil from about one hundred pounds of plant material. Yields will vary according to climate, altitude, and other variables.

If they are labeled "perfume" essential oils, "fragrance" or "potpourri" essential oils, they are of synthetic composition. It does not matter if the words "essential oil" are included; the oil is tainted in an advertising ploy to market a not-so-pure product for a great profit.

When you become more experienced with the true essences and use them regularly instead of all the synthetic fragrances you might have around the house, you will slowly be able to discern what is the "real thing" and what is probably not. Your nose will know. If you can detect a gaseous, harsh, alcohol-like odor from the bottle, the oil may have been stretched with an alcohol. Sometimes an oil is tainted with another essential oil containing similar terpenes. These could cause irritation to sensitive skin.

Genuine and authentic essential oils are the most therapeutic and will have a fuller, sweeter, and milder character. Therefore very little is needed, justifying the higher cost.

I think it's safer to learn the single essential oils before using complex mixtures of many essential oils in one blend. A good rule of thumb is to do a patch test of the single essential oil on yourself or the person for whom you are making the blend. To do this, simply put a drop of the oil on a cotton ball or swab and swipe the inside of your arm adjacent to the elbow. Some experts recommend that you cover the area with a Band-Aid, but I don't think that it's necessary. Check the area within 15 to 20 minutes. Note any redness or itching. If this type of reaction is present, do not include that oil in your aromatherapy preparation.

If you have a known allergy to a plant or fruit, most likely you will be allergic to its essential oil because it is a highly concentrated form of the plant from which it originated. So let's say that you are sensitive to the mint family. You pick up a bottle of body oil labeled Herbal Garden Delight. It boasts a combination of 12 pure essential oils but fails to list every essence contained therein. This poses a risk to you if it contains peppermint, spearmint, or any menthol-related oils. When you have definite allergies or sensitivities, either make your own blends or get a definitive list of ingredients from any highly complex blends.

In some of my workshops I often pass around synthetic versions of lavender or rose scent and let the class experience firsthand the differences between them and the true fine French lavender or Bulgarian rose. Occasionally, the genuine scent surprises them, an indication that we are becoming more familiar with a scented world today. Synthetic aromas are everywhere—from laundry soap, personal care products, household cleansers, and so forth to the new sneakers and women's hosiery we purchase.

Another test for the "real thing" is to put a drop of essential oil on a piece of blotting paper or heavy construction paper and allow it to evaporate for a few minutes. Because they are volatile in nature, the oils tend to evaporate very quickly. The vast majority do not leave an oily ring on the paper, like lavender, all citrus oils, cedarwood, rosemary, all mints, etc. Look for the spot to completely disappear or else it may be diluted in a vegetable oil! Or you can put a drop between two fingers and check for a greasy feel.

Exceptions to this rule are a few essential oils that have a naturally heavy and resinous quality, such as myrrh, patchouli, and most oleoresins, absolutes, and concretes.

How and Where to Purchase Essential Oils

Now that you are aware of the basics for knowing the "real thing" from the rest, the next step is purchasing a few bottles of essential oils for your own. First, decide which essential oils you wish to include in your aromatherapy apothecary. It will not be easy to narrow the choices down to a few, but you are best starting with one, two, or three different ones and really getting to know them well before moving on to a multitude.

Focus on what your intentions are in purchasing them. Are they for a specific recipe, ailment treatment, or a personal favorite scent? There are several I suggest you have in your apothecary because they are very useful both around the house and for personal body preparations. Lavender, Geranium, Peppermint, Lemon, Eucalyptus, Tea Tree, and Cedarwood readily come to mind as examples of common, affordable, safe essential oils to have. Most common in the marketplace are the 1/3-ounce and 1/2-ounce size amber bottles. However, you can order larger sizes directly from most companies if you wish to order in bulk quantities.

You can start by visiting your health food store, local natural grocer, or consumer's cooperative to find out what they may carry. Ask questions about the purity and origin of their essential oils. Test the sample bottles if they have any. You may want to write down the company name and address and write to it directly to get the necessary information before you make any major purchases. Most stores will not accept open bottles for return. If in doubt, ask a salesperson. In the back of this book, under "The Resource Place," you will find mail order information for ordering direct.

I recommend purchasing the typical 1/3- or 1/2-ounce size bottles. This is a reasonable amount to start with and will last quite a while, considering you use only a few drops at a time.

Safekeeping of These Precious Essences

The best way to store your essential oils is in amber, cobalt blue, or other colored glass to protect them from the light. You also want to keep them out of direct sunlight and away from any heat source, preferably in a cool, dark cabinet. I have an antique china closet in my office where I keep over 200 essences. And of course I keep others in the first aid kit, in the kitchen, and the bathroom for convenience.

Because of their potency, please keep oils away from and out of reach of small children. My children are old enough now and respect these precious bottles that hold the scents they have gotten to know so well.

Another idea for keeping your essential oils safe is to keep them well-labeled. There is nothing worse than finding a bottle not labeled and hence not knowing its exact contents. I find using small labels covered with clear tape protects the label from smearing. Do not use rubber stoppers or rubber eye-dropper type lids to store your pure essences long-term. Over time the rubber parts will be softened and destroyed by the essential oils gassing off in the bottle. Always keep the screw tops on tightly, since the oils do evaporate quickly.

For optimum shelf life it is best to re-bottle your oils if they are below half full, since the air inside the vacant space encourages oxidation, or, in other words, a shorter shelf life. Citrus oils are very susceptible to oxidizing and I find if they are kept in half-empty bottles they do not last nearly as long. When these guidelines are kept and storage is ideal, you can expect most of your oils to last 2 to 5 years. (Pots of unguents found in the ancient tombs of Egypt, thousands of years old, remain scented today.)

When an essential oil is mixed with a vegetable oil (carrier), the shelf life of that preparation will equal that of the vegetable oil (carrier). For example, let's say you made a wonderful body oil that consists of lavender and ylang-ylang essential oils in a carrier base of sweet almond oil. The sweet almond oil will determine the shelf life of this aromatherapy blend, not the essential oils. See Chapter 15, *Blending How-To's,* for tips on how to prolong the shelf life of your carrier oils.

You may also want to keep your aromatherapy collection away from homeopathic medicines, since they can be affected by volatile oils such as camphor, eucalyptus, and mints. Also, be cautioned that essential oils can harm some varnished wood surfaces and some plastics, especially Plexiglass. So if you are mixing oils or using them in a diffuser, it would be safest to do so on glass, ceramic, metal, Formica, stone, or natural wood surfaces, just in case of accidental spills.

An Open Invitation—Two Ways Essential Oils Enter the Body

Essential oils penetrate the body in two ways: through the nose and the skin. The olfactory system, the nose-brain association, is the most direct connection we have with the environment. Think about how sensitive our sense of smell is—approximately 10,000 times more sensitive than any other sensory organ we possess. The fact that our sense of smell is linked directly to the limbic brain where emotions, memory, and certain regulatory functions are seated makes me realize how this important route of absorption is neglected in everyday life. I think in the near future we will begin to see medicine given more and more via this route.

> The dominant nostril of a person correlates with the dominant hand.

Have you ever experienced déja-vu? When that familiar, sometimes vivid memory all of a sudden comes flooding back from your childhood or recent past and you don't know why? It may be because of this nose-brain link we're talking about. Perhaps you smelled something that brought back a memory tied to a certain scent. Like when I smell lilacs or peonies I am reminded, or should I say "carried back," to my childhood days with visions of my mother's perennial flower garden. Lavender scent may bring back a memory of your grandmother's linen closet, or perhaps an after-shave cologne may remind you of a boyfriend you once had.

These scent-memory linkages may not always engender a positive effect. For example, a student in one of my classes once shared that she had an uncle whom she strongly disliked growing up as a child. He had smoked a cigar, and reeked of the smell always. To this day when she smells that familiar cigar scent, which is so unpleasant to her, she is reminded of this uncle. As a matter of fact, some leading-edge psychotherapists are exploring this relationship between scent and memory, by using specific scents, like vanilla, to bring back childhood memories.

Because our experiences are so very different, these scent-memory bonds will be unique to us. I will share a personal story to demonstrate. I grew up on a farm in the Berkshires. We had the typical farm animals— cows, pigs, chickens, rabbits, etc. My husband, on the other hand, grew up on the southern tip of Florida, where there were few farms. Now picture us driving in the countryside, car windows down, on a wonderfully warm summer day and driving past a dairy farm. I take a deep breath and am reminded of long summer days on the farm, and remember my favorite cow, Red Riding Hood. The smell of cow manure somehow smells good to me. Even when I use it in the gardens every spring, it doesn't have a negative effect on me. But can you imagine what my husband's reaction is? "Hurry! Roll the windows up! There's a dairy farm ahead!"

> Coho Salmon's olfactory bulb expands almost 70% when it's time to head downstream. It is survival of the species that they are able to "smell" their way home.

There are several variables involved in this route of entry. How keen one's sense of smell is, whether someone smokes or not, will affect that person's ability to smell; some head injuries or a stroke can cause dysfunction in this area as well. It is between the ages of 20 and 40 when our ability to smell is at its peak. And although the rhythm of our bodies and the time of day affect this sense, nighttime is when it is most sensitive. Women have the greatest acuity when scent is involved, especially during ovulation. Studies have shown that women who live together, as in college dormitories, etc., experience synchronized menstrual cycles over a period of time.

Both dogs and pigs are known for their keen sense of smell. It is their long nose structure that helps them in this. The longer the nose, the greater amount of scent molecules can be captured and held in the nasal cavity where the olfactory hairs can "pick up" the scent.

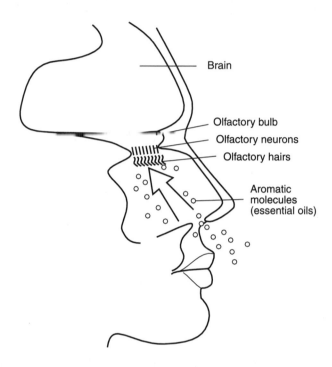

Olfactory System

Incoming **aromatic molecules** enter the body via the nose with every breath inhaled. The nose is structured in such a way as to capture and hold aromatic molecules and to keep the olfactory hairs (cilia) moist.

The **olfactory hairs** pick up the odor molecules and bind them to receptors. Messages are sent along neurons to the **olfactory bulb** and directly to the limbic brain. This ancient area of the brain is where moods, sexual urges, and emotions are seated. And all this takes place within thousandths of a second!

We possess about 5 million **olfactory neuron** cells. These cells are the same type of cells the brain is made of. But unlike brain cells, that last a lifetime, these important cells replace themselves every 1 to 2 months.

The second way for essential oils to penetrate the body is through the skin, our largest organ. Our skin, which is called the integumentary system, is constantly shedding and renewing itself. It helps regulate the body's temperature, by sweating to cool it and by shivering to warm it. It is a two-way structure, which is designed to keep some things in and some out. There are pores, or holes, which allow the free passage of the needed things in, and the no-longer-needed, waste products out.

Because essential oils are organic in nature, and have a very inherently low molecular weight, they are absorbed through the pores and hair follicles of the skin. Unlike synthetic chemicals or drugs, essential oils do not accumulate in the body. They are excreted in the urine, feces, perspiration, and our breath. It takes anywhere from 15 minutes to 12 hours for these essences to be fully absorbed. It takes about 3 to 6 hours to expel or metabolize them in a normal healthy body, and up to 12 to 14 hours for an unhealthy, obese body. One factor that will make this time interval variable is the condition of the skin. Poor circulation, thick toughened skin, or excessive cellulite or fat may slow down the rate of absorption, whereas heat, water, aerobic exercise, and broken or damaged skin will cause increased absorption. Also, the carrier used may affect the absorption rate, since some vegetable oils are heavier than others.

> "The individual can be influenced externally, through the skin, and for this reason all the care which can be given to the latter to make it apt to receive influences and to react are of major importance." (Marguerite Maury)

The method of excretion differs among oils. Some like Juniper and Sandalwood are excreted through the urine, as their aroma can be detected there. Garlic, as you probably know firsthand if you eat a lot of Italian food, exits the body through our breath. Geranium essential oil, which assists in increasing circulatory functions, is detected in the perspiration. Essential oils basically have a low potential to be physically habit-forming because they are eliminated extremely quickly through the skin and organs. Hence, there is no residual or accumulative effect to withdraw from or become "addicted" to.

> Experiment: Cut a fresh garlic clove in half and rub on the sole of your foot. You will detect a garlic odor on your breath within 15 to 30 minutes.

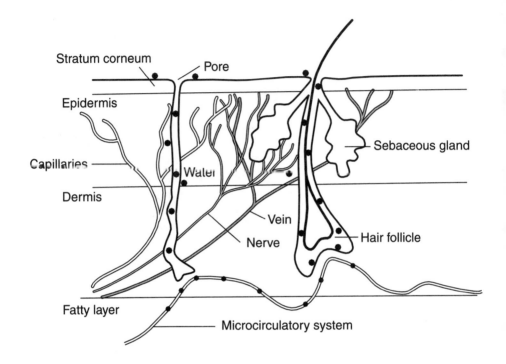

Cross-Section of Skin

The essential oil is applied to the skin, via water, lotion or oil. The essential oil penetrates The skin through the pores and hair follicles, where they are absorbed by tiny
capillaries. They eventually reach the microcirculatory system (bloodstream). Once
in the bloodstream, they can affect adjacent organs and structures and circulate
throughout the entire body, until they are excreted (urine, feces, perspiration, exhalation).

Common-Sense Safety

Not *all* essential oils are beneficial to health as you might expect, just like not *all* herbs are good for you. Something that is "natural" (derived from nature; not artificial) implies a positive effect on health, but does not guarantee it. There are some essential oils that are dangerous to use. Of the hundreds of oils produced and marketed, about 100 are commonly utilized by trained aromatherapists on a regular basis. Of this number you can count on 30 or so to be relatively safe, affordable, and readily available for *you* to use at home with confidence. These are the ones I focus on in the *Essential Oil Reference* section of Chapter 14. Throughout this book I refer to the common names given to essential oils (the plant from which it was derived); however, it is crucial that you refer to the individual listings of each essence in Chapter 14 for the specific botanical name to insure the correct essential oil is used.

I hope you will respect these oils for what they are: highly concentrated plant constituents possessing potent medicinal and cosmetic qualities. Some relax, sedate, balance, rejuvenate, invigorate, and even enhance memory. They have many healthful properties such as being anti-inflammatory, analgesic, anti-bacterial and anti-spasmodic. But there are some that are skin irritants, phototoxic, neurotoxic, or cancer-causing while still others are abortive, or not to be used during pregnancy or on children. That is why this chapter must precede all others.

When using aromatherapy for small children, *always* dilute the normal/adult amount by *half* (or more) to make it safe for the younger ones. This book deals with adult preparations unless otherwise noted, as in the special chapter on children's ailments. Those found in Chapter 8 are already adjusted for children. (Note smaller amounts of essential oils used for the same amount of carrier oil.)

During pregnancy, there are some essential oils *definitely not* to be used. (See list at the end of this section). Because some essential oils can relax muscles, stimulate contractions, or possibly get to the baby, they are strongly advised *not* to be used during pregnancy. A few essential oils are considered abortifacients, meaning they have the potential to cause abortion. Be sure to avoid all essential oils that may be unsafe during this time. I recommend a 1% dilution (of the safe oils), instead of the typical 2% dilution, for body oils and lotions for expectant mothers. This is a conservative approach practiced by many midwives and aromatherapists in England and the United States. Essential oils are best avoided in the first trimester of pregnancy, especially if history of miscarriages is present. Only use the safe oils listed in Chapter 10, in moderation and when necessary.

I will discuss the safest and easiest methods of experiencing the healthful benefits of therapeutic essential oils, through inhalation and skin absorption, as we have discussed earlier. However, in some European countries, like France, essential oils are taken by mouth as a form of phyto-medicine. They can also be found in douches and suppositories prepared for various health conditions. In fact, aromatherapy treatment is a reimbursed therapy in Europe, and is recognized as an alternative, complementary form of natural medicine. It is both effective and cost-efficient.

Because essential oils are highly concentrated, and some are known skin irritants, the best way to use them is in diluted form. There are several essential oils that are skin "friendly" like lavender and Tea Tree. These two oils can be used "straight" or "neat," which means you can put these directly on your skin without diluting them. However, they are an exception, not the rule. Most essential oils you *must* dilute to use. Essential oils do not exist in nature in large quantities; they are tiny, microscopic droplets, unseen by the naked eye within the plant's structure in miniscule quantity. So when you embark on your experiential study of nature's gifts, start by using highly diluted essential oils. In fact, high concentrations of essential oil usage can produce the opposite effect. For example, lavender essential oil can cause restlessness, agitation, and insomnia if too much is used rather than relaxation.

In Chapter 15: Blending How-To's and Helpful Hints, I go into great detail about how to prepare your blends in proper and safe dilution, along with helpful charts. Feel free to go there now and check it out. If you refer to it when preparing your essential oil blends, you will be practicing aromatherapy with safety and peace of mind.

The following lists have been prepared with that utmost safety in mind. There are a few essential oils that fall into gray areas, that is, are debated among health care professionals as to whether or not they are safe. Not only must we consider the differences among essential oils, but also those differences among the individuals who are using them. There is always a risk to generalizing for the "norm" while preparing these guide lists, when in reality we are dealing with people. Painstaking effort has been made in cross-referencing the most recent authoritative journals and publications on the subject to compile this information for you. I have taken the conservative side whenever questionable, for your safety.

Hazardous/Not Recommended for Personal Use

These *essential oils* are not advised for personal use as they can be hazardous to your health. These oils are considered toxic (oral, dermal, kidney, or liver), carcinogenic, or cautionary. Some essential oils have simply not been tested and should be avoided for obvious reasons. (Do not use unless under supervision of an experienced health care professional.)

Ajowan

Arnica

Bitter Almond

Boldo Leaf

Buchu

Calamus

Camphor (yellow or brown)

Caraway

Cassia

Cinnamon

Clove

Elecampane root

Horseradish

Jaborandi

Mugwort

Mustard

Parsley Seed

Pennyroyal

Peru Balsam

Rue

Sage

Santolina

Sassafras

Savin

Savory

Southernwood

Tansy

Thuja

Tonka bean

Wintergreen

Wormseed

Wormwood

Phototoxic Essential Oils

Increases sunburn reaction of skin (including tanning booths). Not recommended for regular use on individuals with history of skin cancer, large moles, or extensive dark freckles.

Angelica Root

All absolutes and concretes

Bergamot (expressed)

Cumin

Ginger

Grapefruit

Lemon (expressed)

Lemon verbena

Lime (expressed)

Mandarin

Orange (expressed)

Avoid During Pregnancy

All essential oils in HAZARDOUS list, in addition to the following (also see Chapter 10 for specific listings):

Aniseed

Armois

Basil

Birch

Cornmint

Fennel

Hyssop

Lavender stoechas

Lavender Cotton

Marjoram

Myrrh

Oregano

Pimenta racemosa

Plecanthrus

Star Anise

Tarragon

Irritant-Prone Essential Oils

Can cause irritation to sensitive, inflamed, or allergic skin types.

Aniseed

Basil

Fennel

Lemongrass

Peppermint (when used undiluted will cause skin irritation on all skin types)

Rosemary

Lemon Verbena

Bay

Benzoin

Citronella

Rose (in high concentrations)

Ylang ylang (in high concentrations)

All absolutes and concretes

Camphor

Let's review the Common Sense Safety points :

- Avoid the hazardous essential oils.
- Keep all essential oils out of reach of children.
- Keep away from light and heat sources.
- Do not take orally.
- Dilute. Dilute. Dilute!
- Use 1% (or less) dilution during pregnancy.
- Be aware of individual sensitivities and/or allergies.
- Do not use on the eyes or near eyes.
- Do Skin Patch test if prone to sensitivities.
- Use extra care on broken or damaged skin.
- Avoid the phototoxic essential oils with history of skin cancer.
- Remember essential oils are potent medicine and cosmetic agents.
- Only use therapeutic genuine and authentic essential oils.

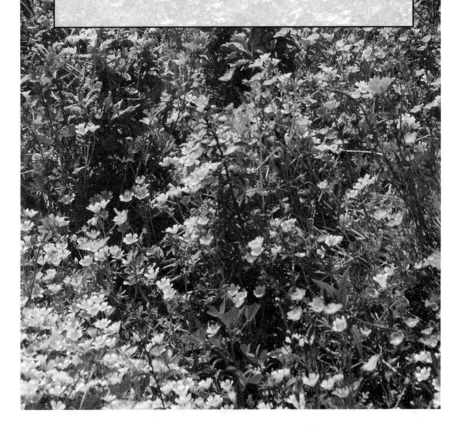

PART TWO

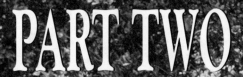

A Self-Help Guide
to Natural Healing
with Essential Oils

This part of the book will give you the tools you will need to begin to heal yourself and your family. While education and prevention are essential, the keys to your success lie in listening to your body and taking responsibility for your personal wellness. You must be prepared to make lifestyle changes and decisions around natural health, and choose safe alternatives over unnatural or toxic medications to demonstrate your commitment to complete wellness. Aromatherapy supports a healthy lifestyle and addresses many common ailments and health challenges.

This compilation of aromatherapy, herbal remedies, and recommended lifestyle changes is based on years of personal and client-based case histories and observation, as well as traditional and historical usage. The ailments or conditions discussed in the following nine chapters are not isolated circumstances, but rather a sign that the holistic health system is unbalanced, or in need of support. For simplicity and easy reference, however, the material is organized according to body systems, common ailment categories, special populations, and mental-emotional health challenges. *Before using any of the recipes included in this section, please reference the essential oil safety precautions by reviewing their individual listings in Chapter 14.*

In other words, I believe our state of health must be addressed holistically to be truly wellness-centered, as opposed to the classic Western way of thinking which attacks the symptom and ignores the cause of the disease process. A very basic interpretation of the holistic approach to wellness is to imagine spokes of a wheel. Each spoke plays an important role in the working condition of the entire wheel. If one or more spokes is out of alignment or is weak, the wheel becomes unbalanced and, with time, will no longer work properly. Our diet, lifestyle, work habits, quality of leisure time, environment, emotional support system, and other factors form the holistic view of our individual lives. One or more of these factors in stress will affect the whole, and may result in either adaptation, modification or disease. See Holistic Health Wheel.

Fact-filled descriptions of each health problem and its possible underlying causes, along with simple and convenient information for health promotion, are given prior to all aromatherapy recipes. There are positive lifestyle recommendations for each corresponding ailment where helpful. Aromatherapy recipes along with the recommendations about how to use essential oils are given in a straightforward manner so you will be able to practice this natural healing therapy in your home or workplace with safety and success.

This book is not meant to take the place of a qualified health practitioner's responsibility to diagnose and prescribe. The main purpose of this book is to provide you with the necessary natural tools to prevent and ease common everyday health challenges simply, safely, and effectively.

As a registered nurse who specialized in the treatment and care of cancer patients, I strongly believe we can do more harm than good by self-diagnosing and treating a potentially serious condition without proper and

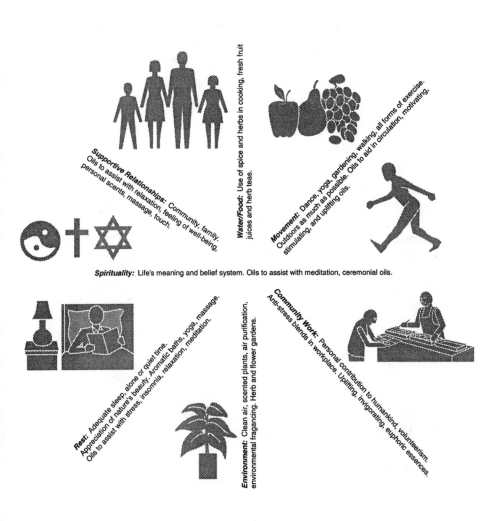

Supportive Relationships: Community, family, personal scents, massage, touch. Oils to assist with relaxation, feeling of well-being.

Water/Food: Use of spice and herbs in cooking, fresh fruit juices and herb teas.

Movement: Dance, yoga, gardening, walking, all forms of exercise. Outdoors as much as possible. Oils to aid in circulation, motivating, stimulating, and uplifting oils.

Spirituality: Life's meaning and belief system. Oils to assist with meditation, ceremonial oils.

Rest: Adequate sleep, alone or quiet time. Appreciation of nature's beauty. Aromatic baths, yoga, massage. Oils to assist with stress, insomnia, relaxation, meditation.

Environment: Clean air, scented plants, air purification, environmental fragancing. Herb and flower gardens.

Community Work: Personal contribution to humankind, volunteerism. Anti-stress blends in workplace. Uplifting, invigorating, euphoric essences.

Holistic Health Wheel

objective physical examination and diagnosis. Where appropriate, I have included cancer warning signs and other potentially serious health problems or symptoms that warrant a doctor's examination and opinion. Please do not overlook chronic problems, out-of-the-ordinary symptoms, or acute changes that could be a warning of something more serious. The several warning signals of cancer are important and are printed here for you to refer to.

Cancer Warning Signals:

1. Unusual bleeding or discharge
2. A lump or thickening
3. A sore that does not heal
4. A change in bowel or bladder habits
5. A persistent cough or hoarseness
6. Difficulty in swallowing or continual indigestion
7. A change in a wart or mole
8. Unexplained weight loss

Although the presence of any of these symptoms does not necessarily mean you have cancer, health care practitioners, along with the American Cancer Society, strongly recommend that you see your doctor immediately if any of these warning signals lasts longer than two weeks.

Symptoms that are considered to be a medical emergency are listed below and are not directly discussed in this book. If any of these conditions are experienced, immediate medical attention is necessary.

- Difficulty breathing or severe wheezing, shortness of breath
- Severe or persistent vomiting or diarrhea
- Sudden dizziness, fainting, or change in vision
- Slurred speech or loss of speech
- Convulsions
- Persistent numbness of extremities
- Temperature of 103° For higher
- Choking that cannot be cleared immediately
- Turning blue for more than a few moments
- Heavy bleeding from any source (mouth, urinary, rectum, lungs)
- Soft spot of infant's head bulging or sinking in
- Sleepiness, confusion or vomiting immediately following head injury, fall, or shock
- Sudden, severe pain in chest or abdomen

CHAPTER 2

Aromatherapy Treatments for the Digestive System

Brief Overview of the Digestive System

The digestive system is a complex interaction of various body organs with the vital function of digesting, assimilating, and eventually eliminating waste from the food we consume. Besides the organs we normally consider to be part of the digestive system (stomach, intestines, etc.), the liver, spleen, pancreas, and gall bladder all make important contributions to digestive function. This system interacts closely with the nervous system, as demonstrated by gastrointestinal symptoms such as diarrhea or stomach upset triggered by stressful experiences. As you might imagine, our emotions can deeply affect how well this system performs.

There is a delicate interrelationship among the various organs of the digestive system which utilizes an abundant amount of energy to facilitate four major steps of digestion. The following is a brief overview of the four processes that take place in the digestive tract:

1. *Ingestion* is a *mechanical* process that involves the intake of various micro- and macro-nutrients for the body to absorb. This includes chewing.

2. *Digestion* is a *chemical* process that utilizes enzymes and various chemicals to break down food even further to be used by the body.

3. *Metabolism* is a *cellular* process which turns nutrients into usable energy and body mass.

4. *Excretion* is the *elimination* process which aids in removing waste from the body in an attempt to keep it clean.

Along with aromatherapy treatments and recommendations, use of the whole herb and spices is suggested throughout this section discussing common ailments of the digestive system. Because this book focuses on skin absorption and inhalation methods for essential oils, oral administration is not discussed or advised (unless where specifically noted). However, I have included a wide variety of herbal tea recipes to take internally, along with the external application of aromatic oils and inhalation of specific essences.

In several instances, I recommend seeking a healthcare professional's opinion. The very best health and wellness approach, which would support a holistic lifestyle, would include several members of a "health care team." A medical doctor, naturopath physician, herbalist, aromatherapist, nutritionist, and chiropractor may all be part of your holistic team. They should be willing to work as a team, to communicate information regarding your health plan with you. Ultimately, however, *your* health is *your* responsibility.

Because this chapter is on common ailments of the digestive system, I have briefly discussed here various medical systems and dietary philosophies that may be helpful to you, which can be used along with aromatherapy. If you find a particular topic of interest to you, I encourage you to get more information on that subject, as it relates to your health challenge.

Natural hygiene and proper food combining: The term "food combining" refers to those combinations of foods that are compatible with each other in the digestive system. The goal is to expedite the digestion of food through the digestive system, without putrefaction or fermentation. Honoring the natural body cycles, in addition to eating foods compatible with each other, are the two major principles of natural hygiene.

The use of food to balance and heal the body: This particular view of healing uses food as medicine, with the principle of the law of opposites. The various qualities of food are considered for their effect on the body and used accordingly.

Ayurveda: A 6,000-year-old science from India. Balance is achieved by maintaining the three mind-body principles (or doshas). Balancing all five senses is important as well. The six tastes and six major food qualities are used to balance the dosha imbalance, along with aromatherapy, daily oil massage, yoga movements, and music.

Refer to the Bibliography for suggested reading on these subjects.

Let us now move on to a discussion of how these principles relate specifically to the digestive processes.

Kiss "Bad Breath" Good-bye

This is one common ailment we have all experienced one time or another. Bad breath or "halitosis" can be a problem if you have poor digestion, a food allergy, a high acid system or simply bacterial overgrowth from poor oral hygiene or infection.

Certain medical systems, such as oriental medicine and Ayurveda, use "breath" odor as a diagnosing tool for determining a patient's state of health. Conditions like diabetes (sugary, sweet odor), kidney-related problems (uric acid or urine odor) as well as digestive problems can produce a change in our breath. Some alternative health practitioners in the U.S., as well as researchers in Great Britain, are employing highly sophisticated equipment that can perform "breath analysis" to diagnose such illnesses as diabetes, cirrhosis of the liver, stomach ulcers, lung cancers, and other diseases known to produce significant changes in breath odor.

An easy and effective mouthwash is all you need for the occasional bad breath or, used daily, for prevention and good oral hygiene. Peppermint essential oil is best known for its beneficial effect on the digestive system, and most notably for bad breath. It is not coincidental that many oral care products, including mouthwashes, breath sprays, toothpaste, and candies, incorporate mint flavorings!

> Of the 300 species of peppermint, only 2 or 3 are used in the commercial industry, with the majority utilized by the dentrifice manufacturers who use peppermint oil to flavor and scent toothpaste, mouthwash, toothpicks, and dental floss.

For daily use and for bad breath use the following mouthwash three to four times daily, preferably after brushing, morning, after meals, and at bedtime. This is also good for morning breath. Your mouth will tingle with freshness. Peppermint essential oil is antibacterial, anti-inflammatory, and has a natural mint flavor and scent.

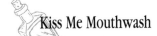

Kiss Me Mouthwash

1 cup distilled water (or Sage herbal tea)
1 teaspoon raw honey (or Sage Honey)
Peppermint essential oil 2 drops
Spearmint essential oil 2 drops
Anise essential oil 1 drop
1 teaspoon fresh lemon juice (optional)

Measure out honey into measuring cup. Add the essential oils, not exceeding 6 drops total. Mix well with the honey. Add a small amount of warm distilled water or herbal tea of sage to the honey until completely dissolved. Add the remaining amount of water. Bottle and label. Shake well before each use and swish for 30 to 60 seconds.

For optimal freshness make weekly.

Time-Saving Tip: If you find you like this mouthwash as much as my family does, and you'll be making it regularly, I recommend mixing up a large amount of the pure essential oils separately in an amber bottle. You can multiply the above essential oil drops by 10, or simply measure them out in full droppers, being sure to keep the same ratios (2:2:1). Then when it's time to make more, just count out the 5 or 6 drops that have been pre-mixed.

In many Eastern and European countries, seeds of specific plants are chewed following a meal to aid in digestion and prevent bad breath. It is the essential oils inherent in the seeds that make them effective. I keep a mix made up in a decorative jar on the counter in the kitchen, that can be passed around after dinner.

Sweet Breath Seed Mix

1 part Anise seed
1 part Fennel seed
1 part Caraway seed

Combine Anise, Fennel, and Caraway seeds in a bowl. Store openly in a dish or small jar. You can also keep them handy in your purse or office drawer. So the next time you go out to that favorite Italian restaurant for a spicy, garlic-laden meal, reach for the Sweet Breath seed mix instead of the candy. Your friends and co-workers will appreciate it.

Traditionally, Garden sage (Salvia officinalis) in tea form was used for a mouthwash. Therefore you can use a weak herbal tea preparation of sage in place of the distilled water in the previous recipe. You can also make a Sage Honey to add in place of plain raw honey. Honey has anti-inflammatory and anti-bacterial properties and acts as the carrier for the essential oils since they do not dissolve in water. A recipe for Sage Honey is given on page 85, where it is referenced as an excellent sore throat remedy.

> In Ayurvedic medicine, part of good oral hygiene includes tongue-scraping with the use of a flat wire instrument. It is believed that the tongue collects a coating of toxins and metabolic waste, especially after a night's rest when many toxins are eliminated. The tongue can also be brushed gently with a toothbrush to get rid of any coating present.

Other helpful essential oils with digestive and anti-bacterial properties include Spearmint, Anise, Nutmeg, and Rosemary. If mouth ulcers are a recurring problem, add 1 drop of Tea Tree essential oil for prevention. Also, consider the anti-stress essential oils discussed in Chapter 9 since there is a strong correlation between stress and mouth ulcers.

Fresh lemon juice is helpful with neutralizing acids and overall detoxification and is a powerful antibacterial agent. It is optional in the mouthwash recipe, yet can be very helpful for those of you who may suffer from a high acid system. If you smoke, drink alcohol, have several cups of coffee per day, or are under considerable stress, you will benefit from the addition of lemon juice to aid in excellent oral health.

> Practical and healthful tip: Rinsing after meals with mouthwash (or water) is the next best thing for good oral hygiene when it is inconvenient to brush. This is a good practice to teach children. Rinse after meals and brush morning and night.

Natural Tooth Polisher

My father always taught me to brush with baking soda and lemon juice. He said it was the best thing you could brush with, especially if you added some finely ground rubbed sage. This combination has many positive effects on the teeth and on the delicate oral mucosa (mucous membranes). Have you noticed how many "new and improved" toothpastes boast this ordinary ingredient? You may never go back to the sugar-sweetened, chemical-packed variety again!

Simply put a few drops of lemon juice on your toothbrush and dip into a small dish of baking soda and brush. The lemon juice reacts with the baking soda, which is a natural abrasive and cleanser, and will bubble. For extra cleaning power add rubbed sage to your baking soda and mix well. Sage has been used for ages in oral care. Next time you're in the garden, pick a fresh sage leaf and rub over your teeth to give them an instant polish; then chew the leaf to freshen your breath!

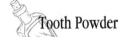

Tooth Powder

4 parts baking soda

1 part sea salt

1 part rubbed sage herb (optional)

lemon juice to moisten toothbrush each time

Combine baking soda, sea salt, and sage in a dish or mortar and pestle if you have one. Carefully check that the sage is finely ground or "rubbed," discarding any large or stick pieces. Store in a wide-mouth jar or covered dish in the bathroom. Moisten toothbrush with lemon juice or tap water and dip into tooth powder (or sprinkle it from a bottle). Brush gently. Rinse thoroughly. Follow with Kiss Me Mouthwash. This dry tooth powder lasts indefinitely.

It takes about 36 hours for a toothbrush to dry completely. By using the same brush daily, germs can easily live on the moist surface. Two options to avoid contamination and bacterial growth: rotate among 3 different toothbrushes, or keep your brush soaking in a baking soda solution.

Healing Help for Canker Sores

Canker sores or mouth ulcers are very painful ulcerations in the mouth, on the tongue, cheeks, or gums, and are red and somewhat swollen. They can be caused by various conditions, but usually are part of a general weakened physical state. Most mouth ulcers result from physical or psychological stress, poor diet, infection (bacterial, viral, or fungal), high acid system, vitamin deficiency, food allergy, immune deficiency (especially after antibiotic use or illness) and simple trauma such as biting your tongue or cheek badly.

Typical canker sores are painful and take one to two weeks to completely heal. They also reoccur frequently. If you observe a reddened area or a sore that does not heal, is not painful, and/or has a white discoloration or patch, you need to get checked by your dentist or doctor as this can be a warning sign of cancer.

Since stress is a major factor in the reoccurrence of canker sores, taking a good stress vitamin high in Vitamin B's and C is a prudent measure. See Chapter 9 for essential oils that are helpful in stress relief, as well as for other helpful coping strategies. Also avoid high-acid foods such as tomato sauce, ketchup, coffee, alcoholic beverages, carbonated cola drinks. Too much pasteurized orange juice and unbuffered Vitamin C can also cause an increase in acid of the mouth and break down the integrity of the mucous membranes.

As with most health problems, prevention is always key to keeping most ailments from occurring. The recipe for Kiss Me Mouthwash can be used on a regular basis with the addition of 1 to 2 drops of Tea Tree essential oil; any of the following essential oils, depending on the cause of ulceration, can be added to the basic mouthwash recipe. Do not add more than a total of 6 drops per 1 cup of distilled water or sage tea. Any combination can be used effectively; however, the mint essential oils taste best. Use for preventative care and also while sores are present and healing.

For *fungal* infections of the mouth (oral thrush, Candida): Chamomile, Tea Tree, Fennel, Geranium, and Lavender have proven useful. Herb tea of Chamomile can be used if you don't have essential oil of Chamomile on hand or can be used in place of the distilled water part of the recipe. It is known for its anti-inflammatory properties.

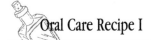

Oral Care Recipe I

for fungal-related infections

1 cup strong Chamomile herbal tea

1 teaspoon raw honey

2 drops Tea Tree essential oil

2 drops Lavender essential oil

1 drop Geranium essential oil

1 drop Fennel essential oil

Brew 1 cup strong herbal tea of Chamomile. In one teaspoon of honey mix the essential oils. Add the medicated honey to the warm tea and mix well. Pour into clean glass bottle and label. Shake bottle well before each use. To use, simply swish vigorously and leave in the mouth for a minute or two before spitting out. Use as needed several times per day following mouth care and meals. Avoid drinking and eating within 20 minutes of use to allow essential oils to be absorbed and affect local fungus growth. For optimal freshness make weekly.

For *bacterial or viral* related infections of the mouth (following a flu, antibiotic use, Herpes Simplex, or poor oral hygiene), Bergamot, Lemon, Tea Tree, Lavender, Peppermint, and Rosemary essential oils are effective. Bergamot is excellent on most mouth infections, including those caused by the Herpes Simplex virus. It negates bad breath because of its antiseptic properties.

Case History: *A young man with a history of Herpes Simplex virus (mouth sores) came to me very upset about their increasing number. He traveled a lot for business, had a very stressful life in sales, drank large amounts of coffee and soda pop, and had a habit of brushing his teeth very harshly. After using the following Oral Care Recipe II for several days, he noticed a shorter healing time and considerably less pain while eating. He now uses this recipe on a preventative basis with minimal outbreaks of mouth sores. As part of his lifestyle change, he needed to cut back on the acid-forming foods and beverages such as coffee, soda pop, and alcohol, especially during stressful times. Stress vitamins with extra B, C, and E were taken. Changing to a softer bristle toothbrush and to a gentler brushing technique was strongly encouraged. The Bergamot essential oil in this recipe helps to balance and regulate the system and is useful as an anti-stress essential oil.*

Oral Care Recipe II

For bacterial or viral related infections

1 cup Rosemary or Sage herbal tea

1 teaspoon fresh lemon juice (optional)

1 teaspoon raw honey

2 drops Peppermint essential oil

2 drops Bergamot essential oil

1 drop Tea Tree essential oil

Brew 1 cup of Rosemary or Sage herbal tea. Add fresh lemon juice. Measure 1 teaspoon of honey and add essential oils to it and mix well. Combine aromatic honey with the warm herb tea and lemon juice. Mix well and bottle in clean glass container. Shake well before each use. To use, simply swish vigorously and leave in the mouth for a minute or two before spitting out. Can be used several times per day. Most beneficial when used following oral care, after meals when the mouth is clean. Avoid drinking and eating within 20 minutes of use to allow essential oils to be absorbed and affect local bacteria. For optimal freshness make weekly.

Plain sage herb tea has been used for centuries as an effective mouthwash and in preventing tooth decay, while the fresh herb was chewed for its healing, soothing, and mouth freshening quality.

For spot treatment of mouth sores, apply Myrrh directly to the sore with a cotton swab by gently dabbing the area several times per day. Myrrh has been used for hundreds of years for mouth problems such as receding gums, bleeding gums, and loose teeth. Calendula succus can also be used as a healing herb to apply directly to open sores and it is very soothing.

Instant Relief for Toothache

Although there are a few excellent remedies for the immediate relief of tooth pain, they do not address the underlying cause of the pain as with an infected tooth. Use these recommendations as needed until you can see your dentist.

Clove is the spice most helpful for the miserable pain of a toothache. Clove contains analgesic properties and Oil of Clove was used in early dentistry for its pain-killing ability. However, today Eugenol is used in modern dental offices, and is a naturally occurring chemical constituent of the natural oil. For toothache, rub ground Clove spice over the area of pain for a minute or two until relief is obtained. Alternately, a few whole cloves can be chewed for more generalized mouth pain or when the ground spice is not available. Note: The whole herb or spice is always more potent than the ground version because more essential oils are contained therein and have not lost their potency by evaporating.

Also, for toothache, a strong herb tea of Sage can be made and used as a mouthwash. For adequate relief, swish the warm tea vigorously and leave in the mouth for longer than usual before rinsing (about a minute or two). A pinch of ground Clove can be added to this wash for added pain relief. I have found the Kiss Me mouthwash to be effective for simple and very mild forms of toothache and gum irritation.

Healthy Treatment for Bleeding Gums

Under normal, healthy conditions our gums do not bleed unless there has been gum trauma of some kind. Bleeding gums result from gingivitis, which is inflammation of the gums. Early signs of this includes redness, swelling, recession, and bleeding. There can be several factors or causes for abnormal bleeding of the gums: bacterial infection, large amounts of

plaque buildup, tobacco smoking, or toothbrush trauma caused by overvig-
orous brushing or an overly stiff toothbrush.

Besides direct trauma, bleeding gums may be a symptom of an underlying weakness in the immune system or a nutritional deficiency. Eating a
variety of foods and basing your diet on whole grains, vegetables, and fruits
is always a good idea. Since digestion begins in the mouth, regular dental
care is essential! While the following remedy is excellent for healing bleeding gums, it is intended as symptomatic treatment only, and the underlying
cause must be addressed for true healing to take place. Note: If you are taking aspirin on a long-term or continual basis, this could possibly be a factor in your gum's bleeding. Please see your health care practitioner for
advice or alternatives.

> **Case History:**   *A seven-year-old boy, with a history of swollen gums with
> occasional bleeding, used this recipe with great success. His mother stated that
> when his gums got red and sore, he refused to brush at all, sometimes for days.
> As soon as he tried the mouth rinse he felt considerable relief from the soreness
> and swelling and the bleeding decreased. By the second and third day he was
> able to brush his teeth, eat without discomfort, and be examined more com-
> pletely by his dentist, which was not possible earlier. When he uses this mouth
> rinse regularly, he has absolutely no complaints and his gums stay strong and
> healthy!*

Mouth and Gum Rescue

a mouth rinse for bleeding gums

1 cup Sage herbal tea

1 Tablespoon distilled Witch Hazel

1 teaspoon raw honey

2 to 3 drops Tincture of Myrrh

1 drop Lemon essential oil

1 drop Eucalyptus essential oil

To the cup of Sage herbal tea add the Witch hazel. Add the Myrrh and
essential oils directly with the honey before combining with the sage tea.
This is best made fresh daily and used warm. Cleanse the mouth well by
gently brushing with a natural toothpaste or my tooth powder recipe, especially following meals to decrease bacterial growth. Thoroughly swish and
rinse with this recipe several times per day. For optimal freshness make
weekly.

Myrrh and Sage have been used traditionally for all mouth and gum disorders. The Sage is healing and astringent in general and helps strengthen the gums. Lemon and Eucalyptus are effective in stopping bleeding, along with Witch Hazel. Sipping Raspberry leaf tea may also work in cases where bleeding is a problem.

Other essential oils and herbs that combat gum disease are Clary Sage, Juniper, Fennel, and Rosemary.

I suggest incorporating more Sage herb in the diet, either as a spice used in food preparation or included as an herbal tea, to be used regularly (daily or several times per week) to strengthen the gums and thereby prevent further symptoms. Also, lemon should be taken daily as fresh juice in hot water every morning before the morning meal. Try 1 to 2 tablespoons per 1 cup of hot water, sweetened with Sage honey or plain honey if desired. See recipe for Sage honey on page 85.

Soothing Treatment for a Simple Sore Throat

For a simple case of sore throat that may be caused by local irritation, trauma or overuse, the following suggestions and recipe will be very helpful. For more serious conditions such as bacterial or viral infections accompanied by fever, nausea, headache, swollen lymph nodes etc., please refer to the following chapter which addresses these topics more fully. See page 84.

This recipe works well for overuse of the throat, or the very early signs of a sore throat. By gargling with this recipe throughout the day, as well as by following a few preventative measures suggested, you will have an excellent chance to stop any further symptoms from occurring. Early treatment is ideal for the prevention of many bacterial infections.

Simple Sore Throat Gargle

1 cup Sage herb tea or water

1 Tablespoon fresh Lemon juice

1 Tablespoon Apple Cider Vinegar (optional)

1 teaspoon Sage Honey or plain honey

2 drops Geranium essential oil

1 drop Ginger essential oil

Brew 1 cup Sage herbal tea or use hot water. Add lemon juice and/or apple cider. Add essential oils to the honey and mix well before adding to herb tea liquid. Gargle with this recipe for 1 to 2 minutes, several times per day. For optimal freshness make weekly.

If fever, swollen lymph nodes, or redness develops, refer to page 84 for bacterial/viral related sore throat infections.

Other helpful essential oils for sore throats include Frankincense, Lemon, Pine, Hyssop, and Tea Tree. Traditional herbs used to treat a variety of throat ailments are garlic, goldenseal, echinacea, agrimony, chamomile, raspberry leaf, fenugreek seeds, and ginger root. Apple cider vinegar has been used for many years as an aid to sore throat simply on its own.

It would be a good idea to keep warm throughout the day and to get more rest. Increase your intake of Vitamin B and C, take garlic and Echinacea herb for prevention, and make sure you eat a balanced diet. Avoid mucus-forming foods such as dairy products, avoid refined sugars, and drink plenty of water and herbal tea.

Easy Recipe for Hiccups

Hiccups are intermittent spasms of the diaphragm which cause the characteristic "hic" sounds. A direct cause can be an overdistended stomach, when too much food has been eaten, as seen frequently at Thanksgiving dinner! Alternately, a reflex can cause hiccups, due to sudden exposure to cold or from drinking very hot or cold liquids. More often than not, hiccups are bothersome and embarrassing, but not serious.

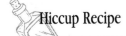

Hiccup Recipe

1 teaspoon vegetable oil

1 drop Chamomile or Basil essential oil

Mix the essential oil in the vegetable oil. Rub on palms and hold over mouth and nose. Inhale very slowly and deeply a few times. Then rub oil over the upper chest area just below the throat, as well as over the solar plexus area (just below the sternum). This main area is directly over several nerves that run through this region. Preferably use your left hand and rub in a counter-clockwise direction. I do not recommend using Basil essential oil for small children; instead use Chamomile or Mandarin essential oil.

Tarragon and Dill weed have been traditionally used for hiccups and can be made in an herbal tea and sipped frequently. There are other essential oils which are anti-spasmodic and can work as well, such as Sandalwood, Fennel, Lavender, Anise, and Mandarin. Breathing into a paper bag is still an old standby remedy, but can be more effective if one of the above essential oils is placed (one drop) inside.

Stimulating the Taste Buds for Loss of Appetite

Experiencing a loss of appetite is often a temporary condition occurring during an illness such as the common cold or the flu, or an infection such as tonsillitis. Our bodies naturally slow down the digestive processes in order for energy to be available to heal and recover. But it is also known that why we taste is closely linked to how well we can smell, and during colds and some other illnesses, the sinuses are blocked. If sinus congestion is a reason for the loss of appetite, use the inhalation methods discussed in Chapter 13, *Breathe Easy,* on page 328 for directions in preparing steam inhalations. I would suggest sinus-clearing essential oils such as Peppermint, Eucalyptus, Pine, or Cedarwood. These notable essences help clear the breathing passages and kill bacteria harbored in these areas. I recommend doing a 5-minute steam inhalation three times per day when your sinuses are congested, and preferably 30 to 45 minutes before mealtime.

Loss of appetite can be caused by a sluggish digestive system in general, or by indigestion. In this case, herbs, spices, and essential oils that are digestive stimulants are called for. Most herbs recommended are in the "bitter" category as they are capable of stimulating the production of saliva, digestive juices, and bile.

One other possible cause of a loss of appetite can be a side-effect of a particular drug or combination of medications you may be taking (the antidepressant drug Prozac is an example). If you suspect this may be a factor, call your doctor or pharmacist to discuss possible alternatives.

If a state of decreased appetite is prolonged, or is accompanied by obsessive thoughts, it could be serious. The medical term given to the extreme inability to eat is called anorexia nervosa, which suggests a psychological component. It is most frequently seen in teenage girls; however, recent information shows a rise in adolescent males as well. This condition is very serious; since professional and prompt help is necessary, it will not be covered in this book.

Case history: *An elderly woman experiencing a loss of appetite caused by a sluggish digestive system, with occasional indigestion, used the following recipe with tremendous results.*

Suggestions on food preparation and use of specific spices were given, along with the recommendation that she take several aromatic baths per week. She particularly liked the Serenity Bath Blend on page 300 which helped with mild bouts of depression and anxiety.

Stimulating Taste-Tea

1/4 teaspoon Caraway seed

1/4 teaspoon Cardamom

1/4" slice fresh ginger root (1/4 tsp. dried)

1/4 teaspoon Gentian root (dried)

Ginger honey or plain honey to taste

Gently boil the above herbs and spices for 5 minutes in 1 cup of water. Strain and sip at least half an hour before meals. All of the above are known to stimulate the appetite. Ginger honey is used the most frequently in our home. It has a delightful taste and a wide variety of uses. Because Ginger is a warming spice, antispasmodic and carminative, it is effective in colds, sore throat and sinus conditions, and even headaches. Put it in warm milk, herbal tea, hot apple cider, or rice pudding. Enjoy.

Ginger Honey

1 1/2 cups raw honey

2-inch piece fresh ginger root, thinly sliced

Heat honey over low setting. Add sliced ginger and heat gently, taking care not to boil. Excessive heat damages the beneficial qualities of the honey; that is the reason for buying raw and not pasteurized honey. In about 20 to 30 minutes, taste the honey. It should be very flavorful and the ginger slices almost dry. The essential oil and juice from the ginger is being extracted out in the honey. Strain with a slotted spoon. If you own a dehydrator, save the ginger slices and sprinkle with sugar and dry to make ginger candy. Although hotter than store bought, it is very appealing during a cold! Store in a clean glass jar and label.

There are many herbs used to aid in digestion and increase the appetite; among the most common are Burdock, Goldenseal and Quassia. Also cooking with the following spices can greatly improve sluggish digestive systems: garlic, lemon, orange, nutmeg, clove, fennel, and ginger.

Before Meal Massage

1 tablespoon vegetable oil

1 drop Bergamot essential oil

1 drop Ginger essential oil

and 1 drop of the following:

Clary sage, Chamomile, or Rose

Mix a total of 3 drops of essential oil in warm vegetable oil. Rub on palms, hold over mouth and nose, and inhale a few seconds. Then rub oil over the solar plexus (just below the sternum), back of hands, and back of neck. When working over the solar plexus area, go in a counterclockwise direction to promote relaxation. Do this 1/2 hour or more prior to your largest meal of the day.

Other essential oils that can be used in massage or aromatic baths to assist in stimulating the digestion are: Bergamot, Coriander, Chamomile, Fennel, Ginger, Juniper, Lemon, and Nutmeg.

Lifestyle and dietary recommendations include the use of fresh and organic foods as much as possible, as well as plentiful use of herbs and spices. If anxiety, nervous tension, or mild depression are factors, see the corresponding sections in Chapter 9 for help. Colorful and visually attractive food presentation may have a positive influence as well. Consider dining options such as eating with friends, fresh cut flowers on the table, candle light or other rituals that will make the experience more pleasant and enjoyable. See Chapter 12 for air purification, environmental fragrancing ideas and fragrant live plant selections.

No More Nausea

There are many causes of nausea, the feeling of sickness from the center of your stomach, that preludes the desire to vomit. Some common causes include putrid odors, hangover, colds/flu, headache, food poisoning, food allergy, poor digestion, emotional or physical stress, jet lag, early pregnancy, drug interactions or side-effects, and motion sickness. Actually it is the latter, travel or motion sickness, that the word 'nausea' is derived from. In Latin it means *seasickness,* and from the Greek translation *sailor.*

Case History: *A few years ago we had a first-hand experience of car sickness when we drove from Massachusetts to the southernmost tip of Florida on a family vacation! The long drive, the medium-size rental car (for 5 people and luggage), the boredom (and the kids' back seat squabbles), humid weather, and the stress of traveling all took their toll. When nausea hit our 7-year-old twin boys, I put a few drops of peppermint essential oil on tissue for each of them to inhale. The effect on us all was immediate! May I also add that for* *car sickness or any other kind of motion sickness, it helps to be out in fresh air. Turn off the air conditioner and open the car windows.*

Helpful hint when traveling: Take along your favorite essential oils on all your travels; include peppermint, eucalyptus, and lavender. In the car they change the environment and air quality quickly, making you feel somewhere other than in a closed vehicle. Essential oils, especially eucalyptus, can also relieve driving stress and encourage alertness.

For most cases of nausea just simply inhaling peppermint works surprisingly well. In more stubborn cases try one of the two recipes below.

No More Nausea Massage Oil

> *5 drops Lavender essential oil*
>
> *2 drops Peppermint essential oil*
>
> *2 drops Mandarin essential oil*
>
> *1 drop Ginger essential oil*
>
> *1 tablespoon vegetable oil*

Count out the essential oils according to recipe into a small amber bottle that holds at least 1/2 ounce. Then add one tablespoon of vegetable oil or unscented body lotion. Shake to combine well. Rub on hands and inhale slowly and deeply a few times. Then massage this blend over the solar plexus (below sternum) in counterclockwise direction with your left hand (promotes relaxation as well). If you know you are prone to travel sickness, do this 30 minutes before traveling. You can mix up the same blend as above, leaving out the vegetable oil, just for inhalation use. Sniff directly from the bottle or put a few drops on a tissue, handkerchief, or cotton balls stored in a plastic bag.

No More Nausea Tea

> *1 teaspoon Raspberry leaf*
>
> *1 teaspoon Peppermint herb*
>
> *1/2 teaspoon Fennel seed—ground*
>
> *1/2 teaspoon Anise seed—ground*
>
> *1 teaspoon Ginger Honey or plain honey*
>
> *1 cup boiling water*

Combine Raspberry leaf, Peppermint, Fennel, and Anise. Put in teapot loose or use tea strainer. Measure 1 teaspoon per cup. Pour boiling water over tea and allow to steep for 5 minutes. Add honey to taste. Sip this tea very slowly, and inhale the anti-nausea aroma from the cup. This blend is especially helpful if nausea is caused by indigestion, overeating, or fried or very rich foods. It is also wonderful for nausea related to colds and flu since the peppermint and ginger help with sinus congestion and stomach upset. The recipe for Ginger honey is on page 38 of this chapter. It is also known to be very effective on nervous tension.

Other useful essential oils to consider for nausea are those that aid in relaxation as well as being carminative, such as Sandalwood and Rose.

Nausea caused by pregnancy is discussed in Chapter 10: *For Women Only,* on page 276.

First Aid for Vomiting

I hope you will not need to turn to this section very often. As a matter of fact, vomiting, the immediate emptying of the stomach contents, is rarely experienced. It is often associated with the flu or food or liquor poisoning, and is our body's natural reaction to get rid of anything that is extremely harmful in our stomach.

If vomiting is projectile in nature, is prolonged, or becomes a symptom following a head injury, seek medical attention at once. It could be indicative of something more serious, such as a blockage, poisoning, or concussion.

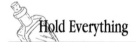

Hold Everything

Relief for vomiting

1 drop Basil essential oil

1 drop Peppermint essential oil

1 drop Lavender essential oil

2 teaspoons vegetable oil

Mix the essential oils in the vegetable oil. Rub in hands to warm and inhale deeply over the nose and mouth area (3 slow, relaxed inhalations). Then massage gently over abdomen in circular motion.

Other helpful essential oils include lemon, anise, and fennel. These oils can simply be inhaled from a tissue on which a drop or two has been placed.

Putting the Intestinal Fire Out—Help for Indigestion

Heartburn and indigestion are health complaints that originate in the stomach, which is responsible for secreting gastric acid (hydrochloric acid), digestive enzymes, and various hormones. Many common ailments relating to the stomach are caused by either too much or too little of these secreted substances. Therefore it is important to identify the exact reasons for the disturbance. Is there too much stomach acid at the wrong time? Or are there not enough gastric juices at the right time? Common symptoms of the latter are discussed here and include bloating, belching, feeling of fullness after eating, indigestion, and flatulence following meals.

Indigestion is commonly caused by both physical and emotional factors. The physical factors can be overeating, overuse of antacids, eating too quickly, or consuming a meal high in fats or dairy products (milk neutralizes stomach acids). The emotional link between digestive problems and stress is evident in the case history that follows, and even more so when ulcers have developed. Whenever difficulty in digestion is a problem, we can assume the food consumed is not being adequately digested, and therefore not properly assimilated into "usable" fuel or energy.

If indigestion lasts longer than two weeks, or if you are experiencing difficulty in swallowing, visit your physician promptly for evaluation.

Case History: *A 30-year-old mother of two young school age children began experiencing an increased number of stomach complaints including indigestion, bloating, and a feeling of "fullness" immediately following meals, especially the evening meal. Upon questioning she said she was very stressed preparing the dinner meal because of her children's negative behavior at this time. She ate quickly and therefore had a tendency to overeat as well. She experienced nervous tension most evenings which unfortunately interfered with her ability to relax before retiring. While she got many recommendations for dealing with the children at this "witching hour," she found the most relief when she addressed her stress and nervous tension. This affected the way in which she ate, helping her to slow down and relax more at meal times. The children, very sensitive to adult emotions, responded favorably to her lower stress level. She was a prime example of how our emotions affect the digestive system. In addition, a diffuser was used in the kitchen and dining area while she prepared the food, with the Slow Down and Relax blend (see Chapter 13, page 335 for recipe). This had a positive effect on the rest of the family, too. She found the Digest-Ease Tea and the Digest-Ease Massage blend were a great help. Feeling more relaxed, she found she had more patience with the children, and her husband noted she was in better spirits when he got home. Within days the indigestion complaints disappeared, and over the following two weeks she noticed she had lost a few pounds! She ate more slowly and as a result did not overeat or overwork her digestive system. Her body was now able to digest the food properly and assimilate the nutrients it needed for good health.*

Digest-Ease Massage Lotion

4 drops Lavender essential oil

3 drops Bergamot essential oil

2 drops Peppermint essential oil

2 drops Basil essential oil

1 drop Neroli (or Chamomile) essential oil

1 tablespoon vegetable oil or lotion

Combine the essential oils in a small amber bottle. Add the vegetable oil to use as the carrier or use a non-scented base lotion. Use this massage lotion 1/2 hour before meals by applying to the stomach area and back of hands. Use sparingly as this is a concentrated blend. Inhale as needed from the back of the hands. This is a massage concentrate and designed to use for specific and localized areas, not the entire body.

The basil and peppermint essential oils both aid in digestion, while the lavender soothes the nervous system in general and is anti-spasmodic. Bergamot and Neroli help with anxiety and nervous tension. Other essential oils that can be beneficial to the digestive system and calming include anise, fennel, ginger, juniper, lemongrass, lemon.

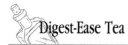

Digest-Ease Tea

2 parts Peppermint herb

1 part Tarragon herb

1 part Lemonbalm herb

1 part Chamomile flowers

1 part Anise or Fennel seed

1/2 part Rosemary herb

Ginger honey or plain honey to taste

Mix herbs, Chamomile flowers, and seeds together in a bowl. Store in glass jar and label with directions for use. To make 1 cup of tea: Add boiling water to 1-2 teaspoons of herb tea mixture. Let steep for 5 minutes. Sip slowly and inhale from cup. Best taken immediately following meals to aid in digestion.

The peppermint, lemonbalm, anise seed, and ginger honey are included in the recipe for their direct beneficial effects on the digestive system. Herbs for nervous tension, tarragon, chamomile and rosemary, are also added in this recipe for their calming effect and anti-spasmodic properties. Rosemary also is helpful in digesting fats and lowering cholesterol levels.

The Sweet Breath Seed Mix given on page 28 of this chapter helps to prevent indigestion and relieves its symptoms if already existing. Simply chew the special mix of digestion-aiding seeds following a meal. This is a typical practice among certain cultures. In Italy, anise is well liked and found in many of the after-dinner liqueurs and desserts. In India and some Asian countries, fennel is used to prepare certain dishes to make them more digestible. Caraway is used also for the same reason.

Some other traditional herbs used in digestive system ailments are licorice, caraway, basil, and savory. Spices used to aid in digestion include cinnamon, clove, coriander, garlic, onion, and sage. Herbs employed for their calming benefits to the nervous system include hops, lavender, valerian, and the aforementioned chamomile, rosemary, and tarragon.

Dietary changes are essential if there is a food allergy, high fat diet, or a large amount of acidic foods or carbonated beverages. Avoiding legumes may be necessary for some. However, there are several ways to make the beans more digestible. Try cooking beans and lentils with a whole onion studded with a few whole cloves, change cooking water frequently or add cumin spice or a piece of Kombu seaweed. Cumin is commonly used in Mexican and Indian dishes that are based on lentils and legumes for this reason.

> Natural Hygiene is a philosophy and lifestyle based both on principles of proper food combinations to aid the digestive process, and following the body's natural cycles of elimination, appropriation, and assimilation.

Lifestyle changes are recommended when emotional factors and the ability to cope with stress are correlated to the digestive distress. The *Slow Down and Relax* inhalation blend was created with this challenge in mind and encourages relaxation and a feeling of wellbeing. You can refer to an in-depth discussion of stress and its effects in Chapter 9 if this is an issue in your own health.

Helpful Tip: In our home at dinnertime we eat by candlelight almost every night. This has a quieting and calming effect, and definitely encourages a relaxing atmosphere. It also demonstrates energy conservation and honors our special family time together. Try it tonight at your dinner table and notice the difference a little thing like this can make.

Is Gas Cramping More Than Your Style?
Abdominal Cramping and Flatulence

Have you ever experienced abdominal cramps and pain associated with gas which have interfered with how you felt and acted out in public? I have heard many funny and somewhat embarrassing stories over the years! Small air or gas pockets trapped in the stomach and small intestines can cause severe pain, sometimes so intense that an ulcer, appendicitis, or worse is suspected. Gas is painful but generally harmless; but be alert for fever, or for sudden or severe abdominal pain not associated with eating food, which might indicate an infection or inflammation. Seek medical attention promptly as this can be more serious.

Some less extreme symptoms related to abdominal cramping and gas are bloating, burping, and flatulence. Gas formation in the stomach can be caused by eating or drinking too fast and literally swallowing air. However, more frequently the cause is a sluggish digestive system which causes undigested food to sit in the stomach where fermentation takes place. Proper food combining can be especially important to some people since certain foods (protein) take hours to digest, and others (fruit) may take only 20 to 30 minutes. So if these two types of food are eaten at the same meal, the fruit will stay in the stomach longer than it should while the proteins are being digested. There are a number of books written on this topic of food combining (also known as "natural hygiene"). Much of the work done in this area is based on Dr. Shelton's studies on the digestive system and its inherent natural rhythms and cycles.

The interaction of specific medications or drugs taken on an empty stomach can produce digestive upset and possibly cramping. Also certain foods such as garlic, onions, legumes, and carbonated drinks produce gas in some people. When gas is trapped in the stomach, spasms and abdominal cramping often result. The body attempts to equalize the pressure in the stomach and esophagus; upper gastrointestinal gas release (burping, belching) is such an attempt and provides some relief of this pressure. Lower down in the digestive tract, gas can be passed by the colon, and flatulence can help to relieve the lower abdominal discomfort.

Case history: *My children are so rarely ill that it sounds strange when I share this story, but it does demonstrate the severity of gas pain in some individuals. Kristopher, one of my 8-year-old twin sons, went to the nurse's office at school with extreme abdominal pain. His temperature was normal, and he had not eaten anything likely to cause cramping. I was called to come and pick Kris up as soon as possible, since he was so uncomfortable. When I got to* *school, Kris was doubled over in pain, and could not walk upright. It looked serious. When we returned home he lay on the couch with a hot water bottle while I confirmed his temperature. I massaged very gently an oil blend for abdominal cramping and gas (given below), and gave him a sugar cube with peppermint essential oil on it to suck on. Within 15 minutes he felt considerably better. After drinking sips of the herb tea I prepared he felt 90% better. In less than one half hour, he had bounced back and appeared perfectly normal! We got to spend a quiet afternoon together, and I wonder if the emotions played a role in Kris' situation. The nervous system interacts closely with the digestive system and is easily affected in children.*

The following massage blend helps to alleviate cramping in the abdominal area caused by gas and spasms. Warming the oil first encourages the muscles to relax. Use a light and gentle clockwise circular massage stroke with the palm of the hands to further stimulate the gas to disperse down the gastrointestinal tract.

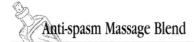

Anti-spasm Massage Blend

for abdominal gas cramping

1 teaspoon vegetable oil

1 drop Chamomile essential oil

1 drop Coriander, Ginger, Lavender, or *Fennel essential oil*

Mix a total of two drops in the teaspoon of vegetable oil. Massage gently over abdominal area with the palm of the hand in clockwise direction. Put hot water bottle or heating pad over abdomen for additional relief and aid to relaxation of muscular spasms. Sometimes lying in a 30-degree angle with head slightly elevated will help as well. Inhale essential oils from hands with slow, deep and full breaths.

Anti-gas Lozenge

1 sugar cube

1 drop Peppermint essential oil

Put one single drop of essential oil of peppermint on the sugar cube. Slowly suck on it to release the essence into the stomach. Peppermint helps to equalize the pressure in the stomach caused by gas and it has an antifoaming action to help prevent further gas formation.

Herb Tea for Tummy Cramping

1/3 teaspoon Cardamom spice

1/3 teaspoon Fennel seed—ground

1/3 teaspoon Caraway seed—ground

1/8-inch slice of fresh ginger root

1 cup water

Heat water to boiling and pour over the above herbs and spices. Let steep for 10 minutes. Strain and sip while still warm. Can be taken whenever gas cramping is present, or 15 minutes before meals to prevent cramping and to relax the stomach. These herbs are digestion aids as well as anti-gas and anti-spasmodic agents.

Among traditional European remedies for colic, gas, and stomach cramping, "gripe water" was and still is an effective syrup to use. It contains dill, anise, fennel, and caraway as the active ingredients. Other herbs traditionally used for gas problems include catnip, chamomile, hyssop, marjoram, sage, savory, tarragon, and thyme. Spices known to help in this area are cinnamon, clove, coriander, ginger and nutmeg.

Many essential oils assist with muscular relaxation (anti-spasmodic properties) and aid digestion; most recognized for these qualities are anise, basil, bergamot, chamomile, fennel, lavender, marjoram, and peppermint. These oils can be used in diluted form as massage oils to be applied over the abdominal area, or used as inhalants on a tissue, from an aroma lamp or simply from the bottle or hands. Peppermint is one of the few essential oils I recommend taking internally (by mouth) for dyspepsia (digestive problems) and only so by a single drop on a sugar cube, which is the medicinal carrier. Other essential oils are too concentrated to be taken this way and carry greater risks; therefore they are not the subject of this book.

Lifestyle and eating patterns that facilitate digestion include eating in a relaxed, slow manner and avoiding situations where you may eat too fast and under stress. Food combining and avoiding gas-producing foods will also help. Proper cooking of beans and legumes (with cumin, for example) will decrease gas formation. Avoid wearing tight clothing, especially around the waist and abdominal area; this can impede both digestion and elimination.

Stomach Ulcers—What's Eating You?

Peptic or stomach ulcers are areas of erosion within the mucous membrane lining of the stomach. More than 12 million people in the United States suffer from gastritis, the inflammation of the stomach's lining, and peptic ulcers. Often there is a characteristic sharp pain experienced in the stomach region, burning, and varying degrees of indigestion.

Possible complications, such as bleeding, perforation, or blockage, that can arise from peptic ulcers mandate continual medical supervision. Discuss with your health care practitioner the following complementary and supportive measures that can be added to your program, or used in prevention.

Several factors can be the underlying cause promoting ulcer formation. Emotional stress, especially extreme feelings of anger, anxiety, and resentment, has been correlated to digestive problems and specifically to stomach ulcers. It appears that it is not necessarily the *amount* of stress that determines digestive problems, but rather how well one manages or *copes* with the stress factors. Aromatherapy is very effective in stress reduction, and is discussed in detail in Chapter 9. I suggest you refer to that chapter after completing this section to get the whole picture of how stress directly affects our physical, mental, and emotional health, and how it ties in with your individual health circumstances.

Overuse of antacids, especially by people who already have low levels of stomach acid, is another major factor to consider. More than $2 billion worth of antacids and related prescription drugs are sold in the United States per year. Irregular eating patterns, eating too quickly, food allergies and eating under stressful conditions also contribute to this ailment. Some drugs, like aspirin, aminophyllin, and non-steroidal analgesics can irritate the stomach lining and may promote ulceration with prolonged usage, especially if a predisposed weakness exists. This is the main reason why such drugs are to be taken with milk or food to buffer this reaction on the stomach lining.

Ingesting acid-producing products like coffee, black tea, and cola beverages, and smoking tobacco are associated with an increased risk of stomach ulcers, in addition to a percentage of those with a genetic predisposition or family history. This last factor may involve a genetic link that indicates an inability of the mucous membrane lining to defend itself and maintain optimal health and integrity, or perhaps there are family-learned behaviors of dealing with stress and venting extreme emotions that factor in the equation.

Up until the last ten years, it has been common medical thought that stomach ulcers were caused by too much acid in the stomach, which eroded the delicate lining. However, more recent thought is that the cause is an infection by the *Helicobacter Pylori* bacteria. As many as 70% of gastric ulcer patients were found to be infected with H. pylori. Some studies have shown that when healthy individuals were infected with the pylori bacteria, they developed pre-ulcer conditions and ulcer formation. The detection of H. pylori can be done by a simple blood test. Treatment for this type of infection of the stomach lining would involve antimicrobial agents in addition to anti-secretory medicine. Several other therapies are currently being investigated to treat this bacteria.

In summation, "what's eating you" could be your inability to cope with stress effectively, the drugs you take, the acid-forming foods you ingest, or the *H. pylori* bacteria.

Case history: *A 47-year-old male with a history of a peptic ulcer, high level of job-related stress, as well as a diet relatively high in acid-forming foods, was interested in alternatives that could support his health condition. Remaining under doctor's care and support, he came to see me for aromatherapy. The main areas that called for immediate attention were his stress-coping mechanisms, his daily intake of highly acid-forming beverages, and herbs and essential oils that would support and encourage healing of his gastric lining. Over a four-month period we modified and re-evaluated different stress reduction plans that worked for him, as well as experimented with various aromatherapy blends. The following aromatherapy massage oil came to be his blend of choice which he used faithfully twice a day in the beginning, then once a day, and now several times per week. His greatest challenge was making time for his stress-relief program and cutting back on his coffee intake. He turned out to be a great advocate for cabbage juice and the massage oil. At this writing, it has been nine months since his initial consultation, and he is off all prescription drugs; his doctor told him his ulcer has totally healed. He continues regular follow-up visits with his physician and is aware of his tendency toward ulcers, should he return to his "old" lifestyle and dietary habits.*

Ulcer Healing Massage Oil

2 tablespoons vegetable oil (preferably calendula infused oil recipe)

10 drops Lavender essential oil

5 drops Geranium essential oil

5 drops Lemon essential oil

4 drops Chamomile essential oil

400IU Vitamin E (contents of 2 200IU gel caps)

Any vegetable oil can be used as the carrier for the essential oils, but since calendula is known in herbal medicine to aid in ulcer healing, I highly recommend using it in this recipe. The Vitamin E is an antioxidant that helps to prolong the shelf life of the vegetable oil, but is added here primarily for its benefit to healing. Count out the recommended amounts of the above essential oils into an empty amber glass bottle. Add Vitamin E, then the vegetable oil. Shake gently to mix. Label contents. This blend is designed to be used as a local treatment (massage concentrate) and applied to the abdomen, concentrating on the upper abdominal region over the stomach. Following application, inhale the essences by cupping your hands over your nose and mouth. Take several long, deep, and relaxed breaths. I suggest you use this massage oil daily, preferably the same time every day, and incorporate its application into your daily regimen, perhaps following your morning shower. This way you will be getting consistent daily absorption of these anti-ulcer plant oils. All the essential oils listed in this recipe help in stressful conditions, in addition to being antimicrobial.

I want to point out here that this aromatherapy blend has been very helpful in supporting overall healing and relaxation in general, and is meant to be part of a dietary and lifestyle plan. As with most chronic or long-term health challenges, overnight recovery is not to be expected. It has taken years for problems such as these to surface, and it will sometimes take months to return to the level of health desired.

Ulcer-healing Herb Tea

1 part Marshmallow root (ground)

1 part Licorice root (ground)

1 part Slippery elm

1/2 part Echinacea angustafolia

1/2 part Geranium

Sage honey to taste

Mix the above tea in a bowl. Pour 1 cup boiling water to 1 teaspoon of herb. Let steep for 15 minutes. Drink on an empty stomach, two or three cups daily. These herbs have been traditionally used for healing stomach ulcers and decreasing stomach acids, as well as for binding proteins. The sage honey and Geranium are recommended for their astringent properties in preventing bleeding.

Other herbs known to be effective in healing ulcers are goldenseal, catnip, meadowsweet, ginger root, and peppermint.

Essential oils not already listed in the recipe that have proven effective in treating ulcers are frankincense and marjoram.

Here are some dietary recommendations that have a direct positive effect on the healing of the stomach lining and on decreasing the formation of ulcers:

- be tested for *H. pylori* by your health care practitioner
- if food allergy is a factor, avoid that reactive food
- avoid alcohol, coffee, black tea, and cola beverages

- quit smoking
- drink fresh lemon juice in warm water every morning (1/2 lemon squeezed)
- drink 2 to 3 cups raw cabbage juice daily (known to heal ulcers)
- increase Vitamin A, E, and Zinc in diet (from foods or supplements)
- increase fiber in diet
- eat more cabbage and okra
- drink peppermint herb tea with ginger honey on ice, instead of cola drinks.

Recommended lifestyle changes primarily involve learning more effective coping strategies for dealing with stress. Refer to Chapter 9 of this book for more information and direction.

Relief for Colitis

Colitis, as the name suggests, is an inflammation of the colon. The cause is not always clear, but seems to be related to the nervous system and the diet. Symptoms alternate between those related to constipation and diarrhea. At times the stools will be "pebble-like," dry and hard and then the next day may be very loose, or mucous-like. Bloating of the abdomen, mild cramping or strong spasms, flatulence, depression, and an overall diminished feeling of vitality can be experienced. High stress levels, presence of infection, disturbance within the immune system, food allergies, and genetic factors all come into play as possible contributors to colitis and other forms of inflammatory bowel disease.

Any sudden change in bowel habits, blood in the stool, or pain with movement of the bowels warrants an examination by your doctor since it could be more than colitis. One of the most ignored symptoms of colon cancer is a change of bowel habits, especially if noted for more than a week or two. Not everyone who experiences any of the above warning signs has cancer, but it is a good idea to rule out the possibility. Ignorance is sometimes much more harmful than the disease itself. Early detection and treatment determine your success in most health problems.

Case history: *A 43-year-old female with a history of colitis since her teenage years asked me to see her about one year ago, during a week of acute symptoms. She has experienced episodes of colitis-related symptoms six to eight times per year. She typically experiences a change in stools, alternating between constipation and diarrhea, with some abdominal bloating and cramping several hours following meals. She is frequently depressed and has*

*gradually been withdrawing from her social life during times of distress relat-
ed to the colitis. She refuses to see a physician for medication, as she is opposed
to taking drugs unless absolutely necessary. She has recognized foods that
seem to aggravate her condition, such as corn, large amounts of raw vegetables, fatty foods (especially fried food), and coffee. According to her, the colitis is not directly related to anything very stressful in her life; however I suspect
she is not fully aware of her stress levels and ability to cope with changes. She
refused any type of stress evaluation, etc., but she was willing to try an aromatherapy lotion and bath regime. I made further recommendations in her
diet which included decreasing other stimulant beverages like cola, chocolate
drinks, and tea blends which contained black tea leaves. She was unaware
these had almost as much caffeine as coffee. She used the massage lotion
recipe given below (which she called her "Chill Out" lotion) and drank the
herb tea occasionally. She has had but two episodes in the last six months, and
she attributes her improvement to the essential oils. Besides these recipes, she
would not be without the depression blend on pages 241–242 (Chapter 9)
which she uses whenever she feels down or blue.*

Colitis Relief Lotion

---

4 oz. unscented body lotion or vegetable oil

30 drops Lavender essential oil

10 drops Ylang- ylang essential oil

5 drops Bergamot essential oil

3 drops Chamomile essential oil

Add the essential oils to your base lotion or vegetable oil. Shake well to
mix thoroughly. Apply daily to the lower half of the abdomen area with
gentle massage with palm of hands. Inhale essences from hands afterwards.

Colitis Relief Tea

---

1 part Lemonbalm herb

1 part Catnip herb

1 part Calendula flower tops

1 part Chamomile flowers

Honey to taste

Combine the dried herbs in a bowl. Store in a clean glass jar and label. Use
1 teaspoon per cup of hot water. Steep for 5 minutes, then strain. Drink as
often as desired. The lemonbalm, peppermint, and chamomile herbs are

anti-spasmodic, while the calendula is added for its healing benefits. This tea happens to be very soothing, slightly cooling, and makes a great refreshing ice tea for the summer months. You don't have to have colitis to enjoy it!

Some additional herbs not mentioned up until now include the use of fenugreek seeds, marshmallow root, meadowsweet, slippery elm, hyssop and Mexican wild yam. Typically you would want to avoid highly spiced foods if they caused more complaints; however, these spices of cinnamon, garlic, thyme, and anise seed have proven of help with colitis symptoms.

Other essential oils used for this condition are basil, geranium, lemongrass, rosemary, pine, and peppermint. Most relaxing-type oils will also be useful for their calming effect on the nervous system. Anti-stress essences as well as depression-lifting oils can be used successfully and are given in Chapter 9 under related subjects. The use of aromatic baths is also extremely effective (see Chapter 11 for recipes and instruction). In England, Peppermint essential oil is used frequently in irritable bowel syndrome. As a matter of fact, doctors there incorporate Peppermint oil in preparations when patients need examination of the rectum and colon (endoscopy) because it has proven useful for colon spasms.

Gentle Stimulation for Sluggish Bowels and Constipation

This is probably the least exciting subject in this entire book. Nonetheless it is a common complaint among many, and fairly simple to rectify. Constipation is the name usually given to the lack of a bowel movement over a period of time, for most people about 24 hours. In general, it involves some difficulty in passing stools, which are often hard and dry in consistency. Sometimes there can be pain in the lower abdomen, and chronic constipation can lead to hemorrhoids as well. Although herbs are mostly recommended in this section, there are a few essential oils that can be supportive in stimulating peristalsis (the wave-like contractions of the intestinal walls that support the movement of materials through the bowels).

If you are elderly, and have had normal movements for most of your life and suddenly find yourself constipated, you need to get checked by your doctor, as changes in bowel habits can be a warning sign of a serious problem such as physical blockage.

Some of the causes of sluggish bowels and constipation are nervous tension, a diet consistently low in roughage (fiber), dehydration, and a sedentary lifestyle. In recent years, constipation has been increasing related to overuse of laxatives which may promote "lazy" bowels because the body loses the ability to regulate the passage of stools. Even herbal laxatives can have a negative effect if used too frequently. Laxatives should be used on an occasional basis. If you find yourself reaching for a laxative more than once a month, consider dietary and lifestyle changes to support your body regulating function.

> **Case history:**   *An elderly woman experiencing occasional bouts of constipation asked for my advice while visiting family during the summer. After further evaluation, it appeared to be a simple case of constipation due to lack of exercise, the stress of traveling, and a change in her typical eating patterns. She was curious to give herbs and aromatherapy a try since this was entirely new to her. She was one of the most conscientious clients I have ever worked with! She did everything that was recommended to her and called with questions and feedback. She made dietary changes which called for increasing fiber and liquids. She looked forward to her bran muffin every day, and she enjoyed her "special potion," as she called her aromatherapy blend. It was so funny because her favorite aromatic bath is the Woodstock recipe (in Chapter 11). We joked about that every time we saw each other!*

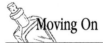

Moving On

a massage oil for sluggish bowels

2 tablespoons vegetable oil

7 drops Rosemary essential oil

5 drops Fennel essential oil

Mix the essential oils with the vegetable oil in a small amber bottle. Massage a small amount to the lower abdomen and sacrum area (lower back over spine) on a daily basis. These oils help to stimulate sluggish bowels.

Herbal Laxative Tea

1/8" slice fresh ginger root

1/2 teaspoon Fennel seed

1/2 teaspoon Licorice root

Honey to taste (preferably ginger honey, see recipe page 38)

Pour 1 cup boiling water over herbs and allow to steep for 5 to 10 minutes. Drink this tea for occasional constipation as needed. Best taken at bedtime. Since dehydration is the most common cause of constipation, a laxative tea provides both extra liquid and gentle stimulation.

Guaranteed-to-Work Bran Muffins

Donna-Jean's favorite

1 cup Bran

1/2 cup Oat bran

1 1/2 cup whole wheat flour

1 teaspoon Baking soda

1/2 cup chopped prune pieces

2 egg whites

1 banana

1/2 cup molasses

2 tbls. safflower oil

3/4 cup nonfat milk

12 Walnut halves (optional)

Preheat oven to 400 degrees. Combine all the dry ingredients in a bowl. Add prune pieces. In a food processor or blender, mix together the egg whites, banana, molasses, oil and milk. Add the wet mixture to the dry ingredients. Just fold together until moist (don't overstir). Spray muffin tins with oil or use paper cups. Fill muffin tins 3/4ths full and top with a walnut half. Bake for 15 to 18 minutes. Do not overbake them or they will turn out dry. Enjoy one of these muffins every day. These freeze well so you can make a batch or two and store them 7 per bag for a week's supply. Be sure to drink a full glass of liquid with your muffin. Try warm milk with the ginger honey! Bran works best when taken with plenty of fluids; otherwise it can cause more constipation if the bowels are lacking adequate hydration. Makes one dozen.

Other herbs that are helpful in alleviating constipation are ginger, fennel, licorice, marshmallow root, rhubarb root, slippery elm, and psyllium husk.

Dietary modifications include increasing fluid intake (at least 8 glasses of pure water, herb tea, mineral water, or diluted fresh fruit juice per day). Increase fiber in your diet by adding a little bran to almost everything (rather than all at once); try sprinkling 1/2 teaspoon or more on whole- grain cereal and baking with it. Incorporating more whole grains into your diet will provide a source of natural fiber. And don't forget you can always eat one bran muffin a day—the guaranteed-to-work kind. For mild forms of constipation, many find relief in drinking a cup of hot tea (Herbal Laxative Tea or other herbal varieties) every morning upon rising and developing a routine of sitting in the bathroom until the bowels have moved. Remember not to strain. It is really true how establishing a routine can help in this area.

A look into your lifestyle and habits may enlighten you as to whether or not stress plays a part in your problem. If you tend to be a nervous type or get anxious easily, don't worry because there are many excellent recipes and suggestions in Chapter 9 under the related subjects that may apply to you. So go there now and review the areas you think you might need help in as they relate to the stress, emotional challenges, and the nervous system. If you suspect you have been overusing the laxatives, consult with your doctor if s/he has prescribed them and look at the options we have discussed here.

Natural Remedy for Diarrhea

Diarrhea is the abnormal frequency of emptying the bowels. The degree of looseness and frequency can vary from mild to severe and may be accompanied by abdominal cramping and bloating. In the most severe cases the stool is watery and frequently passed; extreme or prolonged diarrhea can result in dehydration, bleeding, malnutrition, and overall weakness. Common causes include food poisoning, water contamination, viral infection, inflammation (as in colitis and diverticulitis), and nervous conditions (fear, extreme anxiety).

If the reason for the diarrhea is viral infection or food poisoning, it is a naturally protective response by the body to try to expel as much of the "harmful" organisms or poison as possible. Therefore, if you suspect this is the case, let the body run its course for 12 hours before getting concerned. Sometimes this is all that is needed to get rid of the offending organism. Keep in mind that our bodies, and in particular our digestive systems, are constantly dealing with germs and (unfortunately) chemicals. It is only when our immunity is compromised or our defenses are overwhelmed that we experience symptoms.

If your infant is having diarrhea, or if diarrhea has been present for more than 24 hours and the person cannot hold down liquids (vomiting), there is a very real danger of dehydration. This can happen quickly, especially in small children, so you must get them to the doctor immediately. Also, whenever there is bleeding involved, see your doctor for examination.

Diarrhea Remedy Rub

massage oil for abdomen

2 tablespoons vegetable oil

8 drops Lavender essential oil

2 drops Ginger essential oil

1 drop Chamomile essential oil

1 drop Peppermint essential oil

Measure essential oils into a glass amber bottle. Add the vegetable oil and shake gently to mix.

Massage this over lower abdomen and lower back area with palm of hand. Inhale essences from hands with several slow deep breaths following massage. Be careful not to massage too deeply as this can further stimulate the bowels. Lie quietly for 15 to 20 minutes. Apply twice per day.

Other essential oils that can help to calm the spasms and irritability of the bowels include geranium, juniper, lemon, and rosemary. If diarrhea has been chronic, neroli and sandalwood essential oils are advised.

The following drink is similar to the Indian drink called "lassi" which is primarily yogurt and water. It is made sweet with honey or sugar, or a sour version is prepared with salt. Salt helps the body to hold onto fluids; therefore it is added to this recipe for diarrhea. Actually, our family makes many versions of this drink in the summer months using rose water, ginger honey, or fresh mint leaves as different flavorings along with crushed ice; we whip it up in the blender to make a very refreshing beverage. Here's my version that decreases the trips to the bathroom when diarrhea is present.

Lassi for Diarrhea

a drink to counteract diarrhea

1/2 cup natural plain yogurt

1/2 cup cold water

1 teaspoon finely grated fresh ginger root

1/4 teaspoon sea salt

pinch of nutmeg

pinch of cinnamon

Use natural yogurt that contains live cultures of acidophilus and lactobacillus to help restore the "good" flora being lost through the bowels with diarrhea. Combine in the blender all the ingredients listed above. Frappe on high.

Some other spices and herbs noted for combatting diarrhea are clove, garlic, onion, sage, and nutmeg. The latter has been used to treat diarrhea with much success. Eucalyptus, chamomile, marshmallow root, meadowsweet, catnip, and slippery elm are also very beneficial herbs. Lemon is antiseptic and antibacterial, so the fresh juice can be added to water that needs further purification, or drink bottled water when traveling in countries where there are questionable health risks.

Dietary changes are made during times of recuperation because the bowels have been overworking and over-stimulated. Eating bland foods and drinking more liquids is the best plan of action. Avoid fruits, sweets, high roughage foods, stimulants such as caffeinated drinks, and highly spiced foods at this time. Nutmeg in warm milk may also calm diarrheal episodes.

Be sure to make space in your life to get more rest and allow your body to heal. I suggest you diffuse cleansing and purifying essences in the air to help with disinfecting and deodorizing the environment. Pure for Sure inhalation recipe is on page 335 in Chapter 13 and would be ideal to use at this time. If you are feeling anxious, or think your nervous system needs some soothing scents, try the Slow Down and Relax blend or take an aromatic bath. Serenity or the Undress-De-Stress bath recipes are given on page 301 of Chapter 11.

Soothing Help for Hemorrhoids

Also known as piles, hemorrhoids are swollen varicose veins in the anal walls. They can vary from pea size to large clusters and may be internal or external. Hemorrhoids can cause itching, pain, and bleeding. Factors that contribute to the problem are straining from constipation, lifting, sitting for long periods of time, lack of exercise, being overweight and/or eating a low fiber diet. They can also present themselves during the last trimester of pregnancy when there is additional weight and pressure on bowels and pelvis.

Hemorrhoids are relatively easy to take care of and prevent. First, you will want to shrink and tone the swollen varicosities with an astringent to help with the immediate pain, swelling, and resultant itching. But to completely treat the problem you must address some elemental dietary and lifestyle habits that are contributing to this ailment. And, yes, it is a common ailment. Millions suffer from this condition. You cannot watch television without seeing an advertisement for hemorrhoid remedies—wipes, pads, creams. The following recipes will help prevent hemorrhoids from forming, and shrink them down if they are already present.

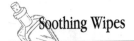 **Soothing Wipes**

to soothe and heal hemorrhoids

8 oz. bottle distilled Witch hazel

5 drops Cypress essential oil

5 drops Lavender essential oil

1 - 2 tablespoons Aloe vera gel (optional)

To the Witch hazel, which is the basic ingredient of these "natural" and very effective hemorrhoid treatment wipes, add the recommended amounts of essential oils. Label the bottle. Shake contents well before each use. To use, dampen a cotton pad with this lotion, and gently pat the affected area. This area is very vascular, and responds quickly to these essential oils, aloe vera gel, and witch hazel, which assist in shrinking, soothing, and healing the swollen varicose tissues. I recommend you use a pad following each bowel movement and a few times during the day if you are experiencing any of the annoying symptoms (burning, itching) that accompany this ailment.

I suggest you buy the round, all-cotton, cosmetic-type swipes or pads that are sold in pharmacies. 100% cotton is the least irritating to the delicate swollen tissues. Many so-called cotton balls are not made of cotton any more, but of all synthetic fibers which may be irritating and are not absorptive.

Helpful Tip: You can make pads up ahead of time by moistening them with this lotion and storing them in a zip-lock plastic bag for convenience. They are especially soothing when stored in the refrigerator.

Other helpful essential oils you can use that will provide similar results in toning vessels and decreasing inflammation are bergamot and myrrh.

Some of the herbs that are traditionally used for hemorrhoids are Pilewort (*Ranunculus ficaria* or lesser celandine), dandelion root, goldenseal, and yarrow. Aloe vera, garlic, and onion have also been proven useful.

Lifestyle and dietary modifications that can assist in prevention are:

- Increase dietary roughage to avoid constipation, and keep bowels healthy
- Increase fluids, at least 8 glasses of pure water, herb tea, fresh fruit and vegetable juices per day
- Avoid sitting for long periods of time—take intermittent breaks.
- Exercise regularly
- Avoid caffeine and alcohol.

Avoid harsh toilet soaps on this area until the hemorrhoids have healed. Most soaps are very drying and cause further itching and irritation because they contain chemical deodorants and fragrances. Also, sitz baths can be very soothing for this ailment. Use the suggested essential oils in a shallow bath tub of lukewarm water and sit and soak. Avoid using hot water on hemorrhoids because it encourages the dilation of blood vessels. Alternatively, you can use calendula oil or ointment with these essential oils as well for direct application and spot treatment. See recipe for calendula oil page 372 and the directions for making your own ointment on page 378.

CHAPTER 3

Aromatherapy Treatments for Eye, Ear, Nose, and Throat Problems

Brief Overview of Eye, Ear, Nose, and Throat

Most of this chapter pertains to the very early signs of illness related to the eye, ear, nose, and throat areas. Generally, these ailments are a result of infections, allergic reactions, and traumas. The eyes are briefly addressed in this chapter, with major emphasis on upper respiratory infections of the sinuses (the four cavities of the face), earaches, and minor throat irritations, inflammation, and infection. Where there is a risk of complications or more serious conditions, I have made note to seek professional attention for accurate diagnosis and treatment.

The following anatomical portions of the body are discussed as they relate to the common ailments associated with them.

The *eyes,* including the conjunctiva (the membranous covering of the sclera) and the upper and lower lids. This covering is transparent and contains red blood vessels which can become dilated and produce the characteristic "bloodshot" eye appearance. Under healthy conditions this covering is clear, and there is no presence of drainage or crusting.

The *ears,* specifically the outer portion, auditory canal, and ear drum, are reviewed in regard to earache. Primarily seen in children, earaches usually are a result of head colds, fever, and pressure. The ears are often affected by other ailments such as swollen tonsils, sore throat, and coughing.

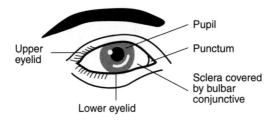

The Eye

Most often, when one of these underlying conditions is present, the Eustachian tubes that drain the inner ear become blocked and change the inner ear pressure, causing a buildup of fluid. The ears are responsible for our sense of balance as well as hearing.

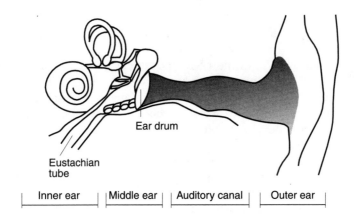

The Ear

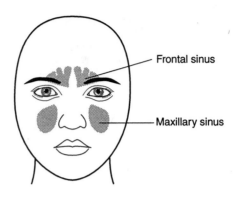

Frontal sinus

Maxillary sinus

The Sinuses

The *nose* and *sinuses* are discussed, as well as ailments of the upper respiratory tract. The four sinus cavities are located in the front and maxillary areas of the face. Under healthy conditions the nasal membranes are pink and moist, with no drainage present. Dry nose, bleeding, and sinus infections are common ailments addressed in this section.

The *throat,* including the tonsils, vocal cords, and larynx, will be discussed in addition to the local lymph glands (nodes) which may be involved in upper respiratory infections.

The general health of the body, the strength of the immune system, and the body's ability to ward off and resist outside pathogens, such as bacteria and viruses, are the underlying factors in how ailments of the eye, ear, nose, and throat present themselves in the above mentioned areas of the body. The average person is constantly exposed everyday to germs, both airborne and by direct contact. Children who attend school or day-care centers are at greater risk for exposure to these germs, since they are still developing their immune systems. Our defense against all microbes begins with our overall health and especially the strength of our immune system. The Holistic Health Wheel, which incorporates into a whole some of the diverse forces that affect our health, provides a good visual reminder of the need for balance in our lives. You may wish to review the wheel again at this time. Our ability to cope with stress is one of the most important factors in determining the state of our immune system. Chapter 9 which covers stress-related aromatherapy, will be an essential companion to this chapter.

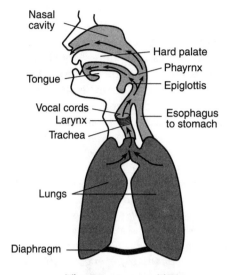

Nasal cavity

Hard palate

Phayrnx

Tongue

Epiglottis

Vocal cords

Larynx

Trachea

Esophagus to stomach

Lungs

Diaphragm

The Respiratory Tract

Why Are Essential Oils So Effective for Treating Infection?

- Essential Oils are less toxic to the body than synthetic antibiotics.
- Essential Oils do not create bacterial resistance as do antibiotics.
- Essential Oils effectively stimulate the Immune System.
- Essential Oils act directly on bacteria.
- Essential Oils support life, whereby antibiotics destroy healthy intestinal flora.
- Essential Oils do not accumulate in the body with continued use.

Based on *The Pacific Institute of Aromatherapy,* Aromatherapy Course, Second Edition, Dr. Kurt Schnaubelt

Relieving Conjunctivitis

Conjunctivitis is an inflammation of the transparent tissue covering the sclera of the eye and the lids. It is very common and is typically characterized by redness, swelling, itching, burning, and possibly tearing. The conjunctival tissue becomes inflamed and red, hence its common name of "pink eye." Conjunctivitis is most often caused by a bacterial infection and is seen frequently among preschool-age children. This condition is contagious and can spread to the other eye quite easily, as well as to other children, if care is not taken. Discharge is common and is a result of the inflammatory process. If the tearing matter is clear and watery, chances are it is of viral origin. The bacterial-type infection produces a yellowish or green-colored discharge. Often upon awakening in the morning, the person will have a crusted discharge around the eye. Conjunctivitis typically does not cause visual changes. It is associated with allergies or environmental irritants such as exposure to smoke and chlorine (in swimming pools, for example).

Case history: *A 5-year-old girl who developed conjunctivitis was succcess-fully treated with aromatherapy in the form of an eye wash and compress. She initially complained of itching, dry eyes and her conjunctiva was the typical red-colored "pink eye." In the morning she awoke with yellow dry matter crust-ed around the eye corners. Over the two days during which she received eye wash and compress treatments, she felt immediate relief from the dryness. Although there were no symptoms present after the initial two days of treat-ment, the regimen was continued for another two days. Her eye infection remained isolated to the one eye.* '

 Eye Wash

for conjunctivitis

1 cup boiled tepid water (or distilled bottled water)

1/4 teaspoon sea salt

Dissolve salt in water. With inflamed tissue, such as conjunctivitis, always use cool or tepid water temperatures to encourage a decrease in the swelling. Fill an eye wash cup, or a shot glass, with the salt water solution. Bend over onto the eye cup and fit as snugly as you can over the eye area, trying to prevent any leakage. Tilt head backwards, and blink several times, washing the eyeball and lids with the liquid. Tilt head back to the forward and down position and empty eye cup contents into sink. Refill, and wash several times. Pat eye area gently. Wash eye cup well with soap and water, as well as your hands. Do not re-use towels, as this can spread to other members of the family, or to the other eye. Follow with compress recipe.

The following recipe is for an eye compress that can be used for any inflamed eye condition. A compress is an external application (usually a cotton pad or cotton balls) moistened with a lotion of water, herb tea, and essential oils. The eyes *must* stay closed during this treatment to avoid irritation from the essential oils. The herbal and aromatic properties of the compress will be absorbed through the eyelids. This treatment makes a great follow up to the eye wash (salt water solution). A cool temperature is recommended for the compress, so you can make this ahead of time and let it cool in the refrigerator before using it.

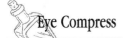 ## Eye Compress

for inflamed eye conditions

2 cups boiled water (or distilled bottled water)

1 teaspoon distilled witch hazel (optional)

2 teaspoons of one of the following herbs:

Chamomile, eyebright, or calendula petals

several 2-inch round cosmetic cotton pads/wipes (or cotton balls)

Heat two cups of water to boil. Then add the herb and let steep for 5 to 10 minutes. Strain through a paper coffee filter or several layers of cheese cloth. Pour into clean glass jar. Add witch hazel. Close jar and shake well. Refrigerate to cool. When ready to use, shake contents well and pour over cotton pads. Wring out the pads and lie down in a relaxing place. Apply the moist compress to the affected eye for 5 to 10 minutes. Do this two or three times per day. Remember to keep eyes closed during application! Do not use this application on small children who are unable to follow directions.

The particular herbs chosen for this eye compress recipe are ones that are good for inflammation and irritations of the delicate and sensitive eye areas. Eyebright (Euphrasia) is particularly known for its benefit to the eyes (as reflected by the name). The witch hazel is an astringent and helps with swelling.

Other herbs traditionally used in the treatment of eye disorders such as conjunctivitis are quince, elderflower, goldenseal and ginseng. Boric acid has been widely used by traditional western medicine for washing the eye, but must be very well diluted and care must be taken in its use.

Hydrosols or floral waters are recommended rather than essential oils. Chamomile, Rose and Lavender floral waters are excellent choices for eye compress usage. However, I find that Chamomile floral water is the finest choice for this condition and is the mildest for the delicate tissues.

Since conjunctivitis is contagious, good hygiene is required. Clean towels and utensils along with meticulous handwashing are very important. Eye symptoms may be exacerbated by irritants; therefore exposure to the causative factors should be avoided as much as possible (chlorine pools, environmental irritants, contaminated eye products, such as mascara).

Save Your Eyes—Preventing Eye Strain

Eye strain frequently occurs among computer operators, TV watchers, and avid book readers. Possible symptoms include difficulty in focusing, watery or itchy eyes, tiredness, headaches, blurred vision, or seeing spots. It equates to visual stress from constantly overworking these sensory organs and is generally preventable. Finding the cause of the problem, such as poor lighting, glaring light, computer screens, night driving, and wearing eyeware with an incorrect prescription, will help in its prevention.

A cool compress over the eyes will be of great help in relieving eye strain after a long day. Use the eye compress recipe on the previous page for inflamed eye conditions. Lie quietly for 10 minutes or longer with the eye compresses over the eyes. Because eye strain usually has an emotional or physical stress component, you will also benefit from anti-stress blends for your bath and from inhalation methods. I highly recommend the *TGIF* aromatic bath recipe for sensory overload found on page 300 of Chapter 11.

Eyebright (Euphrasia herb) tea can be taken internally for general weakness of the eyes and eye strain. Commercial eye packs made of gel-filled plastic can be purchased and stored in the refrigerator for future use. You can also make a handmade eye pillow for eye strain and stress. I have included a recipe for making an eye pillow on page 332.

Lifestyle changes in the workplace may include installing full spectrum lighting. The ideal lighting arrangement for reading or detailed work is bright lighting at shoulder level, placed behind you and off to one side. Anti-glare computer screen frames are available to cut down on glare and light reflection. And let's not forget to take breaks! Get up and walk around periodically. Allow your eyes to rest and adjust. Under less optimal conditions, look up every so often to focus on a corner of a room, or distant object to rest your eyes. Being kind to your eyes is the long-term answer to this common ailment.

How to Cure Earaches

First, let me clarify: we are talking about earaches of the external ear and auditory canal. Middle ear infections (otitis media) can be serious if left untreated, leading to more severe complications, such as mastoiditis, brain abscesses, or meningitis. See warning symptoms following.

Symptoms of a typical external earache are often seen during a cold or flu, when the Eustachian tubes become blocked from swelling and/or irritation. They are common among young children whose tubes are more horizontal in position than in an adult.

Warning: There are several symptoms that should be evaluated promptly by a physician if they develop. These include a sudden hearing loss, severe headache or nausea and vomiting, dizziness, chills, fever, and persistent pain in and around the ear, and discharge. When ear infections are a chronic problem, constitutional treatment is recommended.

Aching or pain in the ear can be caused by a bacterial or fungal infection, or trauma to the ear canal. If the earache is accompanied by congestion, then alleviating the mucous accumulation will prove helpful and is discussed on page 70, "Incredible Relief for Congestion." Since ear pain often accompanies other conditions, it is important to treat the whole person.

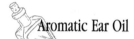 Aromatic Ear Oil

for earaches

1/2 teaspoon Mullein infused oil*

1/2 teaspoon Garlic infused oil*

1 drop Lavender essential oil

1 drop Chamomile essential oil

Cotton for inserting in the ear

Combine mullein and garlic oils in a small dish. Add essential oils and mix well. Gently warm in hot water bath. Apply 2-3 drops of aromatic ear oil into the ear canal with an eye dropper. Plug ear with cotton to protect clothes or bedding.

*If these oils are not available, use extra virgin olive oil or sesame oil. Refer to page 372 on infused oils to make on your own.

Mullein flowers, with strong antibacterial properties, have been widely used for treating the nerve-type pain associated with earaches. Garlic oil is used for its natural antibiotic effects as well. Chamomile and lavender essential oils are gentle enough for use in the ear, and possess anti-inflammatory and analgesic properties. Other essential oils that have been successful in alleviating ear pain are basil, tea tree, and hyssop.

In traditional folk medicine a small muslin bag or sock filled with sea salt, flax seeds, or buckwheat was heated and placed over the affected ear, to draw moisture from the ear canal. Similarly, mothers would instinctively rock their babies with their "bad" ear against their bosoms. A hot water bottle works well too!

There are a few lifestyle alterations you can make to prevent earaches. Keep the ear dry, especially following showers, swimming, or shampooing. If allergies are a factor, which is often the case in recurrent chronic earaches, then identifying the allergen is important and may be facilitated by a nutritionist. A large number of children's earaches and infections, for example, stem from an allergic reaction to dairy or wheat products.

Sniffing Out Relief for Dry Nasal Passages

A dry nose can be an uncomfortable nuisance that may set the stage for other problems, such as nosebleeds and infection. It is a symptom that you are not taking in enough liquids, and/or your environment is too dry. This condition presents itself most often during the mid-winter months, when the central heating is on, the house is closed up, and the outside air can also be dry and cold.

> **Case history:**   *A 40-year-old woman who was very physically active became distressed when she began to experience a very dry nose with tiny scab-like sores. She had recently begun working full-time indoors at a new job. She was impressed with the results after using this nasal oil remedy. The warm sesame oil gave her instant relief and she later added Tea Tree essential oil to help heal the tiny scabs that had developed. She used room mists and left windows cracked open as much as possible to increase the moisture content of the air in her home, and increased her fluid intake.*

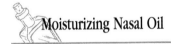 Moisturizing Nasal Oil

for dry nose conditions

1 Tablespoon natural sesame oil (warmed)

Put a small amount of sesame oil in a shallow dish or saucer. A ramekin is perfect for this. Warm the oil in a hot water bath or use at room temperature. Every morning upon waking, and several times per day as needed, sniff the oil by dipping your little finger in the oil and inserting it into one nostril. Close the other nostril with your index finger, and sniff or inhale the oil from your finger. Repeat the same procedure for the other nostril. The further you can insert your little finger the better. You will want to do this in the privacy of your bathroom for obvious reasons!

According to Ayurvedic medicine, sesame oil is very balancing to the nervous system and moisturizing to the skin; sniffing sesame oil is also known to balance Vata body types, one of the three Ayurvedic constitutional types. This ancient healing art believes as well that total body massage with sesame oil is very grounding, healthful, and balancing.

The following recipe includes Tea Tree essential oil and can be used for more severe nasal dryness and irritation, in addition to healing scab-like sores in the nose.

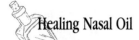

Healing Nasal Oil

for nasal sores

1 tablespoon natural sesame oil

1 tablespoon calendula infused oil

1 – 2 drops Tea Tree essential oil

Vitamin E (400IU)

Mix the sesame and calendula oil in a small dish or wide-mouth amber bottle. If you do not have calendula oil, use sesame oil (2 tablespoons total). Cut the end of the Vitamin E gel cap or capsule and squeeze the contents into the sesame oil. Add the Tea Tree essential oil and mix thoroughly. Use this nasal oil several times per day until sores heal. Use the same directions for sniffing the oil into the nose as stated for the Moisturizing Nasal Oil recipe given previously.

Calendula infusion oil is extremely healing and moisturizing. Directions are given on page 372 to make your own at home. Use the finest olive oil you can get to make this oil; you can't find a better remedy for healing the skin and mucous membranes. Tea tree is very healing, antibacterial and anti-fungal, so it is a good choice to prevent infection.

Lifestyle recommendations include any or all attempts to increase the moisture content of your living and working environment. These may include:

- cracking windows open to allow air exchange
- lowering the central heating temperature
- placing pans of water on radiators, stovetops, etc.
- using a humidifier (put on timer to go off automatically)
- use more indoor plants, preferably the clean air plants suggested in Chapter 13
- use room mists to add moisture and purify the air (see Chapter 13 for recipes)
- spend more time outdoors in the fresh air

A dry nose can also be a sign of dehydration within the body, so increase your fluid intake. Pure water, herbal teas, and diluted fresh fruit and vegetable juices are best! Coffee, black tea, alcohol, and cola drinks will aggravate the problem, since they are dehydrating. As a matter of fact, you should be drinking 2 or 3 glasses of water for every glass of the above concentrated beverages you consume.

You can also use steam inhalations for a dry nose condition. I recommend warm or hot water. Be careful not to overheat the water as this can be drying and could cause harm to the already compromised lining of the nasal passages. Add 1 or 2 drops of the Tea Tree essential oil to your steam inhalation treatment, following the directions given in Chapter 13, and modify the water temperature.

Incredible Relief for Congestion— Loosening Up the Mucus

Catarrh is the term given to the formation and accumulation of mucus in the nose and throat. When you experience a quick onset of nasal congestion, it is called *acute rhinitis*. Aromatherapy is particularly well applied in this area, since volatile oils are the most natural and best remedial treatment for catarrhal conditions. Most infections involving the mucous membranes of the nasal cavity are caused by viruses. Another common cause is an allergic reaction to food allergens, environmental pollutants, etc. The result is inflammation and congestion. The severity can range from mild catarrh to excessive mucus discharge. If drainage is colored yellowish-green, then a bacterial infection may be present. See "sinusitis" for treatment of this type.

> **Case history:** *A 12-year-old girl suffering from congestion with clear mucus used the following steam inhalation recipe for consistent improvement and ease in breathing. After the very first steam treatment she felt her nasal passages opening up, which she described as "crackling" sounds in her nose. She opted not to use the chest rub during the day because of its medicinal smell, so she applied it after school and at night. She carried Eucalyptus oil with her throughout the school day to inhale as needed when her stuffy nose became a problem. (A plastic baggie holding a few cotton balls with several drops of essential oil on them makes an easy inhalation method for travel.) Normally with acute rhinitis, a fever and a decrease in energy levels would occur. With some of these simple steps, neither of these conditions existed. Her runny nose was almost gone after two days of therapeutic essential oil inhalations. She was delighted both with her quick recovery and the simple methods.*

Steam Inhalation for Catarrh

to loosen and expectorate excessive mucus

ceramic or glass bowl

4 cups hot water

2 drops Eucalyptus essential oil

1 drop Cedarwood essential oil

a towel

Pour hot water into bowl. Add 2 or 3 drops of essential oils listed above. Hold head over bowl (about 8 inches from water) and cover your head with the towel to form a tent. Keep eyes closed during this treatment as the volatile oils can irritate the eyes and cause tearing. Slowly and deeply inhale through the nose and mouth. Allow loosened mucus to drain freely into water bowl. Steam for 5 to 10 minutes for full benefit. Pat face and neck area dry with towel. Keep neck and chest covered and warm following treatment. Follow with chest rub.

Eucalyptus essential oil is the best expectorant (promotes the discharge of mucus from the respiratory tract). Many other essential oils have this property as well, such as cedarwood either used singly or in combination with eucalyptus oil in the steam treatment.

While for catarrh steam inhalation will break up and remove secretions immediately, chest rub oils are best for continual all-day relief, and they help prevent bacterial infections. See Chapter 13, *Healing Treatments for the Respiratory Tract,* for more information on methods that can be employed. This chest rub blend is a favorite for many of my clients. It has a clean, fresh, and herb-like scent unlike the medicinal menthol-smelling ointments on the market. It's 100% natural and extremely effective for nasal congestion. *Caution:* Do not use during pregnancy.

Chest Rub for Catarrh

for stuffy nose

2 ounces vegetable oil

20 drops Eucalyptus essential oil

5 drops Basil essential oil

5 drops Peppermint essential oil

5 drops Cedarwood essential oil

In an amber glass bottle add the above essential oils. Then pour the 2 ounces of vegetable oil into the bottle. Shake well and label. This oil is to be applied to the upper chest area, lower neck, and back (between the shoulder blades and base of neck). Inhale the essential oils from your hands following the application. Use 2 or 3 times per day, preferably in early morning and at bedtime.

Other essential oils that can be used for nasal catarrh are bergamot, fennel, frankincense, hyssop, lavender, lemon, marjoram, myrrh, pine, sandalwood, and rosemary. There are many choices, so if you have particular scent favorites, use them. Remember that fennel, peppermint, rosemary, and basil are possible skin irritants, so use them in small quantities. See Chapter 1, *Common Sense Safety.*

Lifestyle and dietary changes that can hasten recovery are:

- avoid dairy products, which are known to increase mucus production
- drink fresh lemon juice in hot or cold water during the day
- eat more fresh fruit and vegetables
- cook with garlic and onions ; these also help with catarrh
- carry a tissue with a few drops of essential oil on it to inhale during the day
- use a room diffuser to purify the air, and to enhance respiration (expectorant oils)
- get rest and drink more fluids

Is There Help for Anosmia?—How to Stimulate Your Sense of Smell

Unless you have this condition, you probably haven't heard of it before. Anosmia is the inability to smell. Approximately 1 1/2% of the American population (more than 2 million) experiences this unpleasant condition. The numbers are even greater if you include those individuals who experience a reduced ability to smell (hyposmia) or a distorted sense of smell (parosmia).

Some of the major causes that can alter the olfactory senses include head injury, environmental factors, medications, and some medical disorders. Smell is a chemical phenomenon: aromatic molecules attach themselves to the olfactory hairs and are transmitted directly into the brain. See Chapter 1, *Olfactory System* diagram page 14. Our ability to smell also varies with age, gender, genetics, and personal experience, which makes it a difficult area to study. Until recently, the sense of smell has been underrated and practically ignored by mainstream scientific and health researchers.

As much as 90% of what we taste is actually smell-related. We use our sense of smell to fully enjoy life's pleasures and to warn us from danger, such as in the case of food poisoning, fire, gas intoxication, etc. It's a wonder that it has taken so long to recognize its importance! Many people who have lost their sense of smell also suffer from depression, a decreased interest in sex, weight gain, and are at greater risk for accidents. It's hard to realize how important our sense of smell really is because it's impossible to imagine life without it.

First, let's discuss the most frequent cause of altered sense of smell, head injury, which accounts for 35 to 40% of the people who are affected by these conditions. Between 5 and 10% of all major head injuries result in some olfactory dysfunction. These statistics show the importance of prevention, using seat belts, helmets, etc.

Conditions or ailments that can affect the sense of smell are colds, allergies, flu, sinus infections, nasal polyps, overgrowth of adenoids, deviated nasal septum, Vitamin A, B12 or Zinc deficiency. Other medical disorders, more serious in nature, that can alter the sense of smell are tumors, neurological problems, endocrine disorders, cirrhosis of the liver, kidney failure, stroke, acute viral hepatitis, Parkinson's, Alzheimer's disease, surgical side-effects or radiation treatment to the head.

Other causative factors such as cigarette smoking (including inhaling secondary smoke) and recreational drug use (specifically cocaine) have been linked to temporary or permanent damage to the olfactory system. Medications and some dietary supplements like nose drops, antibiotics, blood pressure medications, anticoagulants, antihistamines, and cancer chemotherapy have all been linked to the cause of a decrease in the ability to smell.

Environmental factors include exposure to toxic agents such as silicon, aluminum, arsenic, cadmium, gold, hydrogen sulfide, formaldehyde, lead, mercury, and trichloroethylene. These chemicals cause nasal lining inflammation and destroy nerve tissue which prevents the "smell" message from getting to the brain. *Smell adaptation* is the term given to the temporary loss of ability to perceive an odor, while *olfactory fatigue* is the inability to perceive a particular chemical odor, which can be either temporary or permanent in nature.

If you find that you experience residual loss of smell immediately following a cold or flu, Lecithin or fish oil may help improve the olfactory nerve cell transmission. If you question the possibility of a nutritional deficiency (or excess such as copper) see a qualified physician with expertise in these areas for remedial treatment.

If environmental factors have been a concern, then take charge of your health and remove the potential hazards. Refer to Chapter 13 for information on purifying your environment.

Suggestions that can help stimulate your sense of smell:

- avoid cigarette smoke
- remove chemical pollutants (house cleaners, synthetic scents, etc.)
- purify your environment
- add Lecithin to your diet
- eat more fresh fish (fish oils can be beneficial)
- see your doctor regarding the possibility of a nutritional deficiency (check zinc)
- inquire about the medications you are taking; can they elicit side-effects that are related? See your doctor or ask your pharmacist
- see an ENT (Ear, Nose, and Throat) specialist to rule out nasal deformity (polyps, deviated septum, etc.)
- if chronic catarrh is present, deal with underlying cause and use expectorant essential oils to relieve the congestion; refer to the section addressing catarrh
- avoid use of large amounts of peppermint essential oil (high menthol-containing oils)
- use Sense-able Nasal Oil

After exploring and making the necessary changes, both lifestyle and dietary, use the following nasal oil to nourish the delicate nasal mucous membrane lining and protect nerve endings in this area. The suggested oils are ones that contain vitamins and antioxidant properties. They are gentle in nature and will have a positive effect with long-term use. Frankincense is the essential oil of choice because it has a low evaporation rate (base note), is antiseptic, and is a gentle expectorant. It is most useful in chronic, slow-to-change conditions. Frankincense also is beneficial in states of stress, depression, and obsessive thinking, which may possibly be experienced along with the decreased ability to perceive aromas and enjoy life fully. Of course, this is a supportive measure, and the underlying factors must be taken care of to totally remedy the condition. Where surgical side-effects are involved, little or no change may be possible. Keep in mind, the olfactory system is a neuro-chemical phenomenon.

Sense-able Nasal Oil

as an aid for increasing ability to smell

5 teaspoons natural sesame oil

1 teaspoon wheatgerm oil

1/4 teaspoon hypericum infusion oil (St. John's Wort)

1/4 teaspoon mullein infusion oil

1 drop Frankincense essential oil

Combine all oils, including the one drop of Frankincense, into a clean amber glass bottle. Shake well and label contents. Use daily. Refer to directions for inhaling nasal oil on page 68.

Sesame oil was chosen for its calming and balancing effects according to Ayurvedic medicine. Wheatgerm oil is an antioxidant and rich in vitamins. Hypericum oil has anti-inflammatory qualities and is of benefit to nerve endings. Mullein also has anti-inflammatory properties, as well as being helpful in nerve-related conditions. It has been used for many respiratory ailments such as tuberculosis, asthma, and bronchitis and, added to this oil blend, supports the relationship between the nervous and respiratory systems. The use of frankincense is very conservative since the therapeutic approach is to nourish rather than stimulate.

Potent Remedy for Sinusitis

Our head contains four air pockets, known as sinuses, which lie behind the brow and under the cheeks. Sinusitis is an inflammation of the mucous membrane lining of these sinus cavities. Symptoms are stuffed-up nose, sinus pain, frontal headache, mild fever, thick discharge, tooth and upper jaw pain. See diagram of Location of sinus cavities, page 62.

What are some causes of sinusitis? Among the most common, with or without infection, are nose injury, anatomical deviations, allergies, bacterial or viral infections.

Case history: *A 39-year-old man with a history of chronic sinusitis decided to give aromatherapy a try after he found little success with conventional treatments. He had been on decongestants, analgesics, antibiotics, and anti-inflammatory medications for the past five to six years. He was very dissatisfied both with the results and the complications he experienced long-term. He did the steam inhalations faithfully, along with the nose drops. Occasionally*

*he would need to use the hot compresses for additional pain relief. He has sig-
nificantly reduced his sinus issues over the past year and a half, and feels a
considerable increase in his energy level. He was not aware of how much
energy it required to deal with his chronic problem. Along with the following
aromatherapy treatments, he has also boosted his immune system by eating a
balanced diet, taking anti-oxidants (Pycnogenol, aloe vera concentrate), and
making lifestyle changes which involved his home and working environments.*

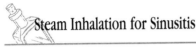 ## Steam Inhalation for Sinusitis

for relief of sinus congestion, a pulmonary antiseptic

ceramic or glass bowl

4 cups hot water

1 drop Eucalyptus essential oil

1 drop Tea Tree essential oil

1 drop Pine essential oil

towel

Pour the hot water in a bowl and add the essential oils. Form a tent over
your head with the towel. Keep your eyes closed and place your head
approximately 8 inches from the water level to prevent a steam burn. Set a
timer for convenience, and inhale slowly and deeply for 10 minutes. This
steam treatment should be done at least twice per day, three times if infection (yellow/green drainage, low-grade fever) is present.

The Eucalyptus, Tea Tree, and Pine essential oils are best for steam
inhalation of the sinuses because these oils are pulmonary antiseptics, anti-
inflammatory, and expectorant. The goal is to drain the sinuses and kill any
germs present. This inhalation remedy will also prevent germs from taking
hold in these swollen, mucus-laden cavities, where they can easily set up
an infection.

For severe cases of sinusitis, or for pain relief associated with blocked
frontal or maxillary sinuses, hot compresses will provide immediate relief.
Hot compresses are local treatment which involves the use of moist heat
and essential oil absorption and inhalation.

Care needs to be taken when applying these compresses to the face.
Avoid the use of extreme heat and keep eyes closed. Do not allow the
compresses to drain into the eye area. Read Chapter 12, *Special Care for
Small Areas,* for detailed information on compress first aid, and Chapter 11
for more information on the use of water temperature for healing
(hydrotherapy).

Hot Compress for Sinusitis

for pain relief associated with sinus infection

1 bowl

1 – 2 cups hot water

4 drops Lavender

4 drops Eucalyptus

1 piece flannel or small face cloth

Pour hot water into bowl. Make sure the temperature is correct (approx. 100–102° F).

Add essential oils. Swish oils to disperse as much as possible. Soak flannel in water. Remove flannel cloth from water/essential oil bath and squeeze out most of the moisture. Lie down on a bed or couch, with head slightly elevated at about a 30-degree angle. This position will further encourage drainage of the sinuses. With eyes closed, apply the compress over the affected sinus areas. With frontal headache and pain between the eyes, apply the compress to the center of the frontal sinuses on the lower forehead just above the eyes. If you are experiencing pain in the cheek, teeth, or upper jaw areas then you will want to apply the compress to the maxillary sinuses on either side of the nose and upper cheeks (below the eyes). Leave the compress on until it dries out, or for a total of 15 or 20 minutes. Cover the bowl of hot water with a lid to keep warm, and re-moisten as necessary.

Applying a massage oil to the face, targeting the sinus areas, can also be helpful. Again, it is important that you avoid the eyes as much as possible, as essential oils are very volatile and can be irritating. This massage oil is especially useful when you do not have the time to do steam inhalation or compresses. It can be used as part of the total sinusitis-relief program or employed as a measure for a mild case of sinusitis and for chronic conditions (for prevention). By applying this oil sparingly over the affected sinuses at night before retiring, you will be receiving a sinus treatment while you sleep.

Open Sesame Sinus Oil

massage oil /nose drops for sinusitis

1 tablespoon sesame oil

3 drops Lavender essential oil

2 drops Eucalyptus essential oil

1 drop Peppermint essential oil

To the sesame oil, add the correct amount of the above essential oils. Mix well.

To use as massage oil: Apply sparingly to the face in the areas of the affected sinuses. Avoid the eyes as much as possible. Massage into the skin until absorbed. Inhale from finger tips before washing hands well. May be used three times per day.

To use as nose drops: Tilt head back and, using an eyedropper, place 1 drop of the above sinus oil mix into each nostril. OR use directions on page 68 to inhale oil from finger. May be used up to three times per day.

Last but not least is the use of a diffuser for therapeutic inhalation. Diffusers are discussed in Chapter 13 *Breathe Easy*, along with recipes for various blends. For sinus conditions I recommend the *Pure For Sure* blend for its antiseptic and bactericidal effects. The *Cold and Flu Relief* blend is useful as an antiseptic for the respiratory tract. Diffuse one of these blends several times during the day and night, for at least 15 minutes each time while you are in the room, to receive the benefits of the essential oils. Regular and consistent use of essences increases your ability to heal or prevent an illness, especially when dealing with ailments of the respiratory tract.

Another option to the diffuser method is the direct inhalation of essential oils from a tissue. Place one or two drops of essential oil on a tissue or handkerchief. Hold up to your nose and mouth and inhale deeply several times. This is the easiest way to take your essential oils while out and about during the day.

Along with the essential oils previously mentioned, others are known to benefit the respiratory system and specifically the sinuses: hyssop, juniper, lavender, lemon, pine, rosemary, tea tree, and sandalwood. Notice many of the oils are ones that are made from trees!

If you suspect an infection, an herb tea will help in fighting it. Garlic capsules are also a natural antibiotic remedy and goldenseal herb tea is very effective.

Some lifestyle changes you can make to help in sinusitis are: get more rest, increase your liquid intake, and avoid dairy products which can encourage mucus formation. If your sinus condition is allergy-related, avoid as much as possible those allergens that you know trigger this condition. Keeping your immune system strong is important as well. When blowing your nose, use equal pressure between both nostrils.

Relieving Symptoms Caused by Colds

The common cold is generally caused by a virus. We are in contact with germs all the time, every day and everywhere we go. When our immune system is lowered, our defense mechanisms are weakened, and we "catch" a cold. It is not the damp, cold weather, as our great grandmothers might have presumed, but our immune system that predetermines whether or not we will get sick. The viral or bacterial organisms only infect the body if our natural defenses have decreased.

As many as 40% of the common cold illnesses are caused by one of the more than 100 varieties of the rhinoviral (*rhino* means *nose*) strains. These organisms enter the body by the mouth or nose. Influenza, the flu virus, accounts for only about 10% of common colds.

Early signs of a cold include a scratchy throat, nasal congestion, slight fever, mild headache, and general feeling of being unwell.

Colds typically reach their peak within 2 or 3 days' time. Early treatment and prevention are the best approach to cold symptoms. The following massage oil is used on lymph glands of the head and neck to help circumvent a cold. This blend has a combination of anti-flu, anti-viral, and anti-bacterial essential oils. They are also pulmonary expectorants and will help the body to expel excess mucus. Because the common cold normally attacks the upper respiratory tract, aromatherapy application is focused on the nose and throat, making steam inhalations a great way to apply essential oils. The remedies given below are for general application of essential oils for the common cold. Because catarrh, sinusitis, and sore throat are ailments that can also be part of the normal cold, please see those ailment sections for specialized treatments.

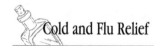 ## Cold and Flu Relief

1st line of defense for combating colds

4 drops Hyssop essential oil

3 drops Rosemary essential oil

3 drops Peppermint essential oil

3 drops Eucalyptus essential oil

3 drops Lemon essential oil

Combine the above essential oils in a small amber bottle. There is a total of 16 drops in this recipe. To use in a steam inhalation, put 3 or 4 drops of the combined oils in a bowl of hot water. See directions for steam inhalation on page 328. Do at least 2 or 3 treatments per day, especially the first day of onset of symptoms, for best results. You can also use half of the recipe above (8 drops total) to use in an aromatic bath. Bathe in a hot tub for at least 15 minutes. Dry yourself completely and wrap up in a cotton terry bathrobe or blanket. Rest for a half hour or more.

This is a very powerful remedy for colds. The combination of warm water, inhalation and skin absorption of essential oils, and increase in body temperature work together to fight the cold from overwhelming the body. A fever or increase in body temperature can help to kill the invading germs. By taking a hot bath with these essences we are encouraging the body to do what it knows how to do naturally!

Warning: Hot baths are not recommended for fevers over 103° F; please see First Aid for Fevers page 219.

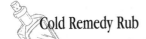 **Cold Remedy Rub**

a massage oil for cold symptoms, swollen glands

1 tablespoon vegetable oil

4 drops Eucalyptus essential oil

4 drops Geranium essential oil

4 drops Rosemary essential oil

Mix the essential oils in the vegetable oil. Store in an amber bottle and label contents. Massage any lymph nodes that may be swollen in the head and neck areas. Use the diagram below for reference. Use small amounts of this oil and inhale from hands after application to the skin. Wash hands well. Cover neck with scarf, towel, or put on a turtleneck sweater or jersey. Apply this oil in the morning, once during the day, and again before retiring at night. See Head and Neck Massage page 105.

Herbal medicine has much to offer in treating the common cold. Herb teas, herb capsules, and herbal tinctures are recommended to aid the body in building the immune system, stimulating the thymus gland, and fighting the germs. A few of these herbs are licorice root, echinacea, goldenseal, and garlic.

Some of the lifestyle and dietary changes recommended to fight a cold include:

- getting more rest
- increasing fluids, especially diluted fresh fruit and vegetable juices, herb teas, pure water
- avoiding dairy products

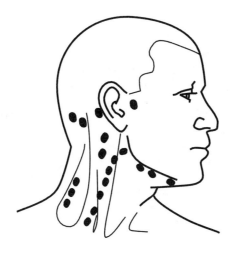

Cervical Lymph Node Locations

- increasing Vitamin C and increasing foods rich in Vitamin C in the diet
- taking aromatic baths
- drinking herbal teas listed for increasing immune system functioning
- frequent hand washing to prevent spread, re-infection

Best Remedy for Coughs

Coughing can be either voluntary, as when air is forced out from the lungs on purpose, or involuntary, such as with a bronchial spasm. Some common conditions that encourage coughing are irritation of the bronchial tubes and lungs by environmental chemicals, bronchial spasm, and cold and flu. In congestion or sinus conditions, a post-nasal drip can be the cause. This is when the sinuses are draining into the back of the throat, and are typically noticed when lying down or when head is in the horizontal position. Post-nasal drip causes a "tickle" in the back of the throat and coughing is the body's reflex attempt to clear it.

Coughs can be moist or dry in nature depending upon how much mucus is present, and whether or not it is related to a cold or irritant exposure. For moist coughs the expectorant and mucolytic essential oils will be best to use. For dry coughs, antispasmolytic and antitussive essential oils will be called for. Antitussive, anti-cough agents are especially good at night if a cough prevents sleep. There are many essential oils that are helpful in relieving coughs; herbal teas and herbal throat drops may also be helpful. The most widely used aromatherapy applications include steam inhalations, chest rubs, and baths.

For persistent cough see your physician for a thorough evaluation, as this can be a warning sign of a serious underlying condition.

Case history: *A 28-year-old flight attendant had been experiencing cold symptoms for about 3 days before I saw her. She had mild rhinitis, with clear drainage. There was no fever, but she did experience general malaise, and a frontal headache. She had just returned to town after a 5-day stretch of consecutive flights. She is usually very healthy and adjusts well to these long work weeks. Her most troublesome complaint was the coughing, which kept her up at night. She followed my suggestions of elevating her head 30–45 degrees with additional pillows, to encourage the nasal drainage. During the day, she did steam inhalations and used the aromatic chest rub. She loved to take baths, and was particularly fond of the* Glad To Be Home *bath blend on page 302, to which she added Hyssop essential oil, which is one of the antitussive (anti-cough) essential oils. She was very happy with the results, and was able to recuperate in time for the following weeks' scheduled flights.*

Aromatic Chest Rub I

for moist coughs

2 tablespoons vegetable oil

12 drops Eucalyptus essential oil

8 drops Hyssop essential oil

4 drops Rosemary essential oil

Mix the essential oils in with the vegetable oil. Store in amber glass bottle and label. Massage upper chest area and lower neck, both front and back. Inhale essences from hands several times before washing them. Use twice per day.

Aromatic Chest Rub II

for dry coughs

2 tablespoons vegetable oil

12 drops Eucalyptus essential oil

6 drops Hyssop essential oil

3 drops Pine essential oil

3 drops Lemon essential oil

Combine the essential oils with the vegetable oil. Store in an amber glass bottle and label. Massage on upper chest and lower neck area on both front and back. Inhale essences from hands before washing them well. Use twice per day. See Chest and Back Massage page 100.

Steam Inhalation for Coughs

for both dry and moist types

ceramic or glass bowl
4 cups hot water
1 drop Cedarwood essential oil
1 drop Eucalyptus essential oil
1 drop Hyssop essential oil
towel

Pour hot water into bowl. Add essential oils. Hold head 8 inches over bowl with towel over head to form tent. Inhale slowly and deeply, keeping eyes closed. Steam for 5 to 10 minutes, two or three times per day. Cover neck and upper chest with warm towel, blanket, or scarf immediately following treatment.

Aromatic Bath

Beth's favorite for coughs

(Glad To Be Home *recipe* + *Hyssop)*
5 drops Lavender essential oil
3 drops Geranium essential oil
2 drops Hyssop essential oil
1/4 cup honey or cream
full bath

Fill bath tub with comfortably hot water. Mix the essential oils in with the honey or cream. These are used as the carrier, since essential oils do not mix with water. Add aromatic honey or cream to bath and stir with your hand to disperse the oils. Soak for 15 to 20 minutes. Inhale deeply; this is an inhalation as well. Wrap up in a warm blanket or robe immediately upon getting out of the bath. Rest for a half hour under blankets. Follow with chest rub before retiring.

Other essential oils that assist with allaying coughing attacks are: cypress, frankincense, juniper, lavender, myrrh, peppermint, and sandalwood.

Lifestyle and dietary alterations that can be made to help with coughs are to avoid dairy products, increase fluids, avoid environmental irritants, and get plenty of rest. Sleeping with a couple of pillows to elevate the head will help with post-nasal drip at night.

Nature's Medicine for Sore Throat

Simple sore throat (relating to local irritation, trauma, and overuse) was covered in the previous chapter on the digestive system. This section addresses sore throats due to viral infections which constitute about 90% of the cases. However, the small number of bacteria-caused sore throats can be serious, as with Streptococcal infection (strep throat). The danger of strep throat is that it can cause rheumatic fever and heart disease; therefore it is best to have a throat culture done by your doctor to rule out this possibility.

Symptoms of a viral sore throat include a rough or raw sensation in back of the throat, fever, general malaise, nausea, headache, red and swollen throat, and tender lymph nodes in neck and under lower jaw. These sore throats usually have a sudden onset, and can be the first sign of a cold, flu, tonsillitis, or laryngitis. Immediate treatment will guarantee the best results for remedy and stave off the possibility of a cold.

> **Case history:** *A strong 16-year-old man had a severe sore throat with a quick onset. He experienced general weakness, headache, and a throat which was red and swollen with tonsil involvement. A throat culture was performed, but while he waited for the results, he did steam inhalations, gargles, and used a throat spray. The irritation and pain made him unable to eat solid food. He was able to take fluids, and an herb tea was taken several times per day. He was advised not to attend school until results came back from the throat culture. (Strep throat had been going around in his high school the previous week.) Three days later he received word from his doctor that the results were negative for streptococcal bacterium; by that time he had reduced most of the symptoms and returned to school.*

Sore Throat Gargle

viral, with swollen lymph nodes

1 cup Sage or Thyme herb tea (or water)

1 tablespoon apple cider vinegar

1 teaspoon Sage honey (recipe follows)

1 drop Geranium essential oil

1 drop Pine essential oil

1 drop Lemon essential oil

Brew the herb tea and strain. Add cider vinegar. Mix the essential oils in the sage honey and then add to warm tea mixture. Stir well. Pour into amber glass bottle and label with directions for use. Shake well before each use. Gargle with this several times as long as you can. Gargle three times per day. Do not eat or drink anything immediately after the gargle.

Use the herbs sage and thyme in this recipe because they are antibacterial and astringent. Apple cider vinegar has been used for ages in alleviating sore throats and colds. Geranium, Pine, and Lemon essential oils are the perfect combination of nature's medicine for sore throats, because they contain anti-inflammatory, antiseptic, antiphlogistic, astringent, and antiviral properties which make them very powerful when used together.

The following recipe is for Sage honey which is very effective for sore throat conditions, colds, and even stomach ulcers, because it is astringent and has drying qualities. It soothes the rough and raw sensations of sore throats and also helps to dry catarrhal conditions where there is an abundance of mucous secretions. I keep a jar full in the pantry cupboard to add to herbal teas when needed. Make a new jarful every year.

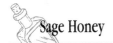

Sage Honey

1 1/2 cups raw honey

1/4 cup fresh sage leaves (salvia officinalis)

Heat honey over low heat. Add sage leaves and heat gently, taking care not to boil (excessive heat destroys the beneficial qualities of the honey). Heat until the sage leaves become dry. Now the herbal qualities and essential oils have been extracted from the sage herb and are contained in the honey. Strain with a slotted spoon or sieve. Pour aromatic honey into a clean glass jar and label. I like to add a fresh sage leaf or two to the final aromatic honey to look nice and for quick identification.

Following is a recipe for a throat spray to be used in sore throat conditions that are severe and necessitate additional medicinals. A spray bottle is needed to deliver the medicine into the back of the throat. There are special glass spray bottles available at the pharmacy, ones with long spray nozzles for reaching the throat. Otherwise, new small spray misters can be used but care must be taken to aim the medicine directly into the mouth and throat, not the eyes or face! The throat spray is easier to use where gargling cannot be the method of choice, for example, traveling or at the work-place.

Intensive Throat Spray

for severe sore throat

1/2 cup Chamomile herb tea

1 tablespoon apple cider vinegar

1 teaspoon Sage honey (or plain raw honey)

2 drops Geranium essential oil

1 drop Lemon essential oil

1 drop Hyssop essential oil

1 drop Tea Tree essential oil

Brew herb tea and strain very well so herb pieces do not plug spray nozzle. Add vinegar. Mix essential oils in with the honey, then add to tea mixture. Pour into spray glass bottle and label. Shake well before each use. To use, spray directly into the back of the throat while breathing in. One to two sprays is equivalent to one single treatment application. The liquid can be swallowed. Do not eat or drink for 15 minutes after using the spray. Take three times daily.

Note the throat spray, more concentrated than the gargle, has a greater number of essential oil drops per volume. Use it like you would any medicine, with discretion and according to directions.

Herbal medicine in the form of herbal teas that can be taken for sore throats are agrimony, sage, chamomile, fenugreek seeds, ginger root and raspberry leaf and berries. Other herbs include those that are helpful in fighting infection: garlic, goldenseal, and echinacea.

Other essential oils that aid in caring for sore throats are frankincense, lemon, pine, hyssop, bergamot, and lavender.

Lifestyle and dietary changes include:

- getting more rest
- increasing fluid intake
- taking sage honey with herb tea
- keeping warm
- avoiding dairy products
- eating a diet composed of soft foods
- eating natural frozen fruit juice popsicles, or homemade fruit ice-cubes
- drinking fresh lemon juice (hot or cold) in water
- increasing foods that contain vitamin B's and C (or take supplements)

- taking garlic capsules and cooking with garlic
- taking echinacea and goldenseal herb to fight infection
- using zinc lozenges
- diffusing antiseptic essential oils and other oils that are helpful during colds (see page 324)

Soothing the Suffering of Tonsillitis

The tonsils are paired structures of lymphatic tissue located in the back of the throat. Under normal conditions the tonsils are flat and pink like the rest of the throat lining. Because they are a common site of infection, they can become swollen and impede swallowing and respiration. Tonsillitis, the inflammation of the tonsils most often seen in children, can range from mild to severe in the degree of swelling and pain associated with the infection. Symptoms include mild to severe throat pain, difficulty swallowing, fever, swollen lymph glands (under the jaw), headache, white or yellow spots on the tonsils, and swollen or reddened tonsils. Sometimes there is also an earache, due to the proximity of the tonsils (and adenoids) to the Eustachian tubes which lead to the ears. Usually a diminished appetite is also a symptom, along with difficulty sleeping.

To observe the tonsils, you will need a flashlight, to look at the back of the throat where the tonsils are located on each side. They will most likely look red, swollen, and may or may not have white or yellow patches.

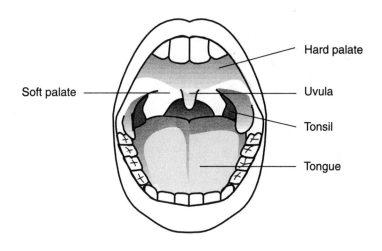

The Tonsils

In the "old" days it was very common to have the tonsils and adenoids removed after an episode of tonsillitis (or several illnesses). Many of
you are without them now. Today, it is common thought that these structures are there for a reason; they are not routinely removed unless in
extreme cases where tonsillitis is a constant and severe problem. All my
children have their tonsils and I intend to keep it that way! The tonsils are
present in our body for good reason: they are part of the body's defense
for "straining" germs. In the next few pages you will discover natural remedies for mild to moderate cases of tonsillitis and sore throat.

For recurrent tonsillitis, I recommend you see your doctor to address
the underlying condition or weakness that may be promoting this condition. If the tonsils are extremely swollen and are interfering with the intake
of air (breathing) and the ability to swallow, seek medical attention immediately.

As you might think, the best forms of aromatherapy that are applied
in this ailment are throat irrigations (gargles), steam inhalations, throat
sprays, and cool compresses. You should read the previous section on sore
throat as the information and the recommendations are quite similar.

Gargle for Tonsillitis

for red and swollen tonsils

1 cup Sage or Thyme herb tea (warm)

1 tablespoon apple cider vinegar

1 tablespoon fresh lemon juice

1 teaspoon Sage or Ginger honey

1 drop Geranium essential oil

1 drop Lemon essential oil

1 drop Ginger essential oil

Brew the herb tea and strain. Add lemon juice and vinegar. To the honey
(recipes on page 85 and 38) add the essential oils and mix well. Add aromatic honey to warm tea. Gargle with this mixture several times, 3 times
per day. Hold in the mouth and gargle for as long as possible before rinsing. Do not swallow the gargle. Do not eat or drink anything immediately
following the remedy.

This gargle has antimicrobial properties and will aid in decreasing the
swelling and local infection. The area in the back of the throat is very vascular, meaning it has a good blood supply. The longer you can hold the
gargle in this area, the more readily absorbed and effective the herbs and
essential oils will be.

A throat spray is very useful for tonsillitis. This herbal and therapeutic essential oil spray provides a direct application of medicine to where it is needed and is a stronger preparation. Please refer to the previous section on sore throat, page 86 for recipe and directions for the throat spray.

Cool compresses are very effective in these cases because there is a great deal of swelling involved, both in the tonsil region as well as in the local lymph nodes in the jaw. Cold temperatures decrease inflammation. In the following aromatic compress recipe used for tonsillitis, essential oils and water work together to achieve the desired outcome—to decrease swelling and to fight infection. Read Chapter 12, *Special Care for Small Areas,* for detailed information on compress first aid, and Chapter 11 for information on the therapeutic use of water (hydrotherapy).

Cool Compress for Tonsillitis

for swollen tonsils and lymph nodes

1 bowl

1 – 2 cups cool water

4 drops Lavender essential oil

2 drops Tea Tree essential oil

1 drop Chamomile essential oil

1 drop Lemon essential oil

1 wash cloth or piece of flannel cloth

Pour cool water into bowl. Make sure the temperature is correct (cool, not cold to the touch). Add essential oils to bowl of water and stir to disperse as much as possible. Soak flannel in water. Remove cloth and squeeze out most of the moisture. Apply to the neck region directly under the lower jaw. The best position for this is the horizontal, lying position, with the head tilted back. Do not use a pillow. Keep the compress on for 15 to 20 minutes. Re-moisten and apply again within a few minutes or when it becomes body temperature (warm).

It is important to note here that treatment of tonsillitis should be continued for two days following the disappearance of symptoms.

Other effective essential oils are geranium, bergamot, lavender, tea tree, lemon, ginger, and chamomile.

Lifestyle and dietary changes would be the same as for the sore throat ailments covered in the previous section, so please refer to page 86 for those recommendations.

Say Good-bye to Laryngitis

The larynx, or voice box, is located in the upper portion of the trachea, and contains the vocal cords. Therefore laryngitis is the inflammation of the larynx, involving the vocal cords. Symptoms are a change in the normal voice; typically a hoarse, rough, or low voice is experienced. Laryngitis can occur with no other symptoms, or with a sore throat.

If you experience persistent hoarseness (4 to 6 weeks), the feeling of a lump in the throat, pain in the Adam's apple region, or difficulty in swallowing, seek a qualified medical evaluation and opinion as to the cause, since these are cancer warning signs.

> **Case history:**   *A 62-year-old man who is an opera singer heard about aromatherapy through a friend who had taken a class of mine. He did not have laryngitis when he consulted with me, but he was in need of information and guidance as to what to do the next time he experienced voice loss or hoarseness. As you might imagine, this was his greatest fear. He took excellent care of his health and was very oriented toward preventive health. He had experienced laryngitis several times in his opera career, and it was disastrous for him. A good year or more passed without hearing a word from him after our meeting. However, a few months ago I received a call from him while he was singing in San Francisco. He had early signs of laryngitis when he tried the recipes I had shared with him. He related to me that he carried the essential oils with him every time he left so he was always prepared for his worst fear! He gargled, and did the cold compresses that are given below. The symptoms decreased in a little less than a day and he was able to sing the following evening, with his best voice.*

Cold Compress for Laryngitis

for voice hoarseness, overuse

1 bowl

1 – 2 cups cold water

4 drops Lavender essential oil

2 drops Geranium essential oil

2 drops Frankincense essential oil

1 piece flannel, or wash cloth

Pour the cold water into a bowl. Temperature should be 60 – 70 F°. Add the essential oils and swish the water to disperse them as much as possible. Soak the cloth in the aromatic water. Remove cloth and wring most of the moisture from it. Apply to the Adam's apple area, in front of the throat. Re-apply after it becomes warm/ body temperature. Leave on a total of 15 to

20 minutes for full benefit. Lie down during the compress application. Repeat 3 times per day.

A cold compress is used to alleviate local swelling that is part of laryngitis. The essential oils chosen are ones that are anti-inflammatory, and work especially well on the throat and larynx. Other helpful essential oils are sandalwood, cypress, chamomile, ginger, and pine.

Additionally, throat drops can be made to soothe swelling in the throat region. Sugar cubes are used as the carrier for the essential oil. The lozenge is a good way to get medicine to the throat, slowly. The following recipe is to be used no more than three times per day, and in conjunction with the other remedies.

Lozenge for Laryngitis

to help with voice hoarseness

1 sugar cube

1 drop Geranium essential oil

Put one single drop of Geranium essential oil on the sugar cube. Gradually melt the lozenge in the mouth, allowing the medicine to slowly soothe the throat. Avoid eating or drinking immediately following. Do not exceed three per day.

If laryngitis is accompanied by a sore throat, or cough, refer to those specific ailments for detailed instruction on aromatherapy remedies.

A gargle of Geranium essential oil in water is another extremely effective and simple treatment for voice hoarseness. Use 1 drop Geranium essential oil mixed in honey and add to a cup of cool water and gargle well, and for as long as possible. This can be performed just prior to any speaking engagement or voice recital.

Some lifestyle and dietary changes that can be done to assist in healing laryngitis are:

- rest your voice
- avoid dairy products; they increase mucus formation
- increase fluid intake; sip on cold liquids (avoid hot temperatures)
- get more rest
- make a big pot of old-fashioned garlic and onion soup and eat freely (page 97)
- refer to sore throat ailment section for more recommendations that may apply

CHAPTER 4

Aromatherapy Treatments for the Respiratory System

Brief Overview of the Respiratory System

The health of the respiratory system is of crucial importance to our survival. Without air we will die. The simple, yet miraculous, process of breathing is automatic and involuntary. Inhalation and exhalation are the two basic rhythms of this system, while a whole host of other chemical exchanges take place with each and every breath we take. The respiratory system (including the olfactory system) is in direct contact with the external environment.

Therefore, the quality of the air that you breathe is extremely important, as is the functioning of this system. Following this section, turn to Chapter 13: *Breathe Easy—The In's and Out's of Inhalation* for additional information relating to the respiratory system, such as inhalation methods and suggestions for air purification.

The respiratory system includes the nose and sinuses (upper respiratory), in addition to the bronchial tubes and lungs (lower respiratory). Basically everything within the respiratory tract above the larynx is referred to as the upper respiratory system, and below the larynx is called the lower respiratory system or tract. Since the nose and sinus ailments have been addressed in the previous chapter, we will now focus on the *lower respiratory system.*

As air is inhaled with each and every breath, it becomes moistened in the nasal cavity and large airways. This inspired moist air comes into contact with the alveoli, where the oxygen and carbon dioxide gas exchange takes place in the lower respiratory tract. Exhaled air then removes this gas waste (carbon dioxide gas) from the body.

The airway passage below the larynx is relatively sterile, which is one major difference between the upper and lower sections of this tract. The secretions present in this lower tract contain natural antimicrobial substances that the body produces under healthy conditions. These substances kill invading micro-organisms, neutralize harmful bacteria and toxins, and activate the immune system. There is a plentiful blood supply that is in close contact with the lining of the lungs. An increase in blood supply in this area means that the immune system's defense, white blood cells, macrophages, and lymph, are readily available when needed.

The function of the *lungs* is the intake of oxygen and the elimination of carbon dioxide. They contain upper and lower lobes (sections) and are protected, along with other vital organs, by the rib cage structure.

The *bronchi* are large airway branches or tubes that transport air to the smaller airway channels and eventually to the alveoli.

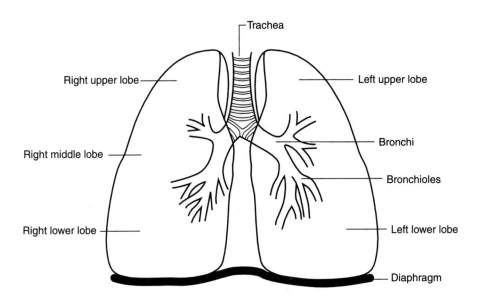

Lungs

The *alveoli* are the functional unit of the lung that are responsible for the gas exchange between the blood supply and the breath. This process is called diffusion. The alveolar-capillary surface comes into direct contact with the atmosphere.

The *central nervous system* controls the diaphragm and thoracic musculature for involuntary breathing to take place. Therefore the nervous system is closely tied to the respiratory system. The relationship between these two systems is demonstrated when you become frightened and your respiration becomes rapid and shallow. In a relaxed state respiration is slow and deep. Aromatherapy can be an effective tool in this area since essential oils aid in relaxation or stimulation and purify the air.

Respiratory-Enhancing Essential Oils

There are many essential oils that are considered to be respiratory enhancers. These essences help the respiratory system because of the specific qualities they possess such as expectorant, mucolytic, anti-spasmodic, anti-inflammatory, anti-allergic or immune stimulants. Essential oils are also beneficial in this area because they have anti-bacterial and anti-viral benefits.

It is very interesting how most essential oils useful in respiratory ailments are those that are distilled from the bark, leaves, berries, and branches of certain trees. Trees purify the air by absorbing the carbon dioxide we exhale (as well as other gases) and produce the oxygen that supports us.

Some of the most important essential oils used for the respiratory tract are those that are considered expectorants and mucolytic. Mucolytic essential oils have the ability to break up and liquefy thick mucus secretions, thereby facilitating their expulsion. Expectorant essential oils activate the cilia along the respiratory mucous membrane to encourage movement and expulsion of secretions. The most well known expectorant in herbal phyto-medicine is Eucalyptus, of which there are approximately 800 species and more than 100 varieties. However, only several chemotypes are used for aromatherapy. The "classic" expectorant essential oils of eucalyptus include the following types which are recommended for all respiratory infections: Eucalyptus *globulus, E. radiata* and *E. smithii.*

They are anti-viral and anti-bacterial, expectorant, mucolytic, and immune stimulating. Extensive work has been done using essential oils of different species of Eucalyptus for various respiratory conditions.

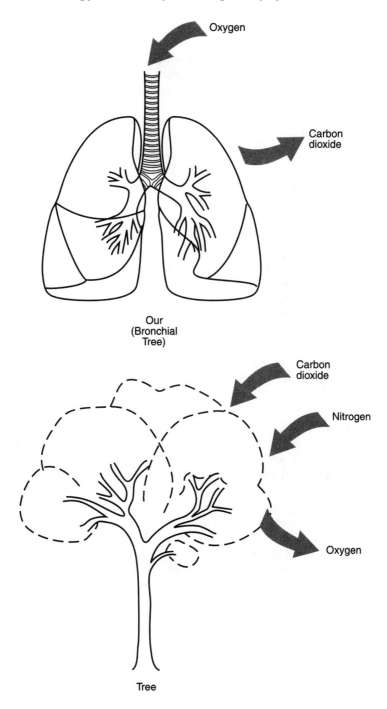

Lung and Tree Illustration

Recovery from Bronchitis

Bronchitis is the inflammation of the bronchi portions of the respiratory tract. Symptoms can be acute (quick onset) or chronic (longstanding condition). Acute bronchitis is categorized by mild fever, chest aches and pains over sternum (of the chest between the ribs), weakness, shortness of breath, increased respiration, lack of appetite, and cough may be present. The cough can vary from mild to severe, with or without production of sputum. This form of bronchitis can follow an upper respiratory infection such as sinusitis or rhinitis, especially in the winter months. Environmental air pollutants can also be a factor. Some examples are inhalation of cigarette smoke, noxious gas fumes or chemicals, or high counts of air pollutants or pollens. Aspiration (when you swallow food or liquid and it goes down the wrong "pipe") can also cause this otherwise sterile area to become contaminated. Unfortunately, hospitalization can also cause respiratory infections, such as bronchitis due to exposure to tenacious pathogens.

Chronic bronchitis, as the name suggests, is a condition that has been present for a length of time, and perhaps has taken years to develop. A productive cough is usually present with a characteristic "musty" odor. This type of bronchitis can be caused by consistent and frequent irritation (such as smoking), or from infection. If you have chronic bronchitis, it is strongly advised that you see a health care practitioner for constitutional treatment.

When the lungs become involved, it is known as pneumonia. Pneumonia means there is fluid and lymph in the lungs. This is dangerous because the fluid is taking up air space, therefore interfering with the delicate gas exchange that normally takes place here. If there are abnormal breath sounds present and shallow breathing with a cough, seek medical care as soon as possible to confirm. Pneumonia is especially dangerous in the elderly population, and is the 5th leading cause of death in the United States. A history of smoking, alcohol or drug use, low immunity or history of taking immuno-suppressive medications are known to be predisposing factors in the development of pneumonia, as well as of chronic bronchitis.

A persistent cough, and difficulty breathing or swallowing are warning signals that should be evaluated by a physician. Often in chronic respiratory conditions, symptoms such as these are overlooked or ignored by the individual.

Case history: *A 54-year-old retired nurse consulted with me for a moderate case of bronchitis that had developed immediately following a bout with the flu this past winter. She presented a mild productive cough, with occasional thick sputum. Mild elevation in body temperature, feeling of fatigue, and mild chest pain with cough were other symptoms she experienced.*

Immediately she increased her daily vitamin C supplementation, along with additional herbs of echinacea and goldenseal. She loved the garlic and onion soup recipe I gave her to make for colds. She found relief from using heat and massage over the chest and back areas, in addition to using the diffuser regularly. In the beginning stages of the bronchitis she followed the recommendations for steam inhalations, but had discontinued them after the third day since she felt much better, and didn't make the time for further inhalation treatments. Regardless of this fact, she improved readily and her energy level increased well within a week's time.

Old-Fashioned Garlic and Onion Soup

for colds, flu, respiratory infections, or for prevention during the winter months

4 large white or yellow onions, thinly sliced

2 whole heads of garlic

2 tsp. thyme

4 tbs. olive oil

6 cups vegetable broth

1/2 c. dry white wine

1 bay leaf

2 tbs. honey

4 tbs. each fresh basil and parsley

1/4 tsp. cayenne pepper (optional)

sea salt, fresh ground pepper to taste

Saute the onions, garlic and thyme in olive oil until golden brown. This step sweetens and mellows the intensity of the garlic and onions. To peel the garlic cloves, smash the individual cloves with the flat side of a chef's knife, then slip out of the skins. Add the garlic and onions to a soup kettle (or slow cooker) to cook with the vegetable broth, white wine and bay leaf. Slowly cook for 2 or 3 hours (or overnight if using a slow cooker). Strain liquid, and then add honey, fresh basil and parsley, sea salt, fresh ground pepper and cayenne. Sip on this hot soup throughout the day, or have for lunch or dinner as a first course.

Roasted garlic used as a spread, garlic powder capsules, garlic oil macerate and aged garlic extract are other ways you can get your garlic. Onions and garlic are both antibacterial in action, as is the herb thyme. Cayene pepper is recommended if there is a fever present, while basil and parsley are cleansing and detoxifying herbs. This is an excellent soup to drink during any type of infection or cold, or to simply prepare during the cold winter months, when colds and flu are more prevalent.

Steam Inhalation for Bronchitis

to loosen mucus, pulmonary antiseptic

ceramic glass or bowl

4 cups hot water

1 drop Eucalyptus essential oil

1 drop Lemon essential oil

1 drop Sandalwood essential oil

towel

Pour hot water into the bowl. Add the essential oils. Hold head about eight inches from the water level, with the towel draped over the head to form a tent. Breathe slowly and deeply with eyes closed. Do this for 5 to 10 minutes each time, three times per day. Pat face and neck area dry following treatment. Wrap a towel or scarf around the neck, or wear a warm turtleneck or sweater to prevent chilling. Follow with bronchitis treatment oils to chest and back areas for optimal benefit.

The next two recipes are for local application of essential oils in a carrier base oil. Choose the recipe that best fits your condition, either for a moist and productive cough, or the one recommended for dry coughs. Because the essences are slowly absorbed into the skin, along with the vegetable oil, this particular method is practical for a continuous treatment throughout the day. It can be applied two or three times per day, in small amounts. To encourage lymphatic drainage and diminish lung congestion, follow the simple chest massage directions on page 100 when applying this oil. Of course if you are using the oils on yourself, it won't be possible to apply them to the back area. However, you will still benefit from this treatment applying the oils to the front chest area.

Chest Treatment Oil I

for bronchitis, moist cough

1 oz. vegetable oil

10 drops Eucalyptus essential oil

5 drops Hyssop essential oil

3 drops Peppermint essential oil

2 drops Cedarwood essential oil

Chest and Back Massage

This encourages lymphatic drainage, draw out fever and to help with lung congestion useful for chest colds, bronchitis and asthma

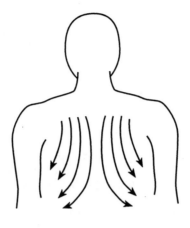

Back

Direction for hand massage

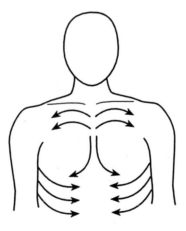

Front

Use double stroke massage technique: 1 hand immediately following the other.

* This technique and massage direction is adapted from Joseph B. Stephenson's work called *Creative Healing*, written by Patricia Bradley, 1994.

Chest Treatment Oil II

for bronchitis, dry, non-productive cough

1 oz. vegetable oil

10 drops Eucalyptus essential oil

5 drops Hyssop essential oil

3 drops Bergamot essential oil

2 drops Sandalwood essential oil

The directions are the same for both recipes given above:

Pour 1 ounce (2 tablespoons) of vegetable oil into an amber glass bottle. Add the essential oils and shake gently to mix. Label contents. To apply, warm a small amount of the blend in your hands before putting it on the skin. Apply the oils to the front and back (upper chest and back). See Chest and Back Massage technique for directions that can increase the success of this aromatherapy treatment. After the oils have been rubbed onto the skin, inhale the essences from the hands by holding them over the mouth and nose area and breathing deeply several times. Wash hands. This chest oil can be applied two or three times per day. Keep chest warm following application of oil treatment.

Essential oils that are useful for respiratory ailments such as bronchitis are cedarwood, eucalyptus, frankincense, fennel, marjoram, myrrh, ginger, nutmeg, bergamot, pine, peppermint, hyssop, juniper, lemon, rosemary, sandalwood, and tea tree. Of the above-listed oils, several are specified for chronic or longstanding bronchial conditions. These are frankincense, cedarwood, sandalwood, and myrrh. To decrease the frequency of bacterial infection any of these essential oils mentioned will be beneficial; however, peppermint and eucalyptus essential oils are the most noted.

A few dietary recommendations can help decrease symptoms and encourage the healing process during an illness like bronchitis. Avoid mucus-producing foods such as dairy products, increase Vitamin C-rich foods and beverages or increase supplementation (1 – 2 grams three times per day), and eat plenty of garlic or drink Old Fashioned Garlic and Onion soup. Remember to drink plenty of liquids, especially herb teas, such as ginger and peppermint tea, or plain hot water with lemon.

Lifestyle recommendations include getting plenty of rest and staying warm. It is important to keep the lungs fully expanded to prevent pneumonia. Perform the breathing exercises on the next page daily. Purify the room air by using a room mist electric diffuser or humidifier. The use of essential oils will keep the bronchial tubes free and clear. See the list of essential oils that aid the respiratory system. Alternatively, inhale essences from a tissue during the day. It would be helpful to refer to Chapter 3, *Aromatherapy Treatments for Eye, Ear, Nose, and Throat Problems* for other related symptoms of the upper respiratory tract if present (catarrh, colds, cough, sore throat).

Breathing Exercises

The following deep breathing exercises help to fully expand the lungs, relax muscles, relieve anxiety, help you fall asleep, as well as enhance vitality and youthfulness as more blood is pumped throughout the body.

General instructions: Clear the nasal passages before beginning these exercises.

1. Stretch the rib cage and spine (overhead arm stretches, side to side, clasp hands in back and lift to fully open the chest area)
2. Inhale through the nose (count of 3)—this allows the air to be filtered, moistened, and warmed.
3. Breath slowly and in a relaxed manner—allow complete exhalation (exhale count of 4)
4. Practice breathing exercises in several position—for varied air distribution.

    Upper chest breathing: Concentrate on filling the upper chest area with your breath. Place your hands on the chest area to focus on this particular area.

    Abdominal breathing: Concentrate on filling the lower lungs with your breath and observe the abdomen rise and fall. Place your hands there to confirm expansion.

    Lateral chest breathing: Concentrate on expanding your lower ribs with each breath. Place your hands on each side to help focus your attention on this area.

How to Use Natural Alternatives to Relieve Allergies— Essences to the Rescue

An allergy is a reactive condition to a substance in the environment or diet which triggers the body to respond in an exaggerated or abnormal way. Persons who experience allergies typically have a dysfunctional immune system. Allergies are often an underlying factor for other ailments, especially inflammations and irritations of the respiratory tract, producing an increased amount of secretions. Because there is a link between allergic conditions and a lowered immune resistance, susceptibility to viral infections is a concern.

A true allergy results from an antibody response to a specific substance. Although this is a protective mechanism by the body, sometimes it actually causes tissue damage. Allergic reactions can be complex and involve several systems such as the lymph, nervous, and digestive systems, in addition to the immune system. The body's reaction to an allergen is to produce extra histamine (a chemical compound made by the body). Over time, repeated exposures, and allergic bodily responses, tissue harm can be the result to several of these involved body systems.

Many symptoms and conditions are considered to be allergy-related. Some include asthma, runny nose, hay fever, cough, tonsillitis, sore throat, sneezing, catarrh, sinusitis, fatigue, hyperactivity, learning disability, ear infections, headaches, as well as skin disorders (eczema, itching, redness, hives). Allergic rhinitis, commonly called hay fever, is usually seasonal and presents a wide variety of symptoms including watery nasal drainage, sneezing, and itchy eyes and nose.

When there is clear drainage without a fever or signs of infection, it is probably the result of an allergy, especially if the symptoms are more pronounced during a seasonal change. Environmental allergens, which trigger allergy attacks, can include paint, solvents, glue, adhesives, heavy metals, smoke, chemical gases, pollen, etc. Food allergens vary greatly from person to person; however, some common ones are wheat, milk, chocolate, citrus, and chemical food additives (dyes, preservatives). Some people are allergic to eggs, fish, shellfish, nuts or peanuts. There is evidence linking low stomach acid conditions and food additives (dyes, preservatives) with allergies.

A person experiencing allergies should seek comprehensive treatment from a health care professional with expertise in this area, to assist with identifying the cause of the allergies and support a holistic approach. Treatment involves avoiding the allergen and strengthening the immune system to decrease the risk of additional allergies. Purifying the air to decrease reactive substances also is critical. General tonics help in conditions associated with allergies, as well as herbs that decrease histamine production and secretion.

When addressing allergies, several important areas can be positively affected by utilizing essential oils, particularly lavender and bergamot, which can be used for their general tonifying properties for allergy-related conditions. Most allergies involve inflammatory responses and will benefit from the anti-inflammatory essential oils such as chamomile and lavender.

Lemon is one essential oil I often include with allergy remedies because it is purifying, anti-toxic and antibacterial. To relieve itching, which is a common symptom in many allergies, use essential oils of lemon, chamomile and peppermint. Rose has been used traditionally for many types of allergy as well. Essential oils use can strengthen your respiratory, immune, and nervous systems when used correctly, and in moderation.

Another consideration is the quantity and frequent use of synthetic fragrances to which an increasing number of people are developing allergies. You don't have to live without the aromatic pleasures of the gentle perfume of a flower or warm fragrance of spice . Just choose the real, nature-produced versions of genuine and authentic, high quality essential oils.

Almost always, stress plays a major role in aggravating allergy conditions. Aromatherapy is extremely effective for relieving stressful states and in prevention; therefore essential oils that promote relaxation are typically included in allergy-related treatment programs.

Caution: People who suffer from allergies must take care when using essential oils (or any other unfamiliar substance). Because you are prone to allergies or are hyper-sensitive in general, it is a good idea to experiment with one "new" essential oil at a time. Always do a skin patch test first when trying an essential oil for the first time. See Chapter 1, page 9 for direction. Also, be sure to remove all traces of cosmetics, perfume, and other body care preparations before applying the natural essential oils, since they could possibly cause a cross-reaction.

For general use in many allergy situations, I recommend a blend of essential oils that can be diffused several times per day and can aid in controlling germs, purifying the air, promoting relaxation and are anti-inflammatory. These are general tonics, anti-toxic and antibacterial in action, while soothing to the nervous system.

Allergy Relief Synergy Blend

for diffuser use

5 parts Lavender essential oil

2 parts Bergamot essential oil

1 part Lemon essential oil

1 part Juniper essential oil

1 part Peppermint essential oil

This recipe is given in "parts" so that large amounts can be made for diffuser use. I suggest you count out the "parts" in eyedroppers or teaspoons, depending on the total amount you wish to prepare. Store in an amber bottle and label. Attach to diffuser according to instructions with the machine, or use in an aroma lamp, potpourri burner, or pan of hot water on the stove or radiator. See Chapter 13 for further options and directions for inhalation methods. Allow this essential oil blend to diffuse three to four times daily, for 10 to 15 minutes duration each time.

For *hay fever*, the sinus congestion and catarrh that often are part of the condition's symptoms can be eased with the recommendations given for related ailments in the previous chapter. If sinusitis, catarrh, or eye irritation is present when you get hay fever, turn to those sections of Chapter 3 for recipes, keeping in mind what we discussed here regarding cautionary measures. Typically eucalyptus essential oil will be the most beneficial for runny nose, catarrh, etc.

To ease most *head-related allergic symptoms*, including headache, congestion, and fatigue, the following essential oil blend can be used with positive results. You can use this blend of essential oils or use Rose by itself. Use the head and neck massage technique on page 105 to assist in clearing the head if congestion is present.

Clear Head Blend

to clear the head, allergy symptoms

1 tbls. olive oil (or arnica infused oil)

1 drop Bulgarian rose oil

1 drop Peppermint essential oil

3 drops Lavender essential oil

In a small amber bottle add the selected essential oils. Add the olive oil and shake gently. Label contents. To use, simply apply a few drops of this blend to your fingertips and massage into the scalp, temples, and cervical neck area. See head and neck massage directions on page 105.

Inhale essences from hands following application. Take a few minutes of quiet time, to relax and close your eyes.

A surprisingly effective remedy for allergy-related symptoms, such as hay fever, is the aromatic foot bath. According to Maurice Messegue, a French herbalist, foot and hand soaks are an easy and effective way of absorbing medicine. He successfully treated many people with a wide variety of ailments, including respiratory problems. The feet are parts of the body which are capable of absorbing herbal and essential oil remedies. For additional benefit, you can also use reflexology of the foot to aid in lung and sinus complaints.

Head and Neck Massage

This facilitates lymphatic drainage useful during colds, tonsillitis, catarrh, and sore throat (follow with chest and back massage technique if lower respiratory tract is involved)

Person should be in upright sitting position for this technique.

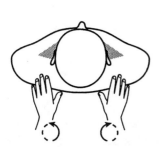 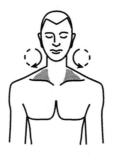 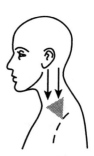

This technique and massage direction is adapted from Joseph B. Stephenson's work called *Creative Healing*. It incorporates these four basic principles:
1. Maintain normal body temperature (to remove or add heat)
2. Create a vacuum (to encourage drainage from glands or organs)
3. Reposition substance (movement of soft tissue)
4. Reposition congestion (to disperse internal fullness)

* This technique and massage direction is adapted from Joseph B. Stephenson's work called *Creative Healing*, written by Patricia Bradley, 1994.

Allergy Relief Formula

a footbath to relieve allergy symptoms

basin or tub

tepid water

2 tbls. Sea salt (or Bath Salts)

3 drops Lavender essential oil

1 drop Rose essential oil

1 drop Geranium essential oil

towel

Fill a foot basin or tub half full with tepid water. Add essential oils to the salts and mix before adding to the water basin. Soak your feet while sitting, for at least 15 to 20 minutes. Pat feet dry and put on warm cotton or wool socks.

This footbath can be done three times per day during allergy attacks, or occasionally when early symptoms begin to surface. Try this footbath daily for prevention when you expect seasonal changes to trigger symptoms, and see if you can observe a more diminished allergic response than usual.

You can apply an oil blend to the feet following the foot bath, or in lieu of the foot soak. Use the recipe given previously for the Clear Head Blend, by adjusting the recipe. To make a larger amount of this oil and to make it more dilute (since you will be covering more skin surface), use 2 tablespoons of olive oil instead of 1 tablespoon, and mix according to instructions. Apply to feet after the footbath if desired.

Dietary recommendations include avoiding the foods which cause problems for you. Drink fresh lemon juice daily in water to purify and detoxify the body. Be sure to drink plenty of pure water too! Anti-oxidants may also help in prevention.

Lifestyle recommendations include relieving the stress in your life, by finding ways to cope better and to prevent stressful situations. Refer to the section on stress in Chapter 9 for additional information, stress test, and suggestions for stress relief. Regular diffuser use would be beneficial in your office and home. Many essences purify the air as well as provide physical relaxation. General air purification is also an area you will want to address, especially if you experience respiratory-related allergies. Read Chapter 13: Breathe Easy after this section for important information and easy ways to purify your environment with aromatherapy and air-filtering plants.

Natural Prescriptions for Asthma

Asthma is an allergic disorder characterized by spasms of the bronchial tubes of the lungs. There is typically an excessive amount of viscous mucus in the bronchial tree causing impairment, or difficulty of breathing. The degree of severity of symptoms is directly related to the extent of airway obstruction; from early or mild episodes of coughing and mild chest tightness, to more severe stages of wheezing, anxiousness, extreme fatigue, and respiratory failure. This characteristic wheezing sound is serious, as it means air intake is being restricted because of the constriction of the airway passages.

Examples of allergic triggers include: springtime tree pollens, summer grasses and weed pollens, animal dander, dust, molds, and fungus. Asthma may also be triggered by chemicals, smoke, cold air, exercise, and respiratory infection. There also seems to be a strong emotional component to asthma.

Major causes of asthma include allergy, hypersensitivity of airways and excessive release of inflammatory chemicals. Some expert health care professionals view asthma as a weakness in the respiratory system. Three percent of the United States population experiences some form of asthma.

Asthma can be caused by a wide variety of factors therefore treatment is highly individualized. There usually is an allergic component, as well as a stress factor, that triggers the asthma attack. Sometimes it can also be of genetic origin. I have seen it related to overexposure to irritants, often chemically related.

There is also evidence linking this condition to emotions and how we deal with them. Studies have been conducted correlating asthma with anxiety, and in China they believe there is a connection between lung problems and grief. I believe we cannot separate the body, mind, and emotions; I honor the belief that health or the elimination of illness must embrace all levels, encompassing a holistic approach. This is why aromatherapy works on such a wide variety of conditions. Some of the essential oils for the respiratory system work on an emotional level, while others are included because they are respiratory-enhancing agents, antibacterial and anti-spasmodic.

The human body is an amazing, magnificent, and wondrous creation. Under normal circumstances and during health and wellness, it is able to compensate and balance much of the negative influences and insults it meets. However, our lifestyle, diet, and attitudes are powerful contributing factors.

Case history: *A 29-year-old woman consulted with me. She had recently developed an asthma condition. Her asthma symptoms were occasional and mild, but her greatest fear was that the symptoms were going to get worse. She requested information on air purification and aromatherapy treatments that could help to prevent and alleviate her symptoms. She was otherwise healthy, and under medical care from her family practitioner. Her aromatherapy regimen included diffusing essential oils during the day at regular intervals. She substituted most of her cleaning products with non-chemical options. She loved the aromatic baths which made her feel more relaxed. She performed breathing exercises daily, as well as cut out dairy products in her diet. She used the aromatic face splash as soon as she felt her chest tightening and breathing becoming slightly more labored. She used the asthma oil blend on her back and feet and found it very helpful. It has been about a year since I have heard from her, but she was continuing with her aromatherapy lifestyle and desired to learn more about "natural medicine" since she experienced such positive results.*

Be slow and cautious when using essential oils with asthmatic persons since they are more prone to sensitivities and allergies. See the previous section of this chapter to review the discussion of essential oil use with allergies.

Aromatherapy is to be used as a complementary or supportive addition to your present medical program designed by your physician; it is not intended to take the place of your medicine! The therapeutic use of essential oils for asthma conditions is very helpful and supportive in many important areas, especially for aiding in relaxation, purifying the air, and generally supporting the respiratory system. You can safely and easily use these recipes along with your present health regime, to ease symptoms and prevent secondary infection and decrease stress. Many people who have asthma and have made lifestyle changes incorporating aromatherapy are able to decrease their medications and continue to enjoy improved health and greater control over their lives.

The asthma aromatherapy and lifestyle prescription includes avoiding possible allergens or triggers, preventing or decreasing spasms, supporting the respiratory system and immune system to prevent progression and infection. Aromatic back rubs, foot and ankle applications, inhalation treatments and breathing exercises are some of the ways to incorporate essential oils into your daily regime. Promoting a clean, healthy living environment is also important. *Note:* Any essential oil has the potential of triggering an attack—so exercise caution and moderation.

For *acute asthmatic attacks*, inhaling the sedative-type and antihistamine-like essential oils can be very effective. These include lavender, chamomile, patchouli, sandalwood, marjoram, neroli and geranium essential oils. You may want to carry a small vial of one of these oils with you for convenience. I have observed people with asthma having more frequent attacks out in public where they have less control over their environment and stress levels. A combination of lavender and neroli essential oil is a favorite for many. The oils in the above list are known for their relaxing effect on the nervous system and are anti-stress oils; choose your favorite.

The following recipe for asthma is a very refreshing, cooling remedy. It is extremely simple yet very effective for mild to moderate asthma conditions as these essences may possess antihistamine-like properties. Remember to keep your eyes closed during the facial splash as all essential oils are volatile and can irritate the eyes; this remedy is not recommended for small children. This recipe can also be made into a facial mist and kept in the refrigerator. See *A User-Friendly Blending Chart,* page 378 for facial mist proportions and Chapter 12 for facial spray instructions.

Aromatic Face Splash

for asthma

sink full of cold water
1 drop Chamomile essential oil
1 drop Lavender essential oil
towel

Fill the bathroom sink or basin with cold water. Add the two drops of essential oil and swish into the water to disperse as much as possible. With the eyes closed at all times, splash the face with the aromatic water several times. Pat face dry with the towel. Wait a minute or two, and then repeat the same process again. This can be done several times during the day.

The recipe for Asthma Oil Blend is to be applied to the entire back area from the base of the spine up to the base of the neck. Also apply these oils to the feet and ankles. Remember the feet are effective areas for application of aromatherapy, especially for respiratory ailments such as bronchitis and asthma.

If there is congestion present, follow the instructions for chest and back massage on page 100 which will help encourage fluid drainage.

The lavender and peppermint essential oils were chosen for this recipe for their general tonic effect on the entire body. Eucalyptus is included for its well known respiratory benefits. I include Ylang ylang essential oil for its effect on the emotions, specifically anger, fear, and anxiety, with which asthma has a strong correlation. Together these essential oils create a synergistic blend which has been very effective for many people.

Asthma Oil Blend

to apply to the back, feet, and ankles

16 drops Lavender essential oil
3 drops Peppermint essential oil
3 drops Eucalyptus essential oil
3 drops Ylang ylang essential oil
2 tablespoons (1 oz.) vegetable oil

In a clean glass amber bottle, add the essential oils and mix. Add the vegetable oil and shake gently to mix thoroughly. Label contents. Apply to upper back area and front of upper chest. Inhale from hands with several deep and relaxed breaths. Apply three times per day.

For inhalation of essential oils an electric diffuser is best since it is the most therapeutic method for inhaling essences. There is no heat involved in the process, which can be an undesirable factor in asthma treatments. I normally do not advise the use of steam inhalation treatment for asthma patients, since it can trigger more symptoms. The following inhalation blend suggested for most mild forms of asthma is intended for a diffuser or aroma lamp. If you have the time, do your breathing exercises while the diffuser is on. This will help to remind you to do them and you will benefit from the deep inhalation of the essential oils. This blend has a very pleasant scent reminiscent of a clean primeval forest rather than the typical medicinal odor one might come to expect of a respiratory blend. Notice all three oils in this recipe are derived from tree sources. You can also put a few drops of this blend on a tissue or a few cotton balls in a plastic bag, to carry with you for inhaling.

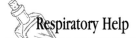 **Respiratory Help**

an asthma inhalation blend

1 part Pine essential oil

1 part Cedarwood essential oil

1 part Sandalwood essential oil

If you can get 1/3-ounce-size bottles of the above essential oils simply add them to a 1-ounce-size amber bottle to hook up to your diffuser. Or to make smaller amounts of this recipe, measure by eyedropper or teaspoons, keeping the equal proportions. Label contents. Diffuse for 10 to 15 minutes, three to four times daily.

Essential oils that are effective in asthma conditions are chamomile, cedarwood, cypress, geranium, patchouli, lemon, lavender, pine, bergamot, peppermint, neroli, eucalyptus, marjoram, mandarin, rosemary, and hyssop.

This herb tea can be taken to support the respiratory system.

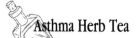 **Asthma Herb Tea**

to strengthen the respiratory and immune system

3 parts Peppermint herb

2 parts Anise seed (ground)

1 part Sweet thyme

1 part Sage

Mix the above herbs together. Store in a clean glass jar, and label with instructions for use.

Use about 1/4 cup per quart of water and simmer for 3 to 5 minutes. Remove from heat and let steep for 10 minutes longer. Strain. Drink warm or at room temperature, up to three cups daily.

Keep stored in refrigerator for later use. Flavor with lemon or honey if desired.

Other herbs that are known to help asthma conditions are elecampane root, grindelia, pleurisy root, marshmallow root, yerba santa leaf, ephedra, licorice, and ginseng.

Lifestyle changes are crucial for the success of any asthma prevention and wellness program. Avoiding the known irritants is an obvious change that must be considered. Here are some of the common irritant and allergen inhalants that should be avoided when possible:

pollens (weeds, grasses, some trees)

house dust, molds, fungal spores (including Athlete Foot Fungus)

feathers, animal hair

paint, gasoline, industrial chemicals

tobacco smoke, cold air, air pollutants

Routine "spring cleaning" of your home on a regular basis is very helpful. Use only natural cleaning products, as many of the chemicals added to commercial brand cleaners are synthetic in origin and irritating to many people in general, but especially to those with a sensitive respiratory tract. Using a vacuum which does not recirculate dust and molds is another suggestion. Remember to ventilate your home regularly, even in the winter months. Additionally, "clean air" plants can be used for their air filtering capability. See Chapter 13 for discussion of different ways of purifying the air with aromatherapy and living plants.

Not all asthma sufferers have an emotional component to their illness; however, it deserves exploration since there is a strong correlation between the two. I recommend that you read Chapter 9 which deals with the emotions. Decreasing levels of stress is beneficial for everyone, and particularly for those with health challenges. Review the holistic health wheel page

23 to determine major areas in need of balancing in your life. Breathing exercises are important to fully expand the lungs, in addition to alleviating stress, so do them daily. See page 101 for breathing exercise instructions.

Dietary recommendations include avoiding any foods to which you are allergic. Avoid dairy products. Use more oregano in your diet as this herb has proven to be useful in asthma-related conditions. Increase your intake of vitamin C, B, and E, eat more foods rich in vitamins B, C, and E or supplement your diet with them. Also essential fatty acids supplementation may be helpful.

CHAPTER 5

Aromatherapy Treatments for the Circulatory System

Brief Overview of the Circulatory System

The circulatory system is one of the most important areas where a person can make a difference in his or her health. Almost all of the factors that increase one's risk for circulatory ailments are caused by things we can change. Lifestyle factors include emotional stress, physical inactivity and sedentary lifestyle, smoking, and taking birth control medication. Dietary factors may involve obesity, high blood cholesterol levels, and high sodium diets. Conditions that can cause circulatory problems are diabetes mellitus, hypertension, pregnancy, and recovery from surgery. There is also a strong link between circulation ailments and genetic predisposition, as family history will show.

Aromatherapy can benefit the circulatory system in many ways, especially where emotional stress is a contributing factor. Stress reduction should be a major component in any wellness program. Stress plays a major role in the development of illness, particularly disorders of the circulatory system, since the heart and great vessels respond to our emotional state.The primary organ of the circulatory system, the heart, as well as the blood vessels, are strongly affected by stresses of the outside world, in addition to internal stress caused by holding emotions in and not expressing them. In-depth coverage on this subject is given in Chapter 9: Psycho-Aromatherapy.

A variety of complaints such as soreness, swelling, numbness, and coldness of the extremities can be the result of poor circulation. If these conditions are allowed to exist long-term, inactivity and decreased movement can further progress into muscle weakness and possible infection.

The lymph system is closely related to the circulatory system. The lymph has a "seek and destroy" mission, in addition to the white blood cells of the circulatory system (blood); it channels the immune defenses by filtering out foreign materials that threaten the health of the body. Lymph nodes can be the site of infection or allergic reactions.

Assistance for Regulating Low Blood Pressure

Many people live a long healthy life with chronic low blood pressure, otherwise know as hypotension. The only true way of diagnosing this condition is by having your blood pressure measured by a blood pressure machine called a sphygmomanometer. This measurement can be performed easily in the comfort of your own home now since these blood pressure appliances are more readily available to the consumer. However, if you have an extremely high or low blood pressure, it's a good idea to get regular checkups by your attending physician, in addition to checking it yourself at home.

Some of the symptoms that may accompany postural or orthostatic hypotension are a reading of 90/60 or below, lightheadedness, dizziness, or fainting. They can occur after you've been sitting or lying down for a long period of time, and the blood pools into your lower limbs. When you stand quickly, lightheadedness is experienced due to the lack of blood circulating to the head. Moving gradually and pacing yourself are important when you have orthostatic hypotension.

Essential oils that can increase blood pressure by stimulating and tonifying the circulatory system are rosemary, lemon, and hyssop. These essences can be inhaled from a tissue or diffused in the room several times per day. Cypress, ginger, black pepper, and peppermint are essential oils which possess vasoconstrictive qualities, and can be used in combination with the cardio-tonic essential oils hyssop and rosemary. This blend has a delightful herbal garden scent which I am very fond of. If running an electric diffuser in the home, I recommend leaving it on for 10 minutes each time. The essential oils will last several hours in the room air, so no need to turn it on again for several hours.

It is important to state here that even though essential oils are pure and natural plant derived substances, they should not be used in large quantity or too frequently. Please refer to Chapter 1: Common Sense Safety, for review. Too much of a good thing can be harmful! Moderation and balance are keys to success with aromatherapy (and other forms of herbal medicine), especially when addressing circulatory ailments.

Inhalation Blend for Hypotension

use in moderation for low blood pressure

2 parts Rosemary essential oil

2 parts Hyssop essential oil

1 part Cypress essential oil

1 part Peppermint essential oil

Mix the above essential oils in drops for inhaling from a tissue, or make it in larger amounts for diffuser use. You can measure in teaspoon amounts or 1/2-ounce bottles purchased from the store.

Aromatic baths and footbaths can have a positive effect on the circulatory system as well. Try *Reviver Blend* or *Tune-Up* bath recipes on pages 300–301 or try the Aromatic bath recipe below to gently stimulate circulation.

Aromatic Bath for Hypotension

for low blood pressure

4 drops Rosemary essential oil

2 drops Geranium essential oil

1 drop Hyssop essential oil

1 drop Eucalyptus essential oil

Carrier (bath salts, Castile soap, honey)

For a very nourishing bath I recommend the Botanical Bath recipe as the carrier choice. The recipe is given on page 298. Subsequently you can use a few tablespoons of honey, bath salts, or Castile liquid soap as a carrier for the essential oils. Simply add the essential oils to the carrier of your choice and mix well before adding to the bath water. For low blood pressure I recommend a tepid water temperature as this is stimulating in general. Stay in and soak for 20 minutes or longer.

This recipe can be used in a foot bath by using half the essential oil amounts recommended above. For a local bath, such as the foot bath, a colder temperature can be used. Cold or tepid water temperature increases circulation by causing local stimulation. This is particularly good for cold feet with poor circulation. These are invigorating and rejuvenating and are meant for shorter periods of time. Refer to the section discussing Hydrotherapy on page 294 of Chapter 11.

Although most herbs have a regulatory effect on blood pressure, ginseng, oats, rosemary, sage, thyme, clove, and cinnamon spices have traditionally been used for hypotension. Cooking with these herbs and spices regularly may help to improve circulation and stimulate blood pressure.

Lifestyle recommendations include regular exercise, such as walking or swimming. Performing the *Breathing Exercises* on page 102 can improve circulation. Yoga has also proven helpful in increasing circulation, and regulating low blood pressure.

Dietary alterations, such as increasing foods rich in Vitamins B and C, can help, as can adopting a generally healthy diet low in animal fats.

Taking the Pressure Off—Help On the Way for High Blood Pressure

A blood pressure reading over 150/90 is considered by many health care practitioners to be "high blood pressure." High blood pressure is considered the medical problem of this century.

Again, blood pressure abnormalities are often silent but may be accompanied by fatigue, headaches, or visual change. Do not take high blood pressure lightly. See your health care practitioner regularly.

Elevated blood pressure is most common in the elderly and overweight populations. Hypertension increases your risk of cardiovascular illness and death. Numerous studies have been conducted with research documenting the fact that it is a disease found primarily in developed countries, so diet and lifestyle changes are essential to treatment.

Anti-hypertensive medications are among the most prescribed prescription drugs in this country and most have serious side effects. Changing your diet and lifestyle are the two most important changes you can make in "taking the pressure off."

It is imperative that you continue the medications prescribed for you by your physician, while you try the recommendations given in this section. Aromatherapy can have a positive and relaxing benefit for your nervous and circulatory systems, although it is not meant to take the place of your medications. Use it to *complement* and *support* your present wellness program. After using these recommendations for several months, visit your physician to be re-evaluated. Or find a physician well versed in natural methods to decrease blood pressure without prescription medications and use aromatherapy as part of a comprehensive program.

For inhalation, using an electric diffuser is the most effective way to introduce healing benefits of essential oils. The following recipe can be used in a diffuser by preparing a greater quantity of blended essential oils. For inhaling from a tissue, or putting a few drops in an aroma lamp, make this recipe in smaller amounts. The essential oils employed for decreasing blood pressure are known for their relaxation and sedating properties. It makes sense that if high blood pressure is a result of too much stress and stimulation of the nervous and circulatory systems, that calming these systems would be appropriate and beneficial. Similarly, relaxation exercises such as breathing exercises, regular and moderate exercise, massage, along with eating a healthy diet, would provide a holistic approach to "taking the pressure off" and are a good complement to aromatherapy. Use this inhalation blend in moderation.

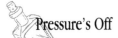

Pressure's Off

an inhalation blend for hypertension

4 parts Lavender essential oil

2 parts Ylang ylang essential oil

1 part Clary Sage essential oil

1 part Nutmeg essential oil

Mix the essential oils in an amber bottle. Use drops if a small amount is needed, and teaspoon- or 1/2-ounce-sized bottle if a large amount is needed for diffuser use. Use in moderation by diffusing 3 or 4 times per day, in 10-minute durations. Practice breathing exercises while the diffuser is on for even more benefit.

Essential oils known to decrease blood pressure by relaxation are chamomile, mandarin, neroli, rose, lavender, clary sage, lemon, marjoram, nutmeg, and ylang ylang. These essential oils can be inhaled by putting a few drops on a tissue. Inhalation is the most advantageous method of using aromatherapy for ailments of the nervous, circulatory, and respiratory systems because the effect can be immediate in comparison to the skin absorption methods.

In addition to inhaling therapeutic essential oils, they can be applied several times per week (or daily) in the form of lotions, oils, and baths. By applying aromatherapy treatments to the skin's surface, a consistent and slow-absorption rate will be achieved. This has several benefits. One is that it's already part of the daily bathing routine, so why not add the essential oils that will benefit your health? Second, if a moisturizing lotion is applied daily, you can add essential oils to this for a regular dose of these relaxing essences. If you like to take baths, then adding aromatics will be easy and an added pleasure for you. However, if you do not know firsthand the benefits a nice, relaxing, warm aromatic bath can bring, you must try it! This can be an excellent way to experience the relaxation that comes with soaking in your very own customized spa.

Did you know that just soaking in a hot tub of water can be relaxing in itself? Imagine adding essential oils that are known to decrease blood pressure, promote relaxation and enhance your feeling of well-being. It's a powerful combination! Sip on a cup of herbal tea made from one of the herbs listed below, and light a candle and play some soft background music. You will feel the stresses of the day melting away. But don't just take my word for it. You cannot experience the benefits by reading about it. Try it yourself. Relax and enjoy this aromatic bath three times per week, or as needed.

Aromatic Bath for Hypertension

for high blood pressure

3 drops Lavender essential oil

2 drops Marjoram essential oil

2 drops Mandarin essential oil

1 drop Geranium essential oil

Carrier of your choice

For a simple carrier, use cream or honey. Recipes for different carrier options are given on page 298. Use warm to hot water temperature to promote relaxation. Soak and relax for 15 to 20 minutes with your favorite relaxing music and candlelight.

Other aromatic baths that have calming and sedative benefits are the *Serenity Blend, Undress-De-Stress, Lover's Bath* and *Child's Play*. These bath recipes can be found in Chapter 11: The Aromatic Bath. You may want to read that chapter in its entirety after reading this section.

To prepare a massage oil to be used on the back (local area) use a massage concentrate. The following recipe is a concentrated oil blend to be applied to the back. This is **not** an all-over body preparation, as it will be too strong.

Massage Oil for Hypertension

for high blood pressure

10 drops Lavender essential oil

6 drops Ylang ylang essential oil

5 drops Sandalwood essential oil

4 drops Marjoram essential oil

2 tbls. sesame oil or vegetable oil

In an amber bottle, add the essential oils. Add 2 tablespoons of vegetable oil, preferably sesame oil, which has a grounding and nurturing quality. Mix well. Label contents. Warm the oil in your hands before applying it to the back in the form of massage. Use gentle easy strokes to encourage relaxation. Inhale the essences from cupped hands during and following the back massage. Simplified directions for aromatherapy massage are given on page 309–311.

You can modify this recipe for a daily lotion blend by tripling (total of 75 drops) the essential oil amounts and adding to 8 full ounces of unscented body lotion. Check the label and be sure it does not contain mineral oil, which is a petroleum product and not good for the skin. To add essential oils to your body lotions refer to Chapter 12 or the *User-Friendly Blending Chart* for exact dilution amounts and ratios.

Breathing exercises are highly recommended since performing these simple exercises encourages relaxation and regulation of the blood pressure. A stress-relief program is essential to any hypertension state. Regular exercise is crucial as well, as it can benefit the nervous system and circulatory system. Walking briskly for just 20 minutes a day is all it takes to get all the benefits of exercise. It doesn't have to be painful or time consuming! Remember, you are worth it!

Dietary recommendations include avoiding salt, fats, and stimulants such as caffeine and alcohol. Caffeine has been shown to contribute to hypertension, and alcohol temporarily raises blood pressure. Deficiencies that can cause hypertension are low calcium, low magnesium and potassium, low essential fatty acids and low vitamin C levels. Increase potassium-rich foods like fruits and vegetables, and be sure to get adequate essential fatty acids by eating avocado or raw nuts and seeds, or fish.

Lifestyle modifications that can greatly reduce hypertension when practiced consistently are meditation, yoga (the corpse pose), breathing exercises, and aromatherapy. Fear, anger, chronic anxiety, psychological and social stress can contribute to hypertension, in addition to job stress. Other contributing factors are smoking and exposure to heavy metals such as lead and cadmium. Nicotine constricts the smaller blood vessels and tends to raise blood pressure, in addition to increasing your risk of heart attack. Avoidance of these substances is crucial in achieving health of this all-important system.

Maintaining an ideal weight allows you to put less pressure on your circulatory system. Drink plenty of pure water. Vegetarians have shown considerably lower risk for hypertension; therefore a diet based on high fiber, low animal fats, and low refined sugar is advantageous to lowering your blood pressure. Also, vitamin C has proven beneficial in regulating blood pressure.

Regular exercise reduces weight, risk of heart disease, strengthens the entire cardiovascular system, and relieves stress. Find what form of exercise turns you on. It can be fun! Try walking with a friend or neighbor three times per week, or meet a co-worker for a lunchtime stroll. Twenty minutes isn't that much time to invest and you reap all the benefits that come with it!

Eat lots of garlic and onions, or make the Old-Fashioned Garlic and Onion Soup on page 97. These two vegetables have been extensively researched and proven to lower blood pressure. Make Guaranteed To Work Bran muffins, and eat at least one daily. They include dietary fiber (bran) in addition to oat bran, which has shown positive results in lowering blood cholesterol.

Diffusing essential oils in the room air, including your bedroom, can be very helpful in stress reduction. Review Chapter 13: Breathe Easy for more information on different methods of using living plants and aromatherapy methods for relaxation, and Chapter 9: Psycho-aromatherapy for anti-stress oils.

Effective Treatment for Palpitations Due to Anxiety

Anxiety is the uneasy feeling of apprehension associated with tight breathing, palpitations, and perspiration. Long-term anxiety can cause digestive disorders (as discussed in Chapter 2), headaches, backaches, and hypertension. Palpitations, the increased awareness or feeling of a strong heartbeat, can be due to stress. They may also follow rheumatic fever or other heart disorders. Mild palpitations due to anxiety and stress, with no history of an abnormal heart condition, are addressed in this section.

Prolonged episodes of palpitations, rapid pulse, chest pain or tightness, shortness of breath, and dizziness are all symptoms that should be evaluated by a health care practitioner immediately, as they are danger signals that the circulatory system is distressed.

Case history: *A 32-year-old mother of two, and full-time office manager at a fast-paced computer software company, consulted with me for aromatherapy. She had recently visited her physician for a complete medical work-up following increasing episodes of palpitations and increased pulse rate. She was found to be in excellent health with a normal blood pressure reading, pulse, and respiratory rate. Her doctor felt the palpitations were caused by stress and recommended a mild tranquilizer, which she did not want to take. She had read about aromatherapy and its usefulness in stress-related conditions, and wanted to give it a try before resorting to prescription drugs. This was her first experience with alternative medicine. She learned new and better ways to deal* *with her stress levels, and incorporated aromatherapy into her lifestyle changes. She also followed other recommendations given in Chapter 9 for stress relief, but found the following recipe for dealing with palpitations proved the most helpful to her with regular and intermittent use. At first it was a challenge for her to avoid stimulants (coffee, chocolate, cola drinks) in her diet, to spend time on herself, to take aromatic baths, to receive massages, and to remember to take the essences to work with her. Eventually (3 weeks after meeting with me), she brought her diffuser to work where it was needed most, and to her surprise was well received by her co-workers. She experiences very few palpitations now, takes time for herself regularly, and never had the need to take the prescription that was first offered to her by the doctor. She sends me magazine articles about stress or aromatherapy every so often, with a little note telling me how she is doing.*

Diffuse *Slow-Down and Relax* essential oil blend in the office or at home, where ever you experience the most amount of stress. The recipe is found on page 335 of Chapter 13. This blend is very helpful for general stress and takes the edge off frazzled nerves. I suggest an electric diffuser for the most therapeutic inhalation benefit. You can turn it on during stressful situations and regularly throughout the day (every 4 hours), for at least 5 to 10 minutes depending on the square footage of the room and ventilation.

A Peaceful Pace

an inhalation blend

4 parts Lavender essential oil

2 parts Ylang ylang essential oil

2 parts Sandalwood essential oil

1 part Lemon essential oil

This blend can be used in a diffuser (in larger proportions) or inhaled from a tissue or small vial for immediate use when palpitations are experienced. Take several deep and relaxed breaths inhaling from the nose for a count of three, and slowly exhale from the nose for a count of 6. Follow the Breathing Exercises outlined on page 102 to enhance the relaxation benefits. If you are in a stressful situation at work, inhaling from a tissue or bottle will be quick and convenient.

The lavender, ylang ylang, and lemon essential oils are recommended for their sedative effects on the nervous system and circulatory balancing effects. Sandalwood essential oil is beneficial for nervous tension and states of anxiety. It also has anti-spasmodic properties which can help to relax and prevent palpitations.

Receiving a relaxing back massage is very nurturing and great for stress, anxiety and episodes of palpitations. Turn to pages 309–311 for a quick review of aromatherapy massage and helpful hints. This massage doesn't have to be complicated or a "big" favor to ask of someone. Simply applying essential oils in a base lotion to the back area is very effective for several reasons. First, the skin on the back is very consistent in thickness and absorbs evenly. Second, the fact that you must lie down and allow someone to give you a back rub is acknowledgment that you are important and deserve attention and a few moments of quiet time. Third, a back massage is very relaxing in itself. Add to that the benefit of inhaling the sedative essential oils, and absorbing them through your skin, and you are receiving a multitude of benefits. This back massage only takes a few minutes, but the benefits will last hours!

Massage Lotion for Palpitations

apply to the back

2 tbls. unscented lotion or vegetable oil

12 drops Lavender essential oil

5 drops Ylang ylang essential oil

4 drops Bergamot essential oil

3 drops Neroli essential oil

Mix the above essential oils in the base lotion or vegetable oil. If using an unscented lotion be sure the ingredients do not include mineral oil or petroleum byproducts as this will interfere with the absorption of the essential oils. Apply to the back with light to medium hand pressure. Work in upward motions toward the heart, while encouraging the person receiving the massage to take slow and relaxed breaths. Allow him or her to inhale the essences from your hands by cupping the hands over the nose and mouth. To get the most from your massage, the environment should be relatively quiet and softly lit. Set up your massage at a time and place where you are unlikely to be interrupted.

Aromatic baths are a very pleasant way to unwind and relax, especially for anyone with a history of anxiety and palpitations. Several excellent recipes given in Chapter 11: *The Aromatic Bath—Your Personal Spa* would be appropriate. Here are a few suggestions from that chapter:

Serenity Blend—a blend of lavender, bergamot, and mandarin

Undress-De-Stress—lavender and clary sage

Glad-to-Be-Home—lavender and geranium

Other essential oils that are useful in relieving anxiety and palpitations are the sedative essences of basil, neroli, geranium, rose, chamomile, lavender, lemon, marjoram, orange, and ylang ylang. Essential oils used for states of anxiety are bergamot, chamomile, cypress, geranium, jasmine, lavender, marjoram, neroli, patchouli, rose, sandalwood and ylang ylang. These essential oils can be inhaled from a tissue for immediate use when palpitations and feelings of anxiety are experienced.

As with most other ailments, prevention is always easier than trying to remedy a symptom that has already manifested itself. When emotional stress is experienced, our heart rate, blood pressure, and muscle tension increase. The nervous system becomes stimulated and goes on alert. Therefore, using essential oils and relaxation techniques should become part of your routine health maintenance, like brushing your teeth or taking vitamins. Since the breath connects the body and mind and produces a general calming effect, it is highly recommended, along with aromatherapy inhalation, to achieve stress reduction. See page 102 for Breathing Exercises.

Dietary changes are for supporting the circulatory system and nervous system. Increase vitamin B- and C-rich foods, or increase supplementation. Avoid stimulants such as alcohol, caffeine, cola drinks, and chocolate to relieve the strain on the nervous system and circulatory system.

Lifestyle recommendations that may be useful are practicing a good stress-release program daily and using relaxation techniques during stressful situations and episodes of palpitations. See Chapter 9 for stress-free recommendations.

How to Alleviate Swelling and Fluid Retention

This is an exciting area in which to apply therapeutic essential oils because you can "see" them working. Swelling of the feet, ankles, and hands is common when there is a condition affecting the circulation. Some conditions that may cause swelling are arthritis, varicose veins, constipation, high blood pressure, and general fluid retention (edema, when the body holds onto fluid). Also, in the last trimester of pregnancy there may be extremity swelling, typically of the hands and feet, due to the additional weight bearing on the pelvic veins. This particular swelling caused by pregnancy will be addressed in Chapter 10: For Women Only where specific essential oils are recommended.

Essential oils help to decrease fluid retention and swelling from the body through the kidneys and the skin. The lungs and digestive system (bowels) also are ways the body uses up water and bodily fluids, but are secondary to skin and kidneys.

Essential oils that are diuretic aid the production of urine and help by encouraging fluids to be excreted via the kidneys and bladder. Diaphoretic essential oils are those which aid the production of sweat, and therefore help the body to secrete bodily fluids via the skin, specifically the sweat glands. See Cross-section of skin illustration on page 16. The diuretic essential oils are most useful; in fact, many diuretic medications prescribed by doctors work in a similar way, by stimulating the kidneys to produce more urine. Essential oils are effective natural alternatives that promote urine production as well, and pose virtually no side-effects or dangers if used within the guidelines stated in this book. The use of aromatherapy in cases of localized swelling is impressive, yet gentle.

Case history: *A 67-year-old woman experiencing ankle and foot swelling for years asked me for recommendations. She has a history of arthritis (in her hands), moderate hypertension, and occasional constipation. She sees her physician regularly for checkups and blood pressure readings. She takes prescription medication, which includes an anti-hypertensive drug and diuretic. However, she is still bothered by moderate to severe swelling of her feet and ankles, especially during hot and humid weather. She continued the advice of her physician, which was to avoid sodium in her diet, and to remain on the drugs she presently takes. Using essential oils in her bath, footbaths and lotion were the only changes she made in alleviating her localized swelling, to achieve positive results. She was amazed at the simplicity of the recommendations and surprised at the tremendous results.*

For generalized swelling and fluid retention, a full aromatic bath is most beneficial. The following bath is best at a warm water temperature, but not too hot. Turn to page 294 for hydrotherapy guidelines. The goal is to encourage circulation and promote sweating, but without undue harm to the tissue and sluggish system. If the temperature is too cool, then the body will not respond as quickly. A full bath is an excellent way to take in essential oils, since a large area of your body's skin surface is absorbing the active ingredients. Following the bath, it is helpful to wrap yourself in a warm bath towel or cotton bathrobe, to encourage sweating further. By sipping cool water or herb tea while in a warm bath you can stimulate the kidneys too! Keep warm and rest by lying down for at least twenty to thirty minutes following the aromatic bath.

The *Cellulite Bath* given on page 303 is extremely effective in ridding the body of excess fluid. You can also make up your own blend by using any of the essential oils listed here for swelling and fluid retention. Remember to follow the guidelines given in Chapter 11: The Aromatic Bath, for the quantity of essential oils used per bath and safety measures. In general, 6 to 10 drops of essential oil per full tub of water is fine. I suggest the bath salt recipe on page 299 to be used as the essential oil carrier as this encourages detoxification and draining effect on the body tissues.

For swelling of the hands or feet, a hand or foot bath can be very soothing, cooling, and an effective relief for localized problems. A cold to tepid water temperature is advantageous to decrease local inflammation and swelling. See page 294 on hydrotherapy guidelines, and refer to Quick N' Easy Shortcuts for directions on foot baths. Try this foot bath for ankle and foot swelling.

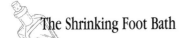 ## The Shrinking Foot Bath

a foot bath for localized swelling

1 – 2 tbls. Castile liquid soap or bath salts (recipe for bath salts on page 299)

2 drops Lemon essential oil

1 drop Cypress essential oil

1 drop Juniper essential oil

bath basin or tub

towel

Castile liquid soap, or bath salts, is used as the carrier for this recipe. Add the correct amount of essential oils to the carrier chosen, then add to the bath basin. Swish the water well to combine. Sit in a comfortable place and allow your feet to soak for at least 15 minutes. Pat the feet dry and elevate them at least 6 to 8 inches above heart level, by lying down for another 15 minutes or more. This further encourages blood return to the heart and decreases local fluid accumulation. While you are lying down and elevating your feet, performing the breathing exercises on page 102 will promote relaxation and good blood circulation.

For local swelling of the extremities, applying cold packs, cold compresses and ice will also ease and diminish swelling, especially during hot weather. For aromatic compress directions turn to page 319. Wearing support hose is helpful for women on their feet all day. I began wearing support hosiery when I was pregnant with my twins while working in the clinic. I remember patients offering their seats to me during my last few weeks before delivery because I was so large. That was my biggest experience with swelling!

Local massage of the feet or hands with an unscented base lotion and essential oils is yet another way to apply aromatherapy for swelling. Or use arnica infusion oil as an excellent carrier for your essential oils in massage blends that involve inflamed (but intact) skin conditions and bruising. A description of this oil is given on page 372; it can be purchased in health stores. Use this concentrated massage oil for local areas, such as the feet or hands, when swelling is a problem due to poor circulation. For chronic problems you can use this preparation daily to help prevent symptoms. Lemongrass is included in this remedy because it tones the skin which has been stretched from frequent swelling of the tissues.

Massage Oil for Swelling

a concentrated blend for local edema

1 tbls. Arnica infusion oil

1 tbls. vegetable oil or unscented lotion

12 drops Lavender essential oil

5 drops Cypress essential oil

4 drops Lemongrass essential oil

4 drops Grapefruit essential oil

In a one-ounce amber bottle, add the essential oils. Then pour in the arnica and vegetable oil in the desired amount. Note: If using a *one-ounce* bottle, simply fill the bottle with the oil; there is no need to measure it. Label contents. This oil can be used daily by massaging it into the affected area (feet, ankles or hands). Always apply with hand strokes and circular massage in the direction towards the heart. This encourages blood flow return and decreases swelling. Use an unscented base lotion (without mineral oil) if you plan on wearing this daily under hosiery. Lotion is water soluble and more readily absorbed by the skin.

Essential oils that are useful for conditions of swelling and fluid retention are Chamomile, Grapefruit, Frankincense, Juniper, Cedarwood, Lavender, Cypress, Lemon, Fennel, Lemongrass, Geranium, Ylang ylang, Mandarin, Hyssop, Rosemary, and Orange.

Lifestyle recommendations include supportive measures that help to prevent conditions of swelling and fluid accumulation due to poor or inadequate circulation. These are avoiding tight-fitting clothing or shoes and wearing support hose or knee highs. Take frequent breaks from continual standing or sitting and elevate the feet as much as possible while sitting (stool under desk, hassock).

Dietary changes are helpful as well and include avoiding salty foods and high-sodium-containing foods (beware of canned and processed foods). Eat a healthy, high-fiber diet to avoid constipation and varicose veins. If arthritis is an underlying factor, refer to that ailment for additional recommendations. Drink fresh-squeezed lemon juice in water as this is a natural diuretic. Eat more onions and garlic as these are diuretic agents; try the soup recipe on page 97. Chew the Sweet Breath seed mix on page 28; these seeds are diuretic too!

Recipes For Varicose Veins

Varicose veins. What exactly are they? Varicosities are dilated, bulging, purple and blue, distorted, and sometimes uncomfortable superficial veins that appear most commonly in the legs. Symptoms include discomfort, itching, heaviness, aches and pains, with varying degrees of discoloration seen through the skin.

Varicose veins can be caused by a weakness in the vein's structure, primarily the wall and valves of the blood vessel. The veins become dilated and filled with blood, which is insufficiently returning to the heart. Women experience the majority of these unappealing, yet relatively harmless vein conditions, up to four times as often as the male population. This is one reason for suspecting a link between varicose veins and varying hormone levels. An increase in venous pressure, straining, vein weakness, prolonged standing, and heavy lifting are all predisposing factors to this ailment. Also there is a strong correlation between low-fiber diets and an increase in varicosities. More than half of the female population over age fifty experiences some form of this condition.

Varicose veins can be anywhere in the body, but are most frequently seen in the lower legs, in addition to the rectal area, where they are known as hemorrhoids. For discussion of this particular ailment, turn to Chapter 2: Aromatherapy Treatments for the Digestive System, where this is addressed. If a varicose vein is deeper in the body, and involves an obstruction of blood flow returning to the heart, it can lead to serious complications and requires the treatment of a health care professional. However, in this section we are directing our attention to the superficial, relatively harmless varicose veins of the legs.

The main purpose of treatment is to tone the vein walls to improve circulation and to support the surrounding tissue. Gentle massage along with application of essential oils will encourage lymphatic drainage and blood return. Astringent and vasoconstrictive agents are utilized as part of compress and massage preparations, in addition to regular exercise, a high-fiber diet and maintaining an optimum weight.

Immediate relief is obtained from the cool compress method, in terms of discomfort and some of the swelling of the vein. However, you must realize that most treatments for varicose veins will take time to remedy. Just as it has taken months, and even years, for this condition to present itself, do not expect miraculous improvement with a few aromatherapy applications. The holistic approach of combining dietary and lifestyle changes will improve the effectiveness of this regimen.

Case History: *Lila, a 62-year-young woman, had taken several of my classes on various aromatherapy subjects. She finally had asked, "What can aromatherapy do for my varicose veins?" Over a three-month period, Lila was committed to following the recommendations I am outlining here, to see whether or not aromatherapy would help alleviate her discomfort. She had several veins that were involved (two on the back of the thigh, above the knee joint and one on her ankle), and had experienced some discomfort after long periods of sitting or standing. She was about 15 or 20 pounds overweight, and was a very active woman with many social activities; however, regular exercise was not part of her lifestyle. She was generally able to walk three to four times per week during the three-month time frame, and was about to embark on a healthier eating plan now since summer was around the corner. The final results were in. She stated she began to see a big change in the vein's appearance after a month or so. After about thirteen weeks, she saw a definite improvement in her skin, specifically directly over the veins; the veins had become smaller and less bulging, she had lost several pounds, her bowels were regular, and she felt "great."*

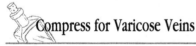

Compress for Varicose Veins

for the immediate relief of discomfort caused by varicose veins

1/2 – 1 cup cold distilled witch hazel lotion

6 drops Cypress essential oil

1 drop Lemon essential oil

1 drop Bergamot essential oil

bowl

piece of flannel, or wash cloth

plastic wrap

towel

Refrigerate the witch hazel lotion so it is cold for application. The cold temperature aids in decreasing local swelling and helps with the aches associated with varicose veins. If you have only one varicose vein to treat, then the 1/2 cup amount will be plenty. If you have several veins to cover, then use more witch hazel, and several pieces of flannel (if in different locations). Add the essential oils to the witch hazel and swish the liquid well to disperse. Turn to page 319 for complete directions on applying compresses. Do this as needed for immediate relief of swollen and aching varicosities. Follow with the aromatic massage oil specifically designed for weak vein walls.

The following recipe is the ultimate daily treatment for varicose vein conditions. The recipe may look complicated due to the various carrier oils I have included, but is really simple and extremely effective if used daily along with the other recommendations given in these pages. If you cannot find the infusion oils, any vegetable oil will suffice, although it will not have the toning, anti-inflammative and healing properties of those oils listed. You can purchase infusion oils in natural health stores, or make your own following the directions for an infusion oil on page 372 in Chapter 15: Blending How-To's and Helpful Hints.

Mullein oil is beneficial in painful or inflamed conditions such as varicose veins. Arnica oil is made from arnica montana flowers which impart a deep red color to the infusion oil. It is a useful first aid oil for bruising and inflammations but use only on unbroken skin. The apricot kernel oil is high in vitamins A and B, and is a light, easily absorbed seed oil which helps heal delicate, damaged, and inflamed skin. You can see how these carriers are doing more than just transporting the essential oils into the skin's surface. They are healing agents in themselves!

Massage Oil for Varicose Veins

use daily to help tone weak veins

1/2 tbls. Mullein infusion oil

1/2 tbls. Arnica infusion oil

1 tbls. Apricot kernel oil

15 drops Cypress essential oil

10 drops Lavender essential oil

5 drops Bergamot essential oil

400 IUs Vitamin E (optional)

In an amber bottle, add the essential oils. Add the various carrier oils and shake gently to mix completely. Label contents. Apply in small amounts to affected areas with gentle upward massage strokes. Use a light touch as we do not want to damage this delicate tissue further. The goal is to encourage blood flow towards the heart, and aid in absorption. Apply twice daily.

Essential oils helpful in varicose conditions are those with vasocon-strictive, anti-inflammatory and slightly diuretic properties. These include essential oils of bergamot, cedarwood, chamomile, cypress, geranium, juniper, patchouli, sandalwood, clary sage, lavender, lemon, neroli, and rosemary. However, essential oil of cypress is most well known for its positive effects on varicose veins.

Dietary recommendations include increasing your dietary fiber to prevent constipation and straining, as there is a strong association between the incidence of varicosities and low fiber diets. Eat more fresh vegetables, fruit, whole grains, and legumes for their fiber content. Fruits high in bioflavinoids are especially helpful for alleviating or preventing this condtion: cherries, black berries, and blueberries. Drink at least the minimum of six to eight glasses of pure water daily.

Lifestyle changes are very important for long standing prevention. Avoid prolonged periods of sitting or standing. By standing (continuously for hours), we can exert more than ten times the pressure on the leg veins! Take frequent breaks and change your posture as much as possible throughout your working routine. Wear support hose, and avoid tight fitting clothes that can impede circulation. Losing those extra pounds can put less stress on the circulatory system too. Get regular exercise, like walking, at least three times per week for 20 minutes or more, to benefit all the systems of the body. Exercise helps push the blood back to the heart and strengthens the entire body. Incorporating yoga exercises, such as the butterfly pose, can help relieve pressure and swelling. Refer to page 280 in Chapter 10 for the Wall Butterfly Exercise instruction. Avoid very hot baths that will dilate the weakened veins even more. And as for many of the other ailments of the circulatory system discussed in this section, adopt stress-relief practices to add to the treatment's end result.

How to Assist Poor Circulation

Poor circulation results in a number of conditions such as low blood pressure, varicose veins, angina pectoris, cramps, or even more serious conditions like thrombosis.

The dangers and possible complications due to poor and inadequate circulation are many. Dangers range from burns, coldness, ulcerations, congested lymph glands, and infection to abnormal blood clotting, heart attack, and stroke. When the "plumbing" isn't working optimally, the entire body is affected. When nutrients and oxygenated blood do not make it to their destination on time, then the tissue cells begin to suffer poor nutrition and work less efficiently. Over time, veins becomes distended (varicose veins), blood pressure is compromised (hypotension), smaller blood vessels in the extremities get less oxygen-rich blood (numbness, coldness), and the greatest muscle of all—the heart—can suffer damage from poor circulation in the form of angina pectoris or heart attack. This is painting a pretty grim picture, isn't it? Yet, it is one of the major areas where we can make a difference in our health! Read on to find out how aromatherapy can benefit poor circulation and aid in prevention of the above conditions.

Ideally, our blood vessels should be clean and in good working condition. There are many books on this topic that can give you detailed information on diet, exercise, relaxation techniques, etc. I will mention some of these subjects briefly too, because they are crucial to a holistic wellness program. Since this book has an aromatherapy focus, we will not give as much attention to those other topics, although I strongly urge you to adjust your entire "holistic health wheel" (see page 23 Chapter 2) to increase your success in this area.

It is unrealistic to expect aromatherapy, or any other complementary medicine, to completely remedy such a system. It is better to do a little in each area (e.g. lifestyle, diet, work, rest) than to put all your energy in one place and neglect the other aspects that play an important role.

The goal is to restore circulation to proper function. A steady routine followed slowly but consistently will benefit this system.

The therapeutic value of essential oils in assisting poor circulation is varied. Those which directly stimulate circulation will be very helpful for local problem areas. General toning of the circulatory system is important, and essential oils can be applied here as well. Aromatherapy is extremely effective in stress-release and stress prevention, which can play a major role in hypertension and heart disease. Herbs and massage, based on essential oil blended applications, support the circulatory system significantly.

A synergy blend is recommended for general poor circulation. This particular blend includes circulation stimulators and toners, nervous system relaxing oils and emotional uplifting essences. This blend can be diffused throughout your living space on a regular basis (3 to 4 times per day) for general use. It will purify the air as well as support your circulation and nervous system. It has a bright and clean natural scent I think you will enjoy.

Good Health Synergy

for poor circulation

3 parts Cypress essential oil

3 parts Lemon essential oil

2 parts Bergamot essential oil

1 part Ginger essential oil

1 part Geranium essential oil

Mix the essential oils in an amber glass bottle. Electric diffusers often come with extra empty bottles that fit onto the machine; use one if you have it. Label contents. You can measure this recipe in eye dropper proportions, or make a large amount using teaspoon measurements.

You can put several drops of this synergy blend in an aroma lamp, potpourri burner, or humidifier. There are many methods in which to utilize inhalation. Turn to Chapter 13: Breathe Easy for other inhalation options. The diffuser is the most effective way to experience aromatherapy, especially for circulation, nervous system, and respiratory benefits. To make sure you get regular exposure to these essential oils and to make it easy, hook up a timer to the diffuser.

Aromatic Bath for Poor Circulation

4 drops Cypress essential oil

3 drops Grapefruit essential oil

1 drop Nutmeg essential oil

Bath salts or Botanical Bath (as carrier)

Choose a carrier (described and recipes given in Chapter 11). I suggest the bath salt or botanical bath recipes for this bath. The bath salts are detoxifying and helpful with sluggish conditions, while the botanical bath is nourishing to the skin. Add the essential oils to the carrier before pouring into the bath water. The water temperature should be very warm (but not hot). Soak for 20 to 30 minutes. For best results, use a dry brush before stepping into the tub to increase circulation on the skin's surface. Or use a loofah sponge in the bath and scrub in circular motion towards the heart. After soaking a while, try elevating your feet above the heart level by resting them on the edge of the tub. Dry briskly with a towel to further stimulate and slough dead skin cells which have become loosened during the soak.

Taking three aromatic baths per week will do wonders to tone and stimulate your body.

A back massage can be another way to apply aromatherapy oils to help with poor circulation.

Massage Oil for Poor Circulation

2 tbls. vegetable oil

12 drops Cypress essential oil

6 drops Rosemary essential oil

4 drops Lemon essential oil

3 drops Nutmeg essential oil

In a clean amber glass bottle add the essential oils. Pour in the 2 tablespoons of vegetable oil and shake gently to mix. Label contents. Apply to the back area with firm upward stroke movements, always working towards the heart, assisting circulation.

Essential oils that are useful in stimulating poor circulation and aid in toning the venous system are bergamot, cypress, eucalyptus, ginger, grapefruit, geranium, lemon, lemongrass, neroli, nutmeg, pine, rose and rosemary. If hypertension and stress are major factors in your poor circulation, then the essential oils that relax and calm the nervous system will be particularly helpful.

Lifestyle recommendations include regular exercise, avoiding alcohol and smoking, and staying at an ideal weight. Be careful when taking baths, showers, washing dishes etc., that the water temperature is not too hot, as persons with poor circulation are more prone to burns. When outside during cold weather conditions, stay warm and keep hands and feet well protected. Easing stress in your life will have positive effects on all aspects, so be sure to address this by reading Chapter 9.

Dietary changes are important as there is mounting evidence for the relationship between food our circulatory health. Adopting a diet that emphasizes fruits, vegetables, and whole grains and limits animal products will have many benefits, such as lower risk of heart disease, obesity, and poor circulation. Decrease refined sugar, and dairy products and avoid salt. Eat plenty of onions and garlic for their health-promoting benefits mentioned earlier. Try the Old-Fashioned Garlic and Onion Soup recipe given on page 97. Taking stress vitamins (B's), vitamin C and E, along with other anti-oxidants like Pycnogenol, zinc, and selenium can be added to your program as well, to assist circulation and to prevent future problems.

Quick 'n' Easy Remedies for Raynaud's Disease

Raynaud's disease is an ailment which affects the circulatory system, specifically the small blood vessels, and most frequently occurs in the hands and feet. It is a hypersensitivity of these blood vessel walls that go into spasm, decreasing blood flow to fingertips and toes, and in severe cases the entire hand or foot. Typically persons who experience this ailment are less sensitive to heat and pressure and are therefore more prone to accidents, cuts, abrasions, burns, etc. It is not a dangerous condition, but may be uncomfortable.

Aromatherapy can be supportive by preventing vasospasm and increasing local circulation.

> **Case history:**   *A 16-year-old young man experiencing hand coldness, white knuckles, and blue fingernail beds, was diagnosed with Raynaud's by his physician. It was becoming more of a bother to him as he participated in outdoor sports during the winter months. He was willing to give the hand oils and hand bath treatments a try. After several weeks, he began noticing a decrease in symptoms, with less sensitivity to the cold weather. He doesn't spend nearly as much effort during the warmer months when his symptoms are less bothersome. But around football and soccer season, he starts up again with the oils and hand baths.*

For the hand bath recipe for Raynaud's disease turn to page 297 in Chapter 11. If the feet are affected by this condition as well, then do foot baths along with the hand bath. Take extreme care in checking the water temperature. I recommend a candy thermometer to measure it accurately, as Raynaud sufferers are definitely prone to burns, and cannot adequately judge the water temperature by using their affected hands. A warm-to-hot bath temperature is optimum (between 98 and 104 F degrees). This bath treatment should be done for 15 to 20 minutes. When the water temperature cools, replace with warmer water. This bath works primarily by dilating the blood vessels to increase local circulation.

This hand (and foot) oil can be applied immediately following the local bath treatment. It can also be made with an unscented lotion rather than an oil base for quicker absorption. It should be applied morning and night for several weeks in order to observe benefits.

Hand Oil for Raynaud's

use daily to help ease symptoms

2 tbls. Wheat germ oil

2 bls. St. John's Wort infusion oil (hypericum)

26 drops Lavender essential oil

10 drops Rosemary essential oil

7 drops Geranium essential oil

7 drops Nutmeg essential oil

800 IUs Vitamin E

In a 2-ounce amber glass bottle, add the essential oils in the above amounts. Add the wheat germ and St.. John's Wort infusion oil. Use Vitamin E capsules by cutting the end of the gel cap and squeezing the contents into the bottle. Shake gently to mix well. Label contents. Use twice daily and more often as necessary during cold weather and attacks.

The wheat germ oil is very high in vitamins A, D, and E and is exceptional for strengthening weakened capillaries. Vitamin E has long been used for skin rejuvenation and healing; in addition, it has anti-oxidant properties. St. John's Wort oil is made by infusing the flower tops of this herb in olive oil. It is very effective in all types of muscular inflammations and nerve- related pain. This combination of carrier oils makes a wonderful hand oil for Raynaud conditions. It must be used regularly and for a length of time to reap the positive benefits.

Other essential oils helpful in easing Raynaud's disease are black pepper, fennel, and nutmeg, in addition to geranium, lavender, and rosemary used in the above recipes.

Decreasing stimulants such as alcohol and caffeine is necessary to ease symptoms of this ailment. Garlic and onions are renowned for aiding in circulatory problems, and Raynaud sufferers can benefit by using more of these in their diets.

Lighten Up with an Incredible Cellulite Program

In some European countries, cellulite is considered a medical condition. The United States, on the other hand, looks upon this condition as a cosmetic circumstance afflicting obese women. It does affect men as well, but not nearly as often as women. Cellulite is fairly common even with women who maintain their ideal weight.

Cellulite is the name given to the unattractive dimpling of the skin, most often appearing on the outer thighs, hips, and buttocks. There is a loss of skin firmness due to the swollen fat cells and fluid and toxin accumulation. There are many theories as to the cause of cellulite. Some include fat cell malfunction, metabolic and circulatory disorders, and hormone imbalance.

Personally, I see the cause as a *combination* of poor circulation, poor elimination, and general toxification. If it was an easy problem to solve, I don't think we would see so many attempts (products, diets, appliances, supplements, drugs) to alleviate it. Of course, you have heard me say it before, prevention is easier and much more effective. There is no simple or easy solution for miraculous results. It takes commitment and consistency on your part, but the end result is well worth it. There are a multitude of products out there claiming to rid you of this unsightly condition. Rub this lotion on, turn this machine on, take this pill, and all your problems will disappear almost overnight. I don't think so! So, friends, I will not disillusion you with any promises. The information here is plain and simple, but takes commitment. For satisfactory treatment of a cellulite condition, diet, exercise, detoxification, excellent elimination, in addition to *caring for yourself* are crucial elements that must be included in your regime. If you give a half-hearted effort, you will achieve the same measure in your results.

Cellulite is a result of poor circulation. There is fluid trapped in between fat cells giving the "cottage cheese" appearance to the skin's surface. Both local stimulation and whole body exercise is necessary. Examples of local methods to stimulate circulation are dry brushing, use of loofahs, massage, hydrotherapy, and body scrubs.

Cellulite is also a result of poor elimination. The body is not removing the toxins and fluids that are being stored in this tissue. Often women who experience this condition also suffer from constipation, inadequate fluid hydration, and general state of toxification. There is a subtle poisoning of the body's tissues taking place, a result of months and years of poor diet choices being made. Our bodies simply cannot handle the doses of chemical-laden preservative additives and colorants we are forcing upon them daily. The body has no easy way of eliminating many of these synthetic chemicals. To detoxify is the only way out.

To discuss dietary changes seems to make the most sense at this time. A diet low in saturated fat and high in fiber is imperative. That means more vegetables, fruit, whole grains, legumes—and organic whenever possible. Drink plenty of pure water to flush out the toxins, at least 6 to 8 glasses per day. Drink hot water with the juice of 1 lemon daily (preferably in the morning) to encourage detoxification and elimination. Lemon is also an effective diuretic, and will stimulate the body to eliminate additional fluid. Eliminate alcohol, coffee, black tea, sugar, and all highly refined and processed food stuffs. Drink herb tea and aloe vera juice (concentrate) to encourage the detoxification process. Increasing vitamins B, C, and E, along with selenium may be helpful. A high-quality oil, such as flax oil, will improve the cellular membranes, helping to eliminate toxins and excess fluid.

Lifestyle recommendations include regular exercise. Movement increases blood flow. Walking at a brisk pace, swinging the arms from side to side, is a great form of exercise you can enjoy outside in the fresh air. Dancing, yoga, hiking, and even sex are considered exercise. Exercise does not have to be (and shouldn't be) painful, boring, difficult, expensive, or inconvenient. Take stretch breaks during your working schedule to avoid long periods of sitting or standing while at the office .

Case history: *A 42- year- old woman with a cellulite condition on her outer thighs came to me for advice. This was her major complaint! She experienced low energy, irregular bowel habits, and a history of sinus problems. She was mildly overweight, and was relatively active. She altered her diet, increased her exercise, and followed the aromatherapy regime outlined below. She took the detox tea and lemon juice daily, and started drinking pure water in the desired amounts. Within a month's time she called with excitement in her voice to say her husband noticed the difference! It was difficult for her to assess her progress; as she said, she never focused so much on herself before. She became aware of every curve, roll, dimple and so forth. But she was elated that her husband made the complimentary observation. She became less ashamed of and shy about her thighs and began wearing shorts more often. All in all she started loving her body again, which, I'm convinced, changed how she presented herself to others.*

The *Cellulite Bath Blend* is given on page 303 in Chapter 11: The Aromatic Bath. Use that recipe with the bath salt recipe on page 299. Epsom and sea salt assist the body in releasing toxins and excess fluids, and makes the best choice for the carrier. You can add the juice of one lemon into the bath water for additional benefits if you desire. Take two to three baths per week. If you do not need to tone and treat the entire body, then a sitz bath can be done in lieu of the full bath, to target the thigh and buttock areas only. Wrap yourself in a warm bathrobe or bath towel to encourage perspiration immediately following the bath. Up to 30 minutes to an hour after an aromatic bath is taken, the body continues to react and respond to the essential oils.

I recommend dry brushing with a good quality, natural bristle brush prior to your aromatherapy treatment bath. See p. 161 in Chapter 7. This will aid in increasing circulation and sloughing dead skin cells. Dry brushing will prepare the skin to more readily absorb the essential oils. Scrubbing with a natural loofah sponge in the bathtub as you soak is another way to target the stubborn areas that need additional attention.

Following the aromatic bath, after your daily shower, it is advised that you end the bathing routine with a cold water application for a few seconds to close the pores, aid in circulation and help firm tissues. See hydrotherapy basics in Chapter 11, page 293 for more detailed discussion on the benefits of using water temperature. This is optional, but an effective tool in promoting excellent circulation and body toning. Try to do it after every shower. Start out slow and work up to a more dramatic temperature change.

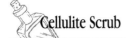 ## Cellulite Scrub

exfoliates and stimulates

1/2 cup medium-ground cornmeal

1/2 cup coarse-ground oatmeal

1 tbls. Sea salt

10 drops Mandarin (or Grapefruit) essential oil

4 drops Juniper essential oil

3 drops Lemon essential oil

3 drops Cypress essential oil

Add the essential oils to the sea salt in a bowl, and mix very well. Add the corn meal and ground oatmeal. Combine very well. Store in a wide-mouthed jar. Use before or after bathing. Simply wet the skin and apply to the affected areas, by rubbing in a circular motion. Do not apply with too firm a hand pressure as this is very coarse. Rinse off and pat dry gently.

The essential oils included in the anti-cellulite lotion recipe given below are the same ones used in the bath recipe. They are natural diuretic agents, which will encourage the kidneys to produce more urine, therefore excreting additional body fluids. The essential oils were chosen for their ability to increase and stimulate circulation and for the firming ability they possess. They work very well together, in both the bath and lotion methods of application. It is advised that you use these two recipes during the day, and not right before retiring, as you may need to empty your bladder more frequently.

The general state of the skin determines how well and efficiently the essential oils will be absorbed. When the skin is congested, thick, or calloused, with poor circulation, expect a slower absorption rate. Another good reason to exfoliate the skin!

The aromatherapy lotion must be prepared with a natural base lotion. If the lotion contains any mineral oil byproducts, the skin will not be able to absorb the essential oils. Mineral oil has a large molecular structure and blocks moisture (and essential oils) from getting in. I once sent a woman the essential oils to add to her lotion to use for cellulite control. I told her to not use any lotion with mineral oil in it, and to also use the lotion in the morning. Due to the diuretic properties of the essential oils used in this recipe, urine production is encouraged. (In other words, if you use this at night, you'll be up going to the bathroom!) I followed up with her two weeks later (by phone), when she indicated that she hadn't noticed much of a difference in her skin, nor was she voiding any more than usual. A closer investigation revealed that there was mineral oil in the "natural" lotion she was using. This was proof for her that mineral oil prevents essential oils from being absorbed.

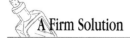

A Firm Solution

anti-cellulite lotion

6 oz. unscented base lotion (no mineral oil)
1 oz. Witch hazel lotion
30 drops Cypress essential oil
30 drops Lemon essential oil
10 drops Juniper essential oil
10 drops Lavender essential oil

Purchase an 8 oz. bottle of your favorite natural unscented base lotion to make this recipe. Refer ahead to Chapter 12 for base lotion options and information. Empty 1/4th of the lotion, or use it up first; we need to have 6 oz. of lotion in an 8 oz. bottle. The extra room is needed to completely blend this in the bottle. (Otherwise you can mix it in a jar or bowl.) In a small cup or dish pour 1 tablespoon of distilled witch hazel lotion. To it add the above essential oils and mix well. Add this mixture to the bottle of lotion. Shake very well and label.

To apply put a small amount on your hand and massage in circular and upward firm strokes towards the heart. Massage until it is completely absorbed. It is best to put this on in the morning after showering.

Essential oils that assist in alleviating cellulite are cypress, cedarwood, tea tree, fennel, grapefruit, juniper, lavender, lemon, lemongrass, mandarin, geranium, rosemary, and patchouli.

Herbs which are diuretic are cayenne, celery, dandelion, fennel, parsley, red clover, and yellow dock. The tea recipe below is useful for detoxification and is recommended during the cellulite regime.

Detox Tea

diuretic, aids in elimination of toxins

4 parts Peppermint herb
1 part Red clover tops
1 part ground Fennel seed
1 part Parsley herb
1 part Dandelion herb/root

Combine the herbs and ground fennel seed together in a jar. Label with directions for use.

Use 1 teaspoon per cup of water. Simmer for 5 to 10 minutes and strain. You can make this tea in larger proportions and keep it in the refrigerator for future use. Drink 1 to 3 cups per day, hot or cold. Flavor with lemon juice if desired.

CHAPTER 6

Aromatherapy Treatments for Muscle and Joint Problems

Brief Overview of the Musculo-Skeletal System

There are over 650 muscles in our body responsible for movement in areas as diverse as the musculo-skeletal system, the heart, and the digestive tract. *Skeletal muscle,* the long muscles that control the head, neck, torso, back, limbs, and fingers and toes, is responsible for movement and control of locomotion and posture and is the subject of this section. Tendons and ligaments anchor muscles to the bones. The nervous system also works very closely with the musculo-skeletal system, directing its movement and sending back signals on position, pain, etc.

Regular exercise is the single most important way to keep the muscular system toned and fit. When muscles are out of shape and circulation is inadequate, cramping, muscular weakness, and aches and pains are experienced as the result of underuse or over-use.

Aromatherapy is a great benefit to the muscular system since specific essential oils can detoxify, relax, and decrease swelling in muscle tissue. A muscle responds to pain with a reflex contraction. Once this occurs and sustains, blood flow to the area is impeded. Less oxygen and glucose are available to the muscle tissue, and the decrease in circulation also means that removal of toxins and waste products are sluggish. Inflammation, muscular soreness, and pain are the result. If this situation continues over any length of time, the nervous system becomes affected, causing nerve-related pain. Essential oils applied directly onto the affected area, via massage, compress, or bath will be absorbed into the muscle and surrounding tissues. Antispasmodic, anti-inflammatory and analgesic essential oils are most effective in this area. Once the therapeutic essential oils have relaxed the muscle and decreased the inflammation, the body will then be able to better handle the situation and heal itself. Essential oils act as agents that go in and aid a compromised condition, putting it in a healthier position to heal itself.

Physical pain triggers a physical response. Muscles tighten, blood vessels constrict, and nerve endings tingle. The nervous system is triggered and we feel pain which results in a protective emotional response of diminishing sensation. Together, these physical, nervous, and emotional responses form a vicious cycle of continued (chronic) pain. Therapeutic use of essential oils can interfere with this pain cycle.

Recently, scientists have discovered that the body naturally produces its own supply of "pain-killer" chemicals, known as neurochemicals. These are opiate-like substances called endorphins and enkephalins produced in the brain and spinal cord. It has been theorized that persons experiencing chronic pain may have below-normal levels of these natural pain-killer substances available. If this theory proves true, then aromatherapy may be very useful in the treatment of chronic pain, but further research is needed. Essential oils may increase levels of endorphins and enkephalins via inhalation, through pituitary and thalamus stimulation. These essential oils have been known traditionally as "euphoric" and "aphrodisiac" essences as they can produce a feeling of wellbeing. For chronic pain sufferers, I suggest incorporating these essential oils into your aromatic lifestyle for their possible benefits in pain control. Those known to stimulate the pituitary, which secretes the neurochemicals called endorphins, are clary sage, jasmine, patchouli, and ylang ylang. Those known to stimulate the thalamus, which produces enkephalins, are clary sage, jasmine, grapefruit, and rose.

Other techniques you can explore to overcome chronic pain are: meditation, visualization, biofeedback, hypnosis, acupuncture, muscle relaxation, chiropractic, and psychotherapeutic support groups. Increasing vitamin intake of calcium and magnesium may help, as they promote muscle relaxation. Vitamins E and C, in addition to carotene, are known to decrease inflammation, and may be increased in the diet or in the form of supplementation. Lowering dietary consumption of meat, dairy, and saturated fats, which can cause an increase in inflammation, may be helpful as well. Caffeine is known to cause tension in many people and should be avoided for this reason.

Soothing Arthritic Pain

There are more than 100 joint disorders, including many forms of arthritis. The most common kinds are osteoarthritis, rheumatoid arthritis, and gout. They possess common characteristics such as pain, swelling, redness, and stiffness of the joints. Sometimes the illness involves several joints or can be localized to just a few, as in the hands.

Osteoarthritis is the most common form of arthritis and will be the focus of this section. It is a degenerative condition of joint cartilage. The cartilage becomes enlarged, swollen, painful, and often deformed as bony outgrowths. Decreased movement of the affected joint results. The most affected joints in the body are the hands and weight-bearing joints such as the knees, ankles, and hips. Symptoms include early morning stiffness, pain that worsens with joint use, local tenderness, soft tissue swelling, creaking or cracking joint noises upon movement, bone swelling, and restricted movement or loss of function.

Several causes are known to influence osteoarthritis. As a degenerative joint disease, osteoarthritis affects the aged population; 80% of persons over 50 years of age suffer from some form of arthritic condition. In general, three times more women are affected than men. From this point on, I will refer to this condition of osteoarthritis as simply "arthritis." It is caused basically from prolonged wear and tear of the joints. Due to strenuous labor and continued use, bone, cartilage, and soft tissue become damaged over time. Obesity influences this condition, but does not cause it. However, extra weight puts unnatural strain on the joints, thus encouraging joint stress. Genetics, inflammatory joint disease, and history of trauma, such as fractures, are known to predispose one to this ailment. Also, over-use and incorrect use (inadequate stretching or warm-up) can also be factors.

> **Case history:** *A 70-year-old man with a history of osteoarthritis had already undergone one total knee replacement in his right leg when he consulted with me for natural alternatives to taking pain medications. He was very active for his age and, though bothered by his arthritic condition, he continued to work in his garden growing flowers, herbs and vegetables to sell to restaurants. He depended on his ability to work the land and needed the function of both legs to get his daily chores completed. He experienced increased pain in his left knee with decreased movement. It was especially stiff in the early morning, and grew increasingly swollen and sore by day's end. He wasn't one to bother with "fancy or complicated" treatments or expensive medicine. He was given dietary recommendations and an herbal tea mixture to drink, in addition to simple massage and bath oils. When he applied the arthritis oil in the morning upon rising, he felt there was considerable easing*

of his pain and stiffness as the morning went on. At night, he enjoyed the arthritis bath; as he said "he was taking his oils and getting clean at the same time!"

If the arthritis condition is localized, as in the case above, then massage oil concentrates, compress or poultices, and local hand or foot baths are the most effective. When the arthritis involves several joints or larger areas, a full aromatic bath is recommended in addition to the local treatments. The following recipe for the Arthritis Rub has several essential oils in its blend which work synergistically to provide safe and effective pain relief. You can make a much simpler version by using two or three different essential oils and omitting the carrot and St. John's Wort oil. Many of these essential oils in the recipe have dual benefits, as anti-inflammative and analgesic agents. The juniper and carrot seed aid in eliminating fluid and toxin accumulation in the joint and surrounding tissue. The carrot seed oil is an essential oil; however, it is used in 10% dilutions in a vegetable oil base, rather than as the carrier. It is very helpful in healing damaged tissue caused by trauma and surgical procedures. (See Chapter 15 for more information on carrot seed oil.)

Many people who have used this recipe proclaim its soothing, pain-relieving and cooling benefits. An avid golfer once told me she would not think of playing a game without it! This is a concentrated oil blend and is designed for local area application only.

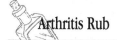 ## Arthritis Rub

for local areas only

14 drops Lavender essential oil

10 drops Rosemary essential oil

8 drops Peppermint essential oil

6 drops Juniper essential oil

1 tsp. Carrot seed oil

2 tbls. St. John's Wort oil

2 tbls. vegetable oil

Add the essential oils to an amber glass bottle that holds at least two ounces. Measure the carrot seed oil and mix well. Add the St. John's Wort infusion oil. Pour in 2 tablespoons of vegetable oil (or fill the remaining space of the two-ounce bottle). Shake gently and label. Use in small amounts by applying to painful or swollen joints. Can be applied two to three times per day.

For additional pain relief a cold compress is ideal. The cool temperature of the compress decreases inflammation and acts as an analgesic temporarily, as it delivers the therapeutic essential oils into the local tissues via absorption through the skin. By elevating the affected joint (above heart level) circulatory drainage will be encouraged. For example, elevate the knee on pillows while lying down, for a compress treatment to the knee. Hands and feet can also be elevated.

 ## Compress for Arthritic Joints

a cold compress to relieve pain and swelling

1 cup cold water
3 drops Chamomile essential oil
3 drops Hyssop essential oil
2 drops Cypress essential oil
piece of flannel or washcloth
plastic wrap
towel
bowl

Add cold water to the bowl. Add the essential oils and stir well to disperse. Soak the flannel cloth in the aromatic water. Wring out the cloth to where it is very moist but not dripping wet. Apply to the affected joint. Lay a sheet of plastic wrap over the moist compress and then the towel. Alternatively, put an ice pack over the plastic wrap to keep it cool longer. Once the compress becomes dry or warm, replace it with a fresh one. Leave the compress on for a duration of 15 to 20 minutes. This may be repeated two or three times per day for severe arthritic pain and swelling.

A poultice is another local treatment, similar to the compress; however, it utilizes fresh or dried ground herb instead of aromatic water as the medicinal agent. I recommend the compress with aromatic water because it is simple and very effective. However, if you have an herb garden or herbs readily available, making a poultice can be very beneficial as well. Refer to page 319 in Chapter 12 for directions on preparing poultices. For arthritis conditions where the joint is red, swollen, and painful, use Comfrey, Yarrow or Calendula herb, singly or in combination. You may want to add 2 to 4 drops (total) of the essential oils helpful with osteoarthritis together with the ground herb.

Hand and foot baths are very soothing pain relief for arthritic conditions of the finger joints or ankles. A recipe for an Arthritis Hand Bath is given on page 305 of Chapter 11: The Aromatic Bath. This recipe is the same for the foot bath. Use warm to tepid water for general aches and pain associated with this condition. If redness or severe swelling is present, use cold water. Refer to the hydrotherapy guidelines written on page 294 for temperatures recommended for various treatments. After a bath treatment, it helps to follow up with a local application of the Arthritis Rub recipe given previously in this section.

For generalized aches and pain related to arthritis, or when a local bath is not appropriate, then a full aromatic bath is the best choice. This bath recipe has been used with favorable results by persons suffering from fibromylagia, an arthritis-related condition that affects the entire body. A warm bath temperature will encourage relaxation of the muscles and increase circulation and absorption of the essential oils. There are several good bath carrier choices that you can use for this recipe. The Bath Salts, Botanical Bath, or Aromatic Honey Bath recipes given in Chapter 11 are beneficial, or simply add a half cup of Epsom salts to the bath to which the essential oils have been added. Epsom salts, magnesium sulfate, aids the body in detoxification and relieves muscular tension.

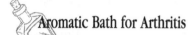

Aromatic Bath for Arthritis

for all-over aches and pain caused by arthritis

4 drops Juniper essential oil

2 drops Lavender essential oil

2 drops Cypress essential oil

2 drops Rosemary essential oil

carrier of choice

Blend the essential oils together and add to the carrier chosen. After the bath has been filled, add the mixture and stir into the bath water. Soak for 20 to 30 minutes. Pat dry and apply the Arthritis Rub to any local areas that need special attention.

Taking an herbal tea daily will be helpful in alleviating pain systemically. The following recipe has natural cider vinegar and fresh lemon juice as the primary cleansing and anti-inflammatory agents. Chamomile, meadowsweet, and bogbean are herbs that are used to make the base tea. If you are allergic to salicylates, omit the meadowsweet. Drink 1 or 2 cups daily.

Arthritis Herbal Drink

1 cup hot water

1 tsp. honey or ginger honey (see recipe page 38)

1 tsp. fresh lemon juice

1 tsp. apple cider vinegar

1/2 tsp. chamomile flowers

1/2 tsp. meadowsweet herb

Pour a cup of hot water over the herb and allow to steep for 5 minutes. Strain and add the lemon and vinegar. Add the honey (more to taste if you wish). Drink warm or cold.

The essential oils beneficial in osteoarthritis are primarily anti-inflammatory and analgesic in physical effects. They include essential oils of chamomile, cypress, cedarwood, eucalyptus, ginger, juniper, lavender, lemon, marjoram, myrrh, pine, peppermint, petitgrain, rosemary, and sandalwood.

Traditional herbs helpful in these conditions are burdock root, cayenne pepper, celery seed, feverfew, kelp, prickly ash, white willow, meadowsweet, thyme, yarrow, and yucca. Garlic and onions also help to relieve symptoms of this ailment because of their effect promotimg circulation. So use them freely in cooking. Alternatively, you can make the soup recipe on page 97.

Dietary recommendations include avoiding tobacco and the vegetables in the nightshade family (tomatoes, potatoes, eggplant, and peppers). Eat fruits rich in flavinoids, such as cherries, blueberries and hawthorn berries, which aid in stabilizing collagen and enhance joint integrity. Increase your intake of high-fiber foods and focus on low-fat foods. Try the bran muffin recipe on page 55. Taking Vitamin C and E, along with other anti-oxidants, may be beneficial as joints need oxygen-rich blood to function properly.

Gentle, non-weight bearing exercise, such as swimming or yoga, is ideal to keep joints flexible. Hand and foot rotation exercises are beneficial as well.

Healing Sprains

A sprain is an injury to the ligamentous structures surrounding a joint. It most often is caused by sudden twisting or wrenching of the joint. Rapid swelling and pain with movement are its two major symptoms. With a severe sprain, when ligaments are torn or dysfunctional, surgical repair may be necessary.

Ligaments themselves do not have a blood supply, but the vessels in the surrounding soft tissue will cause the accumulation of inflammatory products in the joint. Most injuries will benefit from application of heat or cold, and the application of hemostatic, anti-inflammatory and analgesic essential oils and herbs. Typically in the first 24 hours cold application is used to decrease and prevent swelling. After the first 24 hours, mild heat is employed to increase circulation to the traumatized area.

Case history: *A 22-year-old down-hill skier had sprained his knee when he hit a patch of ice on a steep mountain slope. He knew immediately that he had suffered a sprain, as this was his second knee sprain in three seasons. Ice was immediately applied at the ski lodge. He called me that evening to ask for suggestions. I made him a massage oil concentrate to use and gave him the essential oils to use in compresses. They had an immediate effect on the swelling and, after a few days, the extensive bruising became evident. He continued with the massage oil for one week and kept his knee elevated as much as possible. He had expected this sprain to take longer to heal since it was a very bad fall, and his second sprain on that knee. But, to his surprise, he healed in less time and did not need to take any analgesic medication. The doctor recommended a "knee support" to be used when skiing and playing tennis to provide additional support and discourage a recurrence.*

The compress below is to be used on unbroken skin, immediately after an injury. Witch hazel is an astringent and will help stop bleeding and swelling that has occured within the soft tissue. Comfrey tea is suggested for its healing properties, especially on ligaments. Cypress has hemostatic, antispasmodic, and astringent medicinal properties, while the chamomile essential oil is anti-inflammatory and analgesic. The marjoram is also analgesic and antispasmodic, and is useful if there is nerve-related pain.

Cold Compress for Sprains

use the first 24 hours

1/2 cup cold water (or comfrey herb tea)

1/2 cup distilled witch hazel lotion

2 drops Chamomile essential oil

2 drops Marjoram essential oil

2 drops Cypress essential oil

piece of flannel or washcloth

plastic wrap

towel

bowl

In a bowl, add the cold water or cold comfrey tea and witch hazel . Add the essential oils and stir well to disperse. Soak the flannel in the compress solution. Squeeze the cloth and apply to the affected joint. Cover with plastic wrap. If you have an ice pack, lay that over the plastic and cover with a towel. Elevate the sprained joint during the treatment. When the compress becomes dry or warm replace it with a fresh one. Continue the compress for 20 minutes. Do this treatment three times per day.

Following the initial phase of cold treatment should be mild heat to gently encourage circulation and healing. Moist compresses can be utilized, or moist heat. Continue to keep the joint elevated as much as possible, to prevent swelling and encourage blood return back to the heart. The essential oils used in the moist compress are different because the goal of treatment now is to increase circulation and enhance healing, as bruising will have already taken place. Anti-inflammatory agents continue to be included, in addition to analgesic essential oils.

Warm Compress for Sprains

use second day and thereafter following injury

1/2 cup warm water

1/2 cup distilled witch hazel

2 drops Chamomile essential oil

2 drops Rosemary essential oil

1 drop Hyssop essential oil

piece of flannel or washcloth

plastic wrap

towel

In a bowl, pour the water and witch hazel. Add the essential oils and stir well. Soak the compress cloth in the warm solution (98° to 100° F). Wring out and apply to the affected joint. Layer with plastic wrap. Lay over a heating pad set on low to keep compress warm (optional). Wrap with a towel. During compress treatment, elevate the affected limb above heart level, if possible. Replace compress when it becomes dry or cool to body temperature. Leave on for a total of 20 minutes. Do up to three compresses per day to help dissolve bruising and help with soreness.

The following massage oil is very concentrated and is used for local areas, such as sprained joints and bruising. This aromatherapy treatment should be applied several times per day, ideally following compress treatments or cold and heat applications. Massage into the affected joint, in an outward circular direction, and with upward strokes toward the heart, to facilitate drainage and blood return. Use gentle, medium pressure. Wheatgerm oil is ideal for sprains and bruises because it is rich in antioxidant vitamins, aids in strengthening weakened capillaries, and prevents scar tissue. Arnica montana is an herb which is used to make a very healing infusion oil useful for many first aid injuries, including bruises and inflammations.

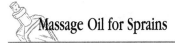
Massage Oil for Sprains

1 tbls. Wheatgerm oil

1 tbls. Arnica infusion oil

10 drops Lavender essential oil

8 drops Rosemary essential oil

4 drops Ginger essential oil

3 drops Peppermint essential oil

In an amber glass bottle, add the essential oils, then the arnica and wheatgerm oils. If these oils are not available, any vegetable oil will do. Shake gently and label. Apply 3 or 4 times daily, preferably after compress treatments, in the morning upon rising and before bedtime.

Poultices, an application of whole herbs, can be made for a sprain treatment. Herbs of turmeric, mullein leaves, comfrey, and even clay, have been used to help heal sprained joints. Refer to Chapter 12, First Aid to the Rescue, for additional information and directions on poultice preparation.

Essential oils useful in treating sprains are marjoram, chamomile, eucalyptus, ginger, jasmine, lavender, pine, peppermint, and rosemary. These can be used singly or in combinations, as recipes show. I like to use a combination of oils for a synergistic effect.

Lifestyle recommendations include staying off the affected limb as much as possible, and keeping it elevated. If chronic discomfort or swelling is present or is a frequent symptom, seek medical advice. Prevention: warmup prior to exercising, and cool down afterwards.

Effective Treatment for Backache

Low back pain is one of the most common ailments reported by employers as the reason for sick-leave. It is a frequent complaint by anyone who does heavy lifting, or prolonged standing. In fact, 8 out of 10 will experience low back pain in their lifetime. Acute low back pain associated with spasms, and sometimes radiating pain, can be caused by several predisposing factors such as muscular strain and spasm (when the muscles are painfully contracted), arthritic conditions, degenerative disc disease, obesity, lack of physical exercise, and poor posture. Pregnancy, another cause of backache, is addressed in Chapter 10.

Warning: If you experience difficulty in controlling your bowels or bladder, numbness, or weakness in your pelvis or lower limbs, seek medical attention as this indicates nerve involvement.

Tension can contribute to spasms of the back muscles. When stress is experienced, either emotional or work-related, tension is often held in the neck or back muscles of the body. Tension headaches can come from neck tension, while low backache can result from back tension. The abdominal muscles serve as a muscular corset, supporting the lower back. This is one of the reasons why poor tone, obesity, and bad posture are contributing factors.

One of the goals in aromatherapy treatment of low backache is to relieve muscle spasm and the inflammation resulting from contracted muscles. Whe the muscles relax, and adequate circulation can resume, inflammation will subside. It can also be eased further by incorporating therapeutic essential oils. Several of these, such as lavender, chamomile, and marjoram, have anti-inflammatory, antispasmodic, and analgesic properties and are considered the basic foundation for problems of the low back musculature.

For acute back pain and spasm, cold application with ice packs or cold compresses is suggested. Cold temperatures decrease swelling and provide local pain relief. But when low back pain is a chronic ailment, caused by consistent stress or poor posture or tight muscles, application of moist heat may provide greater relief of spasm and aches, and increase blood circulation to the area.

Prevention is the best way to treat backache. Lifestyle alterations can reduce and hinder these problems almost entirely and are listed at the end of this ailment section.

Compress for Backache

can use as warm or cold compress

2 to 4 cups water (or more)

3 drops Chamomile essential oil

2 drops Black pepper or Rosemary essential oil

2 drops Clary sage essential oil

1 drop Peppermint essential oil

a bowl

plastic wrap

2 towels

Use cold water temperature for acute and severe spasms. Use warm water temperature for chronic backache or on second day following trauma. In a bowl, add enough water to soak one towel that will cover the size of the area in need of treatment. Add the essential oils and stir well to disperse. Soak the cloth, then wring until just moist. Apply to the low back area where the pain and spasm are experienced. Include the surrounding area to relieve tension in the local area. Cover with plastic wrap and the towel. Leave on for a total of 20 to 30 minutes. Lie with the knees and hips flexed to take pressure off the lower back. Replace the compress as needed. Do the breathing exercises on page 102 while doing this compress treatment to further encourage relaxation and adequate circulation.

A massage oil can be applied on a periodic basis to ease back pain and can be used more regularly for chronic backache . This treatment can be self-applied, although having another person apply it is more effective. Refer to the section on aromatherapy massage in Chapter 12, for helpful directions in giving a massage. It is important to avoid applying pressure directly over the spine.

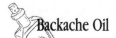 ## Backache Oil

for simple low backache

2 tbls. vegetable oil (or combination of arnica oil)

10 drops Lavender essential oil

6 drops Rosemary essential oil

6 drops Sandalwood essential oil

3 drops Geranium essential oil

Place the essential oils in an amber glass bottle. Mix well. Add the 2 tablespoons of vegetable oil. Shake gently to mix well. Label contents with direction for use. Apply a small amount to the general area of back discomfort. Can be applied prior to strenuous activity that may exacerbate backache, or afterward when pain is experienced.

Essential oils that are antispasmodic and anti-inflammatory are helpful for low backache. These include essential oils of bergamot, chamomile, clary sage, cypress, eucalyptus, fennel, hyssop, juniper, lavender, marjoram, neroli, peppermint, rosemary, and sandalwood.

Lifestyle recommendations include avoiding prolonged sitting, standing, or walking. This includes sitting while driving long hours. Stop and take frequent breaks to walk and stretch. Appropriate shoes with additional cushion and support can be very helpful if you stand for long hours, especially on cement floors. Many companies are investing in preventative back care and are offering classes, in addition to back supports. The fewer work-related injuries experienced benefit both the employee and employer. Rest at regular intervals and take frequent breaks when possible. Lift correctly by bending down, not over! Stretch and exercise regularly to keep the abdominal and back muscles toned, fit, and flexible. Sleeping on a firm mattress or futon can help. My father sleeps on a piece of plywood under the mattress for additional mattress support. If excess weight is a contributing factor, then reducing will help. As mentioned earlier, stress plays a major role in some forms of backache, and a good stress-relief program is needed. Refer to Chapter 9 for stress-free aromatherapy. It would be a good idea to place a diffuser in your work area or inhale relaxing essential oils from a tissue throughout the day for stress prevention.

Relieving Pain Caused by Overworked Muscles

The long day of yard or garden work can take its toll when we have ignored our bodies. Improper or excessive use and tension of muscles can lead to symptoms of overworked muscles hours later. When muscles undergo excessive tension for a length of time, muscle fatigue, swelling, soreness, stiffness, and aches may be experienced. If the muscles are stretched beyond their normal limit, muscle strain occurs. As discussed earlier in this section, sprains occur when ligaments of joints are stretched or twisted excessively.

Local aromatherapy treatment is effective for muscle soreness and stiffness when a specific group of muscles has been affected. If the whole body is sore in general, then a whole body treatment such as an aromatic bath will be the best aromatherapy application. The therapeutic essential oils that will be most useful for overworked muscles are the anti-inflammatory, antispasmodic, and analgesic-containing oils. Besides applying essential oils via skin absorption, plenty of rest and fluids are highly encouraged to heal the body. Chamomile herbal tea is anti-inflammatory and relaxing and can be taken freely following muscular exertion.

Excellent aromatic bath recipes are given on page 298–304 in Chapter 11: The Aromatic Bath. Follow one of the bath blends given there or use this one for a full-body soak that will unwind and relax your entire body. Typically, when muscles have been improperly used and abused, the peak of soreness is up to two days later; therefore I recommend this bath to be taken for two or three consecutive days for best results. Following the bath, you will feel very relaxed. You can apply an aromatic massage oil to any special muscles that need extra attention and then wrap up in a robe and rest. Getting out of the bath and going straight to work will undo some of the "relaxing" benefits of the treatment. Taking the time out to rest is one of the most important steps you can take to reverse the damage and heal your muscles. This bath is totally relaxing, for the mind and for the muscular system.

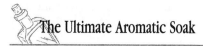

The Ultimate Aromatic Soak

for muscle strain and general body soreness

4 drops Lavender essential oil

2 drops Juniper essential oil

2 drops Rosemary essential oil

2 drops Peppermint essential oil

1 cup Epsom Salt

To one cup of Epsom salt, add the essential oils and mix well. Sprinkle the aromatic bath salts into a full bath of warm to hot water and stir with your hand to disperse. Soak for 20 to 30 minutes. Drink some chamomile tea while in the tub to relax from the inside out too! Pat dry and wrap in a bathrobe or blanket. Lie down to rest with your legs elevated (and arms, if they have been sore and swollen).

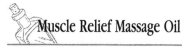

Muscle Relief Massage Oil

for sore and stiff muscles

1 tbls. Arnica oil

1 tbls. vegetable oil

12 drops Lavender essential oil

6 drops Rosemary essential oil

4 drops Juniper essential oil

3 drops Peppermint essential oil

Add the essential oils to an amber glass bottle. Add the carrier oils. Shake gently to combine well. Label with directions for use. This is a concentrated massage oil and should only be used for local areas in need of special attention. Apply a small amount to the affected muscle and massage into the skin. Apply as needed, up to three to four times per day for soreness and stiffness.

Nature's Answer for Cramps

Cramping is a combination of circulatory and muscular system dysfunction, and occurs when muscle tissue has been contracted for a sustained amount of time, resulting in muscle spasm. All muscles can cramp except cardiac muscle (the heart). Out of shape muscles are most apt to experience muscle cramping. Other causes of muscle cramping are fatigue, chilling, muscle tension, poor circulation, pregnancy, and inadequate calcium levels. Some people experience cramping at night, and the most common location is the calf muscle of the leg. Painful muscle spasms, cramps, can range from mild to severe. If muscle cramping is frequent and severe, visit your physician to get advice as to the cause and treatment.

> **Case history:** *A 19-year-old woman began experiencing leg calf muscle cramping while playing soccer, and occasionally at night. She performed mild stretching exercises before her practices, and had just started playing several games per week when the cramping began. She found welcome relief from the aromatic compresses and massage oils. She applied the oils a half hour before practice and games, to encourage muscle relaxation and good circulation. The results were very positive; with regular use, the cramps subsided. She began to focus on a more comprehensive stretching routine before games and at night before retiring to prevent reoccurrences. Cramps were soon a problem of the past.*

Children will often experience night cramping as a part of "growing pains." Keeping a small bottle of aromatic oils next to the bedside (for older children) is handy, should they wake up and need to rub some on. For younger children, applying the oil before bed, or after a bath will help.

Antispasmodic and relaxing essential oils are very helpful for cramps. Heat, in the form of aromatic baths or warm compresses, is also recommended as part of the treatment regime. Aromatherapy massage oils are recommended to encourage circulation and local relaxation of muscle contraction.

 Aromatic Compress for Cramps

---

for muscle cramping and spasm

1/2 cup very warm water

2 drops Lavender essential oil

1 drop Marjoram essential oil

1 drop Hyssop essential oil

piece of flannel or washcloth

a bowl

towel

Pour warm water into a bowl. Add the essential oils and stir. Soak the cloth and wring until moist, but not too wet. Apply to cramping muscle. Cover with a towel. Additionally, St. John's Wort oil can be applied to the skin before applying the compress. This will protect the skin as well as add anti-inflammatory benefits. Reapply the compress when it becomes dry or cool. Leave on for 15 to 20 minutes.

This recipe is a concentrated massage oil intended for small areas only. It is not to be used on the whole body, as it is too concentrated and would be too much for a large area. This oil can also be applied before working out to prevent muscle cramping, or before bedtime if that is when cramping is more apt to happen. Do not leave this or any medicine within reach of small children.

Massage Oil for Cramps

for muscle cramps and spasms

1 tbls. St. John's Wort infusion oil

1 tbls. vegetable oil

8 drops Rosemary essential oil

8 drops Marjoram essential oil

6 drops Lavender essential oil

4 drops Eucalyptus essential oil

In an amber glass bottle, add the essential oils and then the carrier oils. Shake gently to mix well. Label contents with directions for use. Apply a small amount to affected muscles, and massage lightly.

Essential oils used for cramps are bergamot, chamomile, clary sage, cypress, eucalyptus, fennel, grapefruit, hyssop, juniper, lavender, marjoram, neroli, peppermint, rosemary, and sandalwood.

Lifestyle recommendations include adequate stretching of involved muscle groups before and after exercise. Performing a few minutes of stretching before bedtime can help if the calf muscles of the leg cramp frequently. To do this stretch, point the toes up while pushing the back of the knee down against the bed or floor. When done regularly, this both prevents cramping and provides relief for any that occur. Yoga is another form of stretching exercise which is very effective for toning muscles. Keeping the feet elevated will support good circulation, which may also be preventative. Vitamin B-complex may be helpful, in addition to calcium and magnesium, so eat more foods rich in these vitamins and minerals.

How to Alleviate Bursitis Discomfort

Bursitis is the inflammation of the bursae, the serous sac or lubricant of a joint. The shoulder, knee, and elbow joints are the most common affected areas. Symptoms include sharp pain, restricted movement, skin that is hot and tender to the touch, and joint swelling. Causes of this inflammatory joint condition are local trauma, excessive and repeated joint use, and history of inflammatory joint disease.

Resting the affected joint is crucial to alleviate bursitis discomfort and to encourage healing. Essential oils can help with joint swelling and pain, and application of cold compresses and ice will be an important part of treatment. The following cold aromatic compress is recommended for initial treatment of bursitis, followed by local application of therapeutic essential oils in a massage oil preparation.

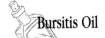 **Bursitis Oil**

to help with swelling and pain

1 tbls. St. John's Wort oil

1 tbls. vegetable oil

1/2 tsp. Carrot seed oil (optional)

10 drops Rosemary essential oil

6 drops Juniper essential oil

5 drops Eucalyptus essential oil

4 drops Chamomile essential oil

Add the essential oils to an amber glass bottle. Add the carrot seed oil, St. John's Wort (hypericum) oil, and vegetable oil. Shake gently to mix well. Label contents and directions for use. Apply to affected areas to help with pain and swelling, up to three times per day. Use a small amount and massage lightly until it is absorbed.

Cold Compress for Bursitis

cooling relief for acute bursitis

1/2 to 1 cup cold water

3 drops Cypress essential oil

2 drops Chamomile essential oil

2 drops Hyssop essential oil

1 drop Juniper essential oil

a bowl

piece of flannel or washcloth

ice pack (optional)

Add the essential oils to a bowl of cold water, and stir well to disperse. Soak the cloth in the aromatic water. Wring cloth and apply to affected joint. Place a cold pack or ice pack (optional) over it to keep it cold. Layer a towel over this. Change the compress when it becomes warm or dry. Leave on for 20 to 30 minutes. Keep joint (limb) elevated if possible. During acute and severe bursitis pain, compress can be done three times per day.

Essential oils helpful with bursitis are chamomile, clary sage, cypress, eucalyptus, geranium, peppermint, pine, hyssop, juniper, lemongrass, marjoram, and rosemary.

Is Tendonitis Affecting Your Game?

Tendonitis, commonly known as tennis elbow, is an inflammation of the tendon sheath of joints. Stiffness, swelling, and pain, in addition to muscle strain surrounding the joint, are typical symptoms of tendonitis. Overuse and trauma of the joint cause this condition. As many as one third of persons over 30 years old who play tennis in the United States will experience tennis elbow, severe pain in the elbow joint and forearm, although they are not the only ones at risk for this ailment. Carpenters, gardeners, as well as other sports enthusiasts (baseball players, golfers, bowlers), and even business professionals who carry heavy briefcases, are prone to this condition. Many of the essential oils that are helpful with arthritis and bursitis are also effective for tendonitis.

In acute painful conditions when tendonitis symptoms occur, immediate application of a cold compress or ice is appropriate. For chronic complaints of tendonitis, daily application of a therapeutic essential oil blend will help to alleviate discomfort and to prevent further swelling and pain. However, rest of the affected joint is crucial for complete remedy of this ailment. Using the heavy-duty *Tennis Elbow Treatment Oil* before your tennis game, and applying ice or cold compresses afterwards, will be effective symptomatic treatment.

Tennis Elbow Treatment Oil

for tendonitis conditions

1 tbls. Arnica oil

1 tbls. St. John's Wort Oil

1/2 tsp. Rosehip Seed Oil

8 drops Rosemary essential oil

8 drops Eucalyptus essential oil

6 drops Peppermint essential oil

2 drops Chamomile essential oil

Mix the essential oils in an amber glass bottle. Add the arnica, St. John's Wort and rosehip seed oils and shake gently to combine. Label contents and directions for use. To use, apply a small amount of this concentrated oil to the affected area. Be sure to apply to the area surrounding the affected joint, as muscle strain can be present as well.

The Cold Compress for Bursitis or Arthritic Joints can be used for this ailment. Both are designed for inflammatory conditions of the joint and local tissue, and employ cold treatment. Alternatively, ice packs or a cold water bath can be utilized for tennis elbow complaints. To prepare a cold water bath, you can fill a basin with cold water and ice cubes and add a few drops of the appropriate essential oils. Submerse the elbow or affected joint into the aromatic water for several minutes at a time for immediate relief of pain and swelling.

Rest and restricted movement of the joint is recommended for complete recovery, in addition to the application of therapeutic essences and cold treatments. Practice good form especially when serving and using your backhand return. You may want to try a lighter racket that is loosely strung to alleviate some of the strain on the arm. You can also ask your doctor to fit you for an elastic support brace. Strengthening the forearm muscles will help. Exercises such as ball squeezing, arm rotation, wrist curls, and finger stretches have been recommended for tennis elbow conditions. Traditional herbal medicine suggests taking turmeric (spice) in the form of capsules three times per day for its anti-inflammatory benefits in easing tendonitis discomfort.

CHAPTER 7

Aromatherapy Treatments for the Skin and Hair

Brief Overview of the Integumentary System

Besides being our largest sensory organ and the body's covering, the skin is the most diverse and most noticeable organ we possess. We are often judged by our appearance; the condition of our skin and hair represents to others our age and lifestyle. Certainly our health and environment affect its condition, as we will discuss shortly. In fact, some health systems are founded on the belief that the skin is a window to internal conditions.

However, let us briefly review some of the very important functions the skin is responsible for. The integumentary system, provides structure for the body and protects underlying tissue that it covers. It prevents dehydration and regulates the body's temperature, either by chilling to increase warmth or by sweating to allow water evaporation and cooling. It eliminates water and toxic waste and manufactures Vitamin D. The skin allows us sensory perception by the sense of touch, by sending neurological information to the brain from heat, cold, vibration, touch, pain, and pressure receptors. The integumentary system also takes in oxygen and eliminates carbon dioxide and other wastes. It protects the internal tissues from external environmental toxins and harmful bacteria. The skin is relatively permeable, allowing substances of 1000m (molecular weight) or below to be absorbed, or various waste products to be eliminated. Essential oils fall within this range of very low molecular weight.

159

About every twenty eight days, new cells from the lower dermal layer of the skin get pushed up to the surface. The top layer of the skin is called the stratum corneum, which is mainly composed of dead cells. This superficial layering of dead skin must be regularly sloughed off or it will block the pores, interfere with absorption and elimination, and give a dull appearance to the skin. Therefore, the skin continually is shedding and renewing itself. See cross section of skin in chapter one.

Our skin contains sebaceous glands that produce sebum, and sweat glands which eliminate water in the form of sweat. These two primary ingredients made by the body form "the film of sebum," a natural moisturizing cream that protects the skin. Basically, all cosmetics are made of these two ingredients - oil and water. Cosmetics are products applied to the skin's surface to help compensate for the decline in sebum which normally diminishes with age. The skin also contains hair follicles which are responsible for hair growth. Americans alone spend on an average of18 billion dollars annually on skin-related products, including hair care.

Beautiful and truly healthy skin is clean, clear, radiant, smooth, moist, firm and resilient. When the body, or shall we say the sebaceous glands of the skin, produce insufficient amounts of sebum, the skin appears dull, dry, rough, cracked and dehydrated. If too much sebum is produced, the opposite condition will exist - skin which is too oily, greasy and shiny. However, there is a benefit to oily skin: people who have oily skin typically wrinkle less and appear more youthful than those who have dry skin.

As you might imagine, healthy and beautiful skin (and hair) are more than skin deep. Many factors are involved in maintaining supple and elastic skin that looks youthful and glowing. The skin is the outermost layer of our bodies, the wrapping or cover, you might say. And unlike many books or gifts you receive, this cover can be judged relatively accurately, because the skin does not lie. If you have spent many years out in the sun, led an unhealthy lifestyle, smoked or overused alcohol, or ate a diet rich in fats (fried foods) and artificial ingredients much of your life, it will be evident in the condition of your skin. Some other contributing factors are chemical pollutants and infection. Interestingly, all of these factors stimulate free radical formation, a key component in the aging process of the entire body as well as the skin. Stress and insomnia will also create a lasting impression on the skin, as will fluctuations in weight and external abuse such as over-cleansing and over- manipulation (pulling, rubbing).

It's a good thing the skin can renew itself! A change in lifestyle, eating patterns and skin care regime will reverse some of the ailments that afflict the integumentary system. Internal cleansing and drinking adequate amounts of pure water, in addition to using purifying herbs, will aid in flushing toxins and waste from the body. You can begin to feed the skin from the inside by eating more foods rich in skin-loving nutrients like vitamins A, B, C, and E and zinc. Include plenty of fresh vegetables, fruit, and whole grains in your daily meals, and make sure you incorporate leafy greens, seafood, and beta-carotene-rich foods. Taking anti-oxidants, which are known to fight free radicals in the body, is another step you can take in preventing future harm from these oxygen-robbers that cause premature aging. Some of the more potent anti-oxidants are pycnogenols and antho-cyanins from pine bark (*Pinus maritima*) and grape seed (*Vitus vinifera*), vitamin C and E, and aloe vera. Some foods rich in antioxidants are carrots, broccoli, collards, and squash.

Regular exercise increases metabolism and circulation, both of which are crucial in good skin integrity. Encouraging blood flow to the skin's surface is important as it carries nutrients and oxygen to the skin cells, and transports waste materials away. The deep breathing exercises described in Chapter 4 are excellent for increasing circulation throughout the entire body, and are beneficial for optimal skin health.

Another way to bring blood flow and vitality to the skin is to perform regular dry skin brushing, which has many benefits. It improves circulation, stimulates the sebaceous glands, increases elimination, has a rejuvenating effect on the nervous system, and removes dead skin cells. Such an easy way to attain so many positive results and it only takes a few minutes! You will need to purchase a natural fiber brush, not nylon or plastic. You can find them in shops that specialize in bath products and natural health stores. Dry skin brushing can be done daily or several times weekly, depending on your skin type and condition. When you begin your dry skin brushing routine, expect some skin sensitivity. Start with a light pressure and work up to firmer pressure as you get accustomed to the stimulation. If you are purchasing a new brush, it can be conditioned by soaking it in hot water to soften the bristles. About every month or so, you will want to clean your brush with mild soap and warm water. For a special treatment, add one or two drops of essential oil on your brush, before using it on your skin. Be sure to use skin-friendly oils like lavender, chamomile, or tea tree essential oil.

The Dry Skin Brushing Technique

Your skin needs to be completely dry, so do this before you get in the shower or bath!

Brush the skin vigorously in a circular or figure eight motion.

Begin at the outermost parts of the body and work towards the heart.

Brush the entire body, including the palms of the hands and soles of the feet.

Give special attention to trouble-prone areas such as the thighs, buttocks, backs of the arms and legs, and the chest.

Do not use the brush on the face. Rather, use a dry wash cloth.

Facial massage is yet another way to boost circulation and metabolism of the facial skin. Typically performed using a warm vegetable oil (with or without essential oils) over a moistened skin surface, massage of the face can be very relaxing for both body and mind. It can help to restore a healthy glow and prevent wrinkling. Skin that has been regularly massaged appears smoother, more toned, flexible and moist, essentially more youthful. Easy instructions are described on page 316 in Chapter 12.

In addition to diet, exercise, dry skin brushing, and massage, you can support the skin by hydrating and nourishing it with external applications of natural plant-based healing agents. Aloe vera, herbs, seaweed, vegetable, nut, and seed oils, and essential oils are among the most natural, gentle and effective healing agents known for healing and maintaining healthy skin. Infusion and plant oils like evening primrose, jojoba, hazelnut, almond, avocado, calendula, St. John's Wort, borage, and black currant are excellent in skin treatments as they are rich in nutrients specific to skin health. Other moisturizing agents used in skin care for their nutrient-rich benefits are Hyaluronic acid, alpha-hydroxy, vitamins A and E and lecithin. You will notice that many of the recipes given in this section that treat skin and hair conditions are made with many of these ingredients. By making your own skin care treatments you will be avoiding chemical preservatives and irritating substances. However, most skin preparations must be freshly made since they do not contain preservatives to extend their shelf life. But essential oils are antibacterial in nature, and will help to preserve the compound they are part of, along with anti-oxidant oils such as wheatgerm, vitamin E, and jojoba oil.

Due to the inherent permeability of the skin, you would not want to use synthetic, unnatural, or irritating agents that could block pores and inhibit respiration of the skin. For these reasons, Vaseline, mineral oil, and paraffin wax are not recommended. These ingredients can make the skin "feel smooth," but they only provide a barrier. They impede anything, including essential oils, from getting absorbed and inhibit elimination of sweat and sebum from the pores, causing blockages known as comedones.

The basics of any skin care regimen will include cleansing, toning, and moisturizing, with occasional "special" treatments such as facial steams, scrubs, and masks. Compresses and poultices are typically used for first-aid treatments like abscesses and boils. To gently cleanse the face use cleansing creams or mild vegetarian-based soaps made with plant oils like olive. The best toners are the simplest ones made of floral waters, witch hazel, apple cider vinegar, or herbal infusions. Do not use alcohol as it is very drying and pulls moisture away from the skin as it evaporates. Occasional treatments might only need to be done 1 to 3 times weekly or monthly, depending on the ailment or condition. Fresh or dried herbs and flowers can be used for facial steam treatments, in addition to a few drops of essential oils specific for your skin type. Natural scrubs can contain grain flours, cornmeal, oatmeal, and herbs. Masks can be made of egg whites, honey, or yogurt as the major ingredients. Chapter 12 discusses body treatments and localized "special" skin treatments in detail. Recipes for facial mists, scrubs, and masks can be found there.

Aesthetic aromatherapy, using essential oils for skin and hair care, is the topic of this chapter as it relates to the many different skin problems. Therapeutic aromatherapy also plays a major role in the topic of discussion as specific essential oils will be recommended for their anti-inflammatory, anti-bacterial, anti-fungal and healing properties. Keep in mind that no matter how beneficial an oil may be for a specific condition, it should at least be agreeable if not pleasurable for the person using it. I give several essential oil options to choose from for each ailment. Many times there are ten or more oils that can do the job effectively, so pick the essences that please you most when you can. *The Essential Oil Reference Guide* will provide you with detailed information on each oil you are considering that will help you to decide which one to include in your recipe. Also do a skin patch test as described in Chapter 1, *Common Sense Safety,* when you are using an essential oil for the first time, particularly when you are prone to allergic reactions or sensitivity. Apply essential oils with great care when using them on damaged skin. Always dilute essential oils in a carrier base lotion or vegetable oil before applying to the skin (unless directed to do so in this book). Lavender and Tea tree are two essential oils that can be applied "neat" or straight on the skin safely. But these are the exceptions to the rule.

The best times to apply essential oils are following a bath or facial steam, when the pores are open and circulation is increased, or during or following a massage when the oils can be readily absorbed. Following exfoliation is also a beneficial time, since the skin pores have been cleaned and circulation is optimal. Examples of exfoliants are dry skin brushing, scrubs, clay masks, and baths. When applying to the skin vegetable oil blends that include essential oils, it is best to warm them slightly to increase absorption into the skin. Use oils that are thinner in consistency for easiest penetration, or when you have an oily skin condition. The heavier oils take a bit longer to absorb, but offer more protection for dry skin types. Refer to Chapter 15 to learn more about carrier oil options and their benefits.

Taking good care of your skin includes looking for signs and symptoms of abnormalities of your skin. Skin cancer, the most common type of all cancers, can be easily detected by those who examine their skin regularly. Most skin cancers are treatable if noticed early, although many people do not take the time to get to know their bodies well enough to spot changes. More than 700,000 Americans are afflicted each year, so it is good practice to look at your skin monthly. Cancer of the skin occurs most often in older and fair skinned people, but anyone who has spent a lot of time in the sun has an increased risk. Most skin cancers occur on the parts of the body that are most often exposed, such as the face, hands, forearms, and ears. Any unusual blemish, lump, or sore, or change in the way the skin feels may be a warning sign of skin cancer. Although most skin problems are not cancerous, it is important to get checked by your doctor if you notice any suspicious skin changes.

Softening Agents for Aging Skin

We are all aging! Recognizing what causes premature aging and what measures can be taken to prevent it are the keys to looking younger than our biological years. If you already are seeing signs of aging, take note as help is on the way. Herbs, flowers, vegetable oils, and essential oils are the perfect softening agents for mature and wrinkled skin. They soften, nourish, moisturize, tone, firm, and protect the skin. Essential oils work at the deepest level by reaching the tiny blood vessels of the skin and feeding new emerging cells.

Some factors that cause premature aging and wrinkling are too much sun, alcohol, and smoking. All of these rob the skin (and the body) of oxygen. Nicotine causes constriction of the blood vessels, which restricts nutrients and oxygen available to the skin. Heavy smokers may be four times as likely to wrinkle as their friends who do not. Sun exposure is the greatest culprit to skin changes, including skin cancer. Although you do not observe changes immediately, over time these factors will take their toll. Fluctuations in weight, a nutrient-deficient diet, and various environmental insults can also play a part in creating wrinkles or dry skin. There is also a genetic factor to consider. Persons who have oily skin, dark complexions, and dark hair will generally retain a more youthful appearance than others who have fair skin, freckles, and light colored hair. Why is this? Typically people with darker skin and hair experience oily skin conditions. More oil (sebum), fewer wrinkles. Wrinkles are basically the skin folding in on itself. The skin's collagen has become hard and criss-crossed, thus greatly diminishing its ability to hold moisture. The areas of the body prone to signs of aging are those parts of the body exposed to sun and weather, such as the face, neck, and hands.

To counteract wrinkles and dry, mature skin, essential oils are combined with vitamin-rich plant oils to soften and nourish the skin. Nutrient packed nut and seed oils are carriers for the essential oils to aid in moisturizing and protecting the delicate tissues. Since skin cells replenish every twenty-eight days or so, I suggest you use these aromatherapy recommendations and lifestyle and diet suggestions for at least a month or longer in order to see improvement. Your skin will begin to appear smoother, firmer, and moist. If you perform regular facial massage, you will multiply the effects. Be careful not to overuse essential oils or overwork the skin and follow the recipes and frequency in accordance with your skin's particular needs.

Floral waters and facial mists are ideal for aging skin, and to prevent signs of aging. The best time to use them is during the day to add moisture to your skin, and as part of your skin care regime, just prior to applying oils. By misting the face you will be adding a layer of moisture to the skin's surface, in addition to gently toning the skin. When applied before moisturizers and facial oils, they provide easy application and glide. This is crucial, especially in aging skin conditions, since we do not want to pull, rub, or overmanipulate the tissues. To make your own aromatic facial sprays refer to Chapter 12. Avoid using alcohol-containing toners which are too harsh.

An excellent facial oil made with light, vitamin-rich plant and seed oils is a necessity. High-quality, cold-pressed oils such as hazel nut, macadamia nut, kikui nut, rosehip seed, carrot seed, and wheatgerm top the list for the benefits they offer to aging skin. Information regarding individual carrier oils can be found in Chapter 15. Additionally, borage, evening primrose, and vitamin E oil can be added as well to facial oils to boost their effectiveness. The recipe given below is a superior blend that is used for aging, dehydrated, and wrinkled skin that has been damaged by the sun and perils of time. When applying oils to the facial area, avoid the eyes and hair line.

After using this recipe for a few months, you may want to start calling it your fountain (or bottle) of youth! Of all the recipes given in this book, this particular blend may be the most costly to make, but it's worth it; it contains some of the finest ingredients known to help with aging skin. You wanted to know what was best for wrinkles; here it is. I consider it the "royal" treatment as it contains both rose (the queen of flowers) and jasmine (the king of flowers) essential oils, renowned since ancient times for possessing anti-aging properties. It just may be the best that aromatherapy has to offer for youthful beauty.

Royal Treatment Oil

a replenishing facial oil for mature skin

2 tsp. Hazelnut oil

1 tsp. Avocado oil

10 drops Carrot seed oil

10 drops Rose hip seed oil

5 drops Evening Primrose oil

3 drops Rose essential oil (Bulgarian preferred)

3 drops Clary sage essential oil

2 drops Jasmine essential oil

2 drops Frankincense essential oil

In a 1-ounce amber glass bottle combine the hazelnut, avocado, carrot seed, rose hip, and evening primrose oils. Cap and shake well. Add the essential oils to the bottle. Cap and shake gently to mix well. Label. To apply place 2 to 4 drops of the blend onto your fingertips. Apply them to a moistened face and neck (use floral water). Always work upwards against gravity when applying oils. Avoid the eye area. Use the facial massage directions on page 316 as a guide to increase circulation. Apply twice daily.

For occasional use, special treatments can be utilized for aging skin. Facial steaming, facial compresses, nourishing masks, and firming masks are most beneficial. I recommend a special treatment up to three times weekly, depending on your skin's needs. Facial steaming is done with gentle, healing, and rejuvenating herbs and flowers. They are listed at the end of this section. Choose one tablespoon of any single herb or combination of herbs to use, or simply add 1 to 2 drops of essential oils known to aid aging skin (also listed here). Directions for facial steaming, compresses and the egg white mask to tone and firm are given in Chapter 12: Local Areas With Special Needs—Made Simple. Here is a recipe for a moisturizing and soothing facial mask perfect for mature skin. Be sure to use plain, natural yogurt with live cultures in order for this mask to be most beneficial for your skin.

For aging and wrinkled skin that is dry and undernourished, replenishing masks that offer moisture and nutrients are important. The Moisture-Balanced Facial Mask given on page 317 in Chapter 12 is the mask base to use for this condition. It contains yogurt, honey, and vitamin E, along with grain flour to thicken it. To that recipe add the following essential oils to aid in softening and rejuvenating mature skin:

- geranium essential oil: supports in balancing and rejuvenating dry skin conditions such as wrinkled and mature skin.
- frankincense and myrrh: both gentle and effective in replenishing moisture.

Together these essential oils work as softening agents.

Facial Mask for Mature Skin

to soften wrinkles and provide moisture

Moisture-Balanced Facial Mask recipe
2 drops Geranium essential oil
2 drops Frankincense essential oil
1 drop Myrrh essential oil

Add the above essential oils to the mask recipe given in Chapter 12. Apply the mask to the entire facial area and neck. Leave on for 20 minutes. Rinse with warm water to remove. Follow with floral water or facial mist.

Essential oils that are useful in mature, aging, and dry skin conditions are carrot seed, clary sage, fennel, frankincense, geranium, jasmine, lavender, mandarin, myrrh, neroli, patchouli, rose, sandalwood, and ylang ylang.

Plant oils beneficial for aging skin, which can be used as carrier oils and anti-oxidant additives, are hazelnut, kikui nut, macadamia nut, evening primrose, rose hip seed, St. John's Wort, vitamin E, and wheatgerm.

Lifestyle recommendations include staying out of the sun and protecting your skin with a good sunblock (see sunburns) and clothing. Getting regular exercise, in addition to performing the deep breathing exercise and facial massage described in this book, will boost circulation and help with stress. Avoid cigarette smoking and overuse of alcohol. Avoid overcleansing your face, and overmanipulation, such as rubbing. Getting a good night's sleep can help too. Review Chapter 9 for insomnia aromatherapy blends if this applies to you. Adapting a stress-relief program, and taking time for yourself is important.

Dietary suggestions include drinking plenty of pure water and eating a healthy diet composed of fresh vegetables, fruits, and whole grains. Be sure to get plenty of fiber which will insure healthy elimination. Taking anti-oxidants and eating foods which contain them naturally would be prudent. All things considered, there is a lot you can do for aging skin.

Adding More Than Moisture—Help for Dry Skin

Dry skin conditions can range in severity from mild dryness to fissured. Chapped, cracked, and scaling skin are some of the telltale signs of dry skin. Particularly a problem in the winter months when the air is dry (and the central heat is on indoors), or if you work in a dehydrated environment, your skin may need extra help to overcome the environmental stress. In addition to the above-mentioned contributing factors, genetics plays a major role. If you are of fair skin and have blond or red hair, you are more likely to experience dry skin conditions.

> **Case history:**   *A 32-year-old stewardess consulted me for help with her dry skin. Areas of her face, hands, and arms seemed to be the driest with some roughness and chapping. She ate a fairly healthy diet, but could stand adding more high-water-content fruits and vegetables. Airplanes are notorious for dehydrated and reconditioned air environments, which spell trouble for dry skin. She used a floral facial mist frequently while traveling; in addition she made a few dietary changes, including drinking more pure water and avoiding concentrated beverages such as soda pop, coffee, and alcohol. She loved using the facial mists most, and she also used an aromatherapy oil blend for dry skin. She had no wrinkles or signs of premature aging, therefore the heavy-duty essential oils (mentioned in the previous section) were not necessary. Within days she began to notice a difference in her skin. Over the next two weeks she was elated to see her skin turn from dry and chapped to moist and healthy.*

Adapting an aromatherapy program early, when symptoms of dryness are first recognized, makes this condition relatively easy to remedy. Chronic and severe cases of dryness that include eczema or dermatitis, however, may take a bit longer to replenish as healing, also needs to take place.

Essential oils provide moisture, healing and nourishment in the dermal layers of the skin and are absorbed into the superficial blood vessels because the skin has the ability to absorb these small molecules. When an aromatherapy oil is applied over moist skin, moisture is naturally held close to the pores of the skin, very important for people with dry skin to know because adding extra moisture is easy. Mist your face (and body) with floral water before applying your moisturizing oils. Most floral waters are excellent for dry skin; chamomile, lavender, neroli (orange blossom), and rose floral waters are best . If you have general dryness over much of your body, try this technique for keeping the skin moist. After taking a bath or shower, do not dry your skin with a towel as usual. Instead, use your hands to rub off excess water from your body. Start at the shoulders and move to the arms and chest, and work downward to the legs. When you're not dripping wet any more, but there remains a nice moist covering on your skin, apply an aromatherapy body oil over your entire body. People with very dry skin should avoid extreme heat, such as hot baths and Jacuzzis. Also, chlorinated swimming pools seem to worsen dry skin, whereas swimming in the ocean will help.

Dry skin conditions needs to be exfoliated like other skin; however it must be done gently and carefully in order not to overcleanse the skin and cause irritation or increased dryness. Dry skin brushing is very helpful as long as it is done correctly. Moisturizing warm baths are a way to slough off dead skin cells gently and effectively too. The Milk Maid's Bath, Bath Oil, and the Botanical Bath are your finest choices for bath carrier options that are emollient and protective (See Chapter 11).

The major factor in many dry skin conditions is that the sebaceous glands are producing insufficient amounts of sebum (natural moisturizer). To stimulate sebum production and circulation, you should do the dry skin brushing described in the front of this chapter. This technique improves circulation to the skin, cleans pores, and triggers the sebaceous glands to manufacture more sebum.. However, you will want to proceed gently and use a light pressure, so you do not cause undue irritation. Finely ground oatmeal-type facial scrubs are great for gently exfoliating the skin. Oats provide moisture in addition to safely sloughing dead skin cells. The recipe for *Farm Fresh Facial Scrub* on page 318 is perfect to use for dry skin. Do this scrub up to three times per week, depending on how your skin feels.

Local or whole body massage, in addition to exercise, helps tremendously to increase circulation to the skin and underlying tissues. Persons with dry skin should not use clay masks, as these remove some of the protective facial "film" and attract moisture, not replenish it. Also, care should be taken not to overcleanse the face, and to avoid using products containing alcohol or other harsh chemicals. Petroleum byproducts such as Vaseline, mineral oil, and baby oil should be avoided as they create a barrier which does not allow moisture or essential oils to get through.

The *Moisture-Balanced Facial Mask* is a special treatment for replenishing the skin with moisture and for soothing minor skin irritations. This recipe can be found in Chapter 12 under the special treatment section. Any of the essential oils listed at the end of this section can be used to treat dry skin conditions. Simply add 4 or 5 drops (total) of these suggested oils to the mask recipe. This mask can be done several times per week.

A very effective, moisture enhancing aromatherapy blend is given below. Use it two to three times daily, as needed. Remember to always apply a floral water or facial mist before using oils on the skin for dryness. You can make this facial oil into a body oil as well; simply refer to the User-Friendly Blending Chart for easy preparation guidelines.

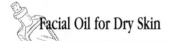

Facial Oil for Dry Skin

moisture and nourishment for dry, chapped skin

1 tsp. Jojoba oil

1 tsp. Calendula infusion oil

1 tsp. Sesame oil

1/4 tsp. Carrot seed oil

6 drops Sandalwood essential oil

4 drops Neroli essential oil

2 drops Geranium essential oil

400 IU's Vitamin E (optional)

In a one-ounce amber glass bottle, add the jojoba, calendula, carrot, and sesame oils. Add the essential oils and vitamin E. Shake well to mix completely. Label. To use: Apply 4 to 6 drops to your finger tips. Apply in upward strokes on moistened skin. Follow the easy facial massage steps on page 316 for additional benefits. Use twice daily or as needed.

Essential oils known to help dry skin conditions are cedarwood, chamomile, carrot seed, frankincense, geranium, jasmine, lavender, myrrh, neroli, patchouli, rose, sandalwood and ylang ylang.

Carrier oil choices include the heavier, vitamin-rich vegetable and seed oils that aid in protection as well as in adding moisture. Infusion oils of calendula and St. John's Wort are two excellent herbal oils. Olive oil contains many vitamins and nourishes dry skin and minor skin irritations. Sesame oil is reputed for its healing and beneficial effects on dry skin conditions. Additional specialty oils are carrot seed, evening primrose, vitamin E, and wheatgerm. Always try to warm your oils before application to encourage absorption.

How to Counteract Oily Skin

Skin that produces an abundance of sebum is called oily. Overactive sebaceous glands are common in the "T" zone across the forehead and midline following the nose and mouth areas. Oily or greasy skin conditions can cause blocked pores and inhibit the skin from performing its many functions, including elimination of waste. If these pores become blocked and infected, then acne will result. Persons who have darker complexions and dark hair tend to experience oily skin most often. The good news is they do not show signs of aging as readily as others, since they have an abundance of moisture.

For oily skin a good all-natural facial cleanser or vegetarian soap is recommended since it dissolves and removes oil, dirt, etc. A good facial toner should be used to remove excess oil from the face and thoroughly clean the skin. Witch hazel, apple cider vinegar, and floral water combine to make a very effective facial toner. Lemon juice, astringent herbs, and infusions are very useful in toning and balancing oily skin types. This facial toner should be applied to the skin with cotton cosmetic pads that will aid in removing excess oils and in balancing the pH of the skin.

Facial Toner for Oily Skin

to remove oil and tone pores

4 ounces herbal infusion (or distilled water)

2 tbs. cider vinegar (or witch hazel)

1 tsp. honey

4 drops Lavender essential oil

2 drops Rosemary essential oil

In an amber bottle add the herbal infusion, or herb tea water. You can use any of the herbs listed on the following page. Sage, yarrow, or rose petals are good choices. Add the vinegar. To one teaspoon of honey add the essential oils and mix well with the end of a spoon. Add the aromatic honey to the toner solution and shake well to mix completely. Shake well again before using. Moisten a cotton pad and wipe face, concentrating on oily areas. Can be used three times per day to remove excess oil.

Ideally you will want to use thin, easily absorbed and light carrier oils or lotions, which are water-based. You can easily add essential oils to your oil-free lotions by following the simple guide given in the User-Friendly Preparation Chart in Chapter 15. Be sure your lotion does not contain any paraffin, mineral oil, or other petroleum byproducts. These will inhibit the essential oils from getting absorbed, and will promote blocked pores and greasy skin. The recipe that follows is made with very light oils and essential oils that are specific to oily skin types. With regular use, this aromatherapy facial preparation will regulate overactive sebaceous glands and diminish oiliness.

Facial Nourishment for Oily Skin

to balance oily skin

2 tsp. hazelnut oil

1 tsp. jojoba oil

1/4 tsp. carrot seed oil

6 drops Rosemary essential oil

2 drops Geranium essential oil

2 drops Basil essential oil

2 drops Cypress essential oil

In a one-ounce amber glass bottle, add the vegetable and seed oils. Add the essential oils and mix well by shaking the bottle. Label. Use twice daily after cleansing the face and use a facial mist just prior to applying. Use 4 to 6 drops and apply to neck and face. Avoid the eye area.

Essential oils useful for oily skin conditions include basil, bergamot, carrot seed, cedarwood, clary sage, cypress, eucalyptus, grapefruit, geranium, juniper, lavender, lemon, rose, lemongrass, mandarin, patchouli, petitgrain, rosemary, sandalwood, tea tree, and ylang ylang.

Carrier oil choices are described fully in Chapter 15 and include apricot kernel, canola, grapeseed, hazelnut, jojoba, kukui nut, and sunflower.

Lifestyle recommendations include using oil-free make-up and foundations or wearing none at all. Avoid using heavy oils on the skin for regular application. Use exfoliants to keep pores clean and open, but take care not to overuse them as they can stimulate oil production when used too frequently. Keeps your hands away from your face to prevent clogged pores and blemishes. Do not use a loofah or any other scrubber on the face.

Dietary changes include decreasing fat in your diet, including dairy. Eat plenty of high-fiber foods such as fruits, vegetables, and whole grains. Incorporate more herbs in your diet, like rosemary, which help with fat (oil) regulation and oily skin conditions.

A Guide to Sensitive Skin

Sensitive skin can be oily, dry, or mature. A person who reacts quickly and easily to certain cosmetics, clothing, etc., or to local irritation is said to have a sensitive skin condition. A reaction may appear red, may itch or swell and be irritated following contact with a "sensitizer." Persons who have sensitive skin are prone to allergic reactions, skin breakouts, and rashes. They may also sunburn easily. Experiencing emotional stress may trigger skin reactions in the form of hives or skin rash.

Mild, gentle, and anti-allergic type skin care products must be used. It is crucial that persons with sensitive skin perform a patch test when using an essential oil, or product, for the first time. Directions on how to do this simple test are in the Common-Sense Safety section of Chapter 1. Avoid complex blends of aromatherapy oils and use simple ingredients. Of course, avoiding cosmetic ingredients known to cause allergic or adverse reactions would be prudent. Some of these include artificially fragranced bath soaps, detergents, deodorants, make-up, hair treatments, moisturizers, and shampoos. Any synthetic fragrance or perfume, chemical preservative or additive, petroleum or lanolin byproduct can cause an adverse reaction in skin that is sensitive. Other oils that are possible sensitizers are coconut, cocoa butter, and corn.

Simplicity and pure ingredients are important in a skin care regime for sensitive skin types. Mild cleansing, kind toners, and delicate moisturizers are the aim. Use a simple floral water, like chamomile or orange blossom, to gently tone and mist the face. Herbal infusions made from mild toning plants can be useful alone, or added to floral waters and a little cider vinegar. A good, safe, and gentle toning lotion may be difficult to find, so make your own using the recipe below. It contains simple ingredients that are effective for toning, balancing the skin's pH, and providing moisture. Chamomile and lavender are the herbs and essential oils that are most often utilized for these sensitive skin types.

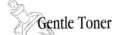 **Gentle Toner**

a skin toning lotion for sensitive skin

7 ounces floral water or herbal infusion (chamomile or lavender)

1 ounce cider vinegar

Make an herbal infusion of chamomile or lavender flowers by pouring near-boiling water over 2 to 3 tablespoons of fresh or dried flower tops. Alternatively, you can purchase pure floral water of the same type to make this recipe. Simply add 1 ounce, or 2 tablespoons, of cider vinegar and mix well. Pour this lotion into a spray bottle or mister for easy application. Use daily after cleansing the skin.

Besides the toner, a good moisture-rich aromatherapy preparation is important to complete the sensitive skin care regime. Hypo-allergenic nut and plant oils along with mild, yet effective, toning essential oils are used in the recipe given below. Carrier choices good for sensitive skin are sweet almond, apricot kernel, avocado, hazelnut, safflower, sesame, and jojoba oil. This oil should be applied twice daily, or after cleansing and toning. The essential oils chosen make this a very emollient, gentle, and light moisturizer oil blend.

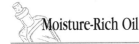 **Moisture-Rich Oil**

for sensitive skin types

2 tsp. Hazelnut oil

1 tsp. Sesame oil

1/4 tsp. Jojoba oil

8 drops Lavender essential oil

2 drops Chamomile essential oil

2 drops Jasmine essential oil

400 IU's Vitamin E (optional)

In an amber glass bottle, add the hazelnut, sesame, and jojoba oil. Add the vitamin E. Capsules can be used by cutting the end and emptying the contents. Add the essential oils and shake to mix well. Label. To use apply to moist skin. Put a few drops on your fingertips and smooth onto the face in upward motion, avoiding the eyes.

Essential oils good for sensitive skin, and soothing to allergic-type reactions, are chamomile, frankincense, jasmine, lavender, neroli, rose, and sandalwood.

Lifestyle and diet recommendations include avoidance of chemical additives, pollutants, and other sensitizers. Incorporating oats, flax seed, and plenty of fresh fruits, vegetables, and whole grain in the diet, drinking plenty of pure water, and supporting the immune system will benefit the body as a whole. Adopting a good stress-relief program will also be a positive change, especially if hives or skin inflammation is experienced during stressful states. Refer to Chapter 9 for help in this area.

How to Use Essential Oils to Relieve Acne

Acne, a condition caused by blocked pores which have become infected, has symptoms ranging from slight blemishes to deep skin infections. It may appear as a local infection of the skin, red sores, pimples, blackheads, or whiteheads and can lead to scarring if poor hygiene, secondary infection, or trauma has complicated this problem. Too much oil (sebum), accumulation of dead skin, and blocked pores all contribute to this condition, as well as taking certain medications such as birth control pills, cosmetic use, puberty, and stress. It is most common among teenagers who are experiencing pubertal hormonal fluctuations. When hormone levels increase, so do oily skin conditions and stress levels. These hormonal changes are the reason for the problem of acne among women who are premenstrual or who take oral contraceptives.

> **Case History:**   *A 14-year-old male with combination skin and experiencing acne wanted to use aromatherapy to help with his condition. Caused by the hormonal changes of puberty, and complicated by a poor diet and teenage stress, he was seeing an increase in blemishes, red inflamed pimples, and whiteheads. He had very dry skin on the forehead and nose, with visibly flaky*

skin. He noted that the medicated soap that was recommended to him for acne helped very little and only made his dry skin worse. His skin condition embarrassed him in front of his peers. He began by decreasing dietary refined sugars and saturated fats (candy, pastries, chips, soda). He also became more aware of how much he handled his face which he learned not to do because this worsened his acne and spread infection. A light facial scrub was used 3 to 4 times weekly, to help exfoliate dead skin cells and clear the whiteheads. A light moisturizing oil blend was used that contained antibacterial and anti-inflammatory essential oils. He was advised to do facial steams weekly as well. The following oil recipe for acne and the facial steam and scrub were part of his skin care regimen. He continued to get occasional breakouts and minor blemishes, but the flaky skin condition and most of the acne had been cleared. For spot treatment of pimples, he used a drop of cedarwood on a Q-tip which helped to decrease inflammation, kill bacteria, and aid in healing the blemish. Showing him the results or scars of mistreated acne skin encouraged him to follow the program closely to avoid such an occurrence.

Facial steams to unblock pores and hair follicles are a key component of any acne treatment program. Keeping the skin very clean and oil free and pores clear is crucial. An antibacterial cleanser to fully clean the skin and an antiseptic toner and light moisturizer with essential oils that are antiseptic and healing are extremely important. Overwashing, over-manipulation and overdrying skin that has acne can complicate the healing process, as well as cause scarring. Additional aromatherapy treatments should be done several times weekly to help exfoliate dead skin cells, and thoroughly clean and balance the skin. These special weekly remedies include facial steaming, deep cleansing, clay masks, and compresses. The aim of these methods is to deeply cleanse, exfoliate and draw out impurities and accumulated sebum. When the pores are kept clear, a healthy diet is maintained, exercise is regular, and stress levels are at a minimum, then acne will diminish or disappear. Healing acne conditions must include diet, lifestyle, and skin care modifications. There is no magic bullet to attack this ailment; a comprehensive approach is required. In this section I have given you recipes for some of the important aspects of this program. Aromatherapy has a lot to offer acne treatment because essential oils are very potent antibacterial and anti-inflammatory agents, unsurpassed by modern acne treatments in the market today. Used correctly, therapeutic essential oils are highly antiseptic without harsh side-effects, such as dryness and peeling, a healing aid, and are safe and gentle to the skin.

A facial steam is an excellent treatment for acne skin conditions because it opens and clears pores and increases circulation by bringing infected pores to a head. It is important not to use boiling-hot water as this may burn the skin. Also, the head should be at least eight inches away from the water level. fifteen to twenty minutes is sufficient for a full facial steam treatment, and can be done 2 or 3 times weekly, depending on individual skin care needs. This recipe can be made with any of the antiseptic and anti-inflammatory essential oils or herbs for acne listed in this section.

Facial Steam Treatment for Acne

4 to 6 cups hot water

1 drop Bergamot essential oil

2 drops Lemon essential oil

a bowl

towel

Pour the hot water into a ceramic bowl. Add the essential oils. Drape the towel over the head, bending over the bowl at least 8 inches from water level, to form a tent. Keep the eyes closed during the steam treatment, for 15 to 20 minutes or until water has cooled. Gently pat face with the towel to dry. Follow with a toner or facial spray (floral mists are good) to close the pores and balance the skin's pH.

For very oily skin with acne, rosemary essential oil and cedarwood can be used. See Oily Skin treatments in this chapter for other recommendations. Lemon essential oil is strongly antibacterial and very cleansing for the skin. Bergamot essential oil is antibacterial as well; however, it is included for its regulating properties. Calendula, peppermint, or lemonbalm herb, fresh or dried, can be used in addition to the essential oils for their healing and antiseptic benefits in this recipe.

Antiseptic Toner for Acne

antibacterial, anti-inflammatory toner

4 ounces herbal infusion (or distilled water)

1 tbls. cider vinegar

1 tbls. Witch hazel lotion

1 tsp. Honey

2 drops Tea Tree essential oil

2 drops Bergamot essential oil

2 drops Juniper essential oil

In a small spray bottle, or glass bottle, add the herbal infusion (see options for herbs at the end of this section) or distilled water. Add the vinegar and witch hazel. Add the essential oils to the honey, in a large spoon or saucer, and mix well. Add the aromatic honey to the bottle and shake very well to mix completely. Label. Mist over the face after cleansing, or moisten a cotton pad and smooth over face to remove oils and dirt during the day.

A good facial nourishment oil specifically made for acne skin conditions and excess oil (sebum) production is very beneficial. Essential oils which have antibacterial properties are used to decrease bacterial growth and prevent infection. If the skin is very dry, then the oils for dry skin are advised. Bergamot and geranium essential oils help to balance and regulate the skin and are often included in either blend. Vitamin E, wheatgerm, or evening primrose can be added to help prevent scarring of the skin.

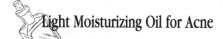

Light Moisturizing Oil for Acne

for oily and blemished skin

2 tsp. Hazelnut oil

1 tsp. Jojoba oil

1/4 tsp. wheatgerm oil

6 drops Rosemary essential oil

2 drops Bergamot essential oil

2 drops Cedarwood essential oil

2 drops Tea Tree essential oil

400 IU's Vitamin E (optional)

In a one-ounce amber glass bottle, add the seed oil, jojoba, and wheatgerm oil. Add the essential oils. Add the vitamin E. If using gel capsules, break open one end and squeeze contents into oils. Shake well to mix completely. Label. Apply to moistened facial skin by pouring a few drops on clean fingertips and spreading over the face. Avoid the eye area. Apply to the neck, back, or shoulders if needed. Can be used twice daily, following cleansing or facial steaming.

The clay facial mask is another good way to draw out impurities, dirt, and oils from acne skin. Clay masks are only recommended for oily skin types, or for occasional use for combination skin. Since clay absorbs many times its weight in moisture, it can be too drying for flaky and dry skin. The recipe in Chapter 12 can be used with the appropriate essential oils given in this section.

A finely ground facial scrub can be used to exfoliate dead skin cells, and deeply clean pores. However, take care not to overly scrub or irritate the skin. If the skin is inflamed, with any open, infected pores, then facial scrubs are contraindicated. If the acne includes flaky dry skin, blackheads and whiteheads, then the facial scrub will be most beneficial. Remember, overstimulation of the skin can cause an increase in sebum production, so don't overdo! The recipe found on page 318 in Chapter 12 is a good grain scrub to use. It contains oatmeal and cornmeal as the abrasive exfoliants, along with honey, yogurt and floral water. Honey is a good antibacterial and anti-inflammatory agent for the skin, and acts as the carrier for the essential oils in the recipe. I recommend you use lavender, chamomile, sandalwood, or bergamot essential oil in this recipe because they are mild enough to use in a scrub preparation. If you want to include peppermint essential oil, do not use more than one drop as it is a skin irritant in higher dilutions.

To treat individual blemishes, use a drop or two of essential oil on a cotton swab to dab onto infected pores. Tea Tree, cedarwood, or lemon essential oils can be used to kill bacterial infections, aid healing, and decrease inflammation. Saturate the cotton swab first with witch hazel or cider vinegar and then apply a drop or two of the listed essential oils. Be sure to just dab the oils onto the infected area only, and not over a large area. This is spot treatment. Used in this way before bedtime, you can often dry up pimples and bring redness and swelling down overnight.

Essential oils known to positively affect acne conditions are numerous, as many are antiseptic, anti-inflammatory and healing. These include bergamot, cedarwood, clary sage, chamomile, eucalyptus, geranium, grapefruit, juniper, lavender, lemon, lemongrass, lime, mandarin, neroli, patchouli, petitgrain, peppermint (in low dilutions), rosemary, sandalwood, tea tree, and ylang ylang.

Carrier oils useful in acne conditions should be light, easily absorbed, anti-inflammatory, and healing. Hazelnut, jojoba, wheatgerm, kikui nut, carrot seed (10% dilution or less), vitamin E, and calendula infusion oil are some useful oils that fit the bill. Avoid mineral oil, petroleum byproducts, lanolin, and Vaseline, as these have been shown to block pores and inhibit skin respiration.

Dietary changes include a diet that is based on fresh fruits, vegetables, and whole grains, and low in animal fats and concentrated sugars. Vitamins and minerals which may be helpful with acne skin are chromium, zinc, selenium, vitamins A, B, and E.

Correcting Eczema

Eczema is a skin ailment which presents symptoms of itching, skin inflammation, dry, thickened skin, red patches, papules, and tiny blisters. Most often the hands, wrists, creases of the knees or elbows, ears, and face are areas which exhibit these conditions.

Eczema is associated with asthma, and is partially an allergic-type reaction of the body. It can be associated with food allergies, family history (asthma, eczema), low stomach acid, dysfunctional immune system, or stress.

The primary goals of aromatherapy treatment are to decrease the sometimes intense itching that accompanies eczema, to increase local circulation, and to promote new healthy skin tissue. Anti-inflammatory agents are useful, in addition to essential oils that ease dry skin conditions. Aromatic compresses and concentrated massage oil preparations are beneficial, but comprehensive treatment by a naturopath or other health care practitioner is necessary to identify the underlying condition (for example, allergies, immune system weakness). Strengthening the immune system is helpful in any case, so steps to build the body's defenses are important.

Cool compresses, such as the following compress recipe, can help with intense itching, swelling, and inflamed skin conditions while concentrated massage oils are applied daily to nourish and heal. Chamomile and lemon essential oils are included for their antipruriginous (itch-relieving) properties. Cool water temperatures are used for inflammations or itching, while hot water helps to increase circulation. See hydrotherapy guidelines in Chapter 11: The Aromatic Bath for more information on the uses of water temperature for healing. Always exercise care when using essential oils on broken or damaged skin as they are more readily absorbed.

Compress Treatment for Eczema

to ease itching and inflammation

8 ounces cool water

2 drops Geranium essential oil

2 drops Lemon essential oil

1 drop Chamomile essential oil

a bowl

a small towel or flannel cloth

large towel

plastic wrap

ice pack (optional)

In a glass or ceramic bowl, add the cool water. See Chapter 11 for water temperature guidelines. Add the essential oils and stir with a spoon or your hands to disperse well. Soak a small towel or flannel cloth large enough to cover the affected area. Wring out the cloth and apply to the skin. Cover with an additional towel, or lay an ice pack over this. When the compress becomes warm or dry, replace with a fresh compress. Do this treatment for 20 minutes.

The massage oil concentrate recipe given below is extremely effective for dry eczema with redness, itching, and swelling present. In most acute cases, healing occurs in 4 to 5 days when it is applied three times daily, in addition to compress treatments. The rose oil is a key component of this recipe as it is known to decrease histamine production and thus helpful in allergy-related skin ailments. Carrot seed and rosehip seed are extremely beneficial in healing and nourishing inflamed and impaired skin tissue.

Healing Oil Concentrate

for dry eczema

1 tbls. Calendula infusion oil

1 tbls. Safflower oil

1/4 tsp. carrot seed oil

1/4 tsp. Rosehip seed oil

12 drops Lavender essential oil

6 drops Bergamot essential oil

3 drops Chamomile essential oil

3 drops Rose essential oil

400 IU's Vitamin E

In an amber glass bottle, add the infusion and vegetable oils. Add the carrot seed and rosehip oil. Add the essential oils and the vitamin E. Shake well and label. Apply in small amounts to affected areas. Massage into the skin until absorbed. Apply three times daily.

Essential oils useful for eczema skin conditions are bergamot, cedarwood, chamomile, carrot seed, geranium, hyssop, juniper, lavender, myrrh, patchouli, rose, and rosemary.

Carrier oils and special additive oils that will increase healing are jojoba, evening primrose, calendula, vitamin E, and rosehip seed oils.

Lifestyle recommendations include using a mild soap for cleansing, and baking soda baths to help with itching. See the Bath Salt recipe in Chapter 11, or refer to the chapter on children's ailments for additional information on baking soda usage for itching skin conditions. Avoid wearing synthetic garments against the affected skin to prevent further irritation and itching. Keeping the fingernails clipped will help to prevent scratching. Adopt a good stress-relief program and see a health care practitioner who has knowledge of natural therapies that can benefit eczema and allergy-related illness.

Dietary recommendations emphasize fresh vegetables, fruits, and whole grains. Taking daily flax seed oil in the diet and eating raw nuts and seeds can help dry skin conditions. Drink plenty of pure water and herbal tea.

Wash Away Body Odor—Natural Germ-Busters

Between our cultural stigmas and our state of health, body odor can have quite a different meaning. A malodorous body smell can be a sign of ill health caused by hormonal imbalances, unhealthy diet, or poor elimination. In fact, the military service in Japan used to disqualify men who presented abnormally strong body odor, believing it an outward sign of general ill health.

Today, our culture is almost obsessed with the idea of body odor, as witnessed by magazine and television advertising. The pendulum has swung from the time when soap was considered unhealthy (England, 1820's), to present day when an obsession with body odor and over-cleansing is the norm. I believe the overuse of skin cleansers is stripping the body's natural protective coating (film of sebum) and washing it right down the drain. This natural moisturizing covering on the skin's surface is crucial for good functioning of the largest sensory organ we possess, the skin. Review of all the important functions of the skin (integumentary system) would be helpful and is discussed in the beginning of this chapter.

Somewhere in between these two scenarios lies the answer to a healthful state. Body odor plays a key role in newborns recognizing their mother and people being attracted to one another (intimate body odors; see aphrodisiacs, Chapter 9). Body odor isn't necessarily a bad thing. Perspiration by itself doesn't cause a problem as long as good health is maintained and adequate hygiene is practiced. Napoleon Bonaparte sent a note requesting that his wife, Antoinette, not wash for the following three days, until his return from the battlefield, as he loved her natural body odor and knew his desire for her was strongest when she did not wash.

Body odor becomes a problem when either improper hygiene, ill health, or abnormally high bacterial growth is present. Bacteria can multiply on the skin's surface, primarily in moist places like the armpits, groin, under the breasts, and feet, and can then cause body odor. It is this type of body odor we are addressing in this section. If the cause of the body odor is poor elimination, read Chapter 2: Aromatherapy Treatments for the Digestive System, and see a health care professional. If an underlying illness is the cause of the body odor, then a visit to your doctor is necessary to find the imbalance or underlying cause.

I think it's good for the skin to sweat and perspire; after all, this is a cleansing effect of the body and skin. I don't recommend the use of anti-perspirants or commercial deodorants. Most of them contain unhealthy chemicals and metals. It is normal for the body to sweat, and we should not interfere with this elimination process. However, there are a few essential oils known to help with excessive perspiration and sweat which do not halt the natural function of the body, but rather aid in regulating over-production and over-stimulation of the sweat glands. These essential oils are cypress, lemongrass, petitgrain, and pine. They are astringent and toning in general. Washing with a mild olive oil-based soap made with antibacterial essential oils is recommended. Various body sprays or body splashes, body lotions or oils, and aromatic baths can be used to alleviate body odor.

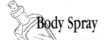 ## Body Spray

a gentle body deodorant spray

7 ounces floral water or herbal infusion

1 ounce cider vinegar

60 drops (total) essential oil

2 tsp. honey

spray bottle

In a fine mist spray bottle, add the herbal infusion (tea) or floral water. Add the vinegar. To the honey, add the essential oils and mix well, before adding to the floral water. Shake bottle well to mix completely. Label. Shake well before each use. After showering or bathing, or for use during the day, simply spray over the entire body, avoiding the eyes and under the arms.

Any of the combinations below can be used for specific scent "themes." Simply add the essential oil recipe chosen to the above Body Spray to make a very pleasant natural deodorizing and mild anti-perspirant mist.

 ## Soft Floral

Rose floral water

40 drops Lavender essential oil

14 drops Mandarin essential oil

4 drops Clary sage essential oil

2 drops Patchouli essential oil

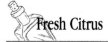
Fresh Citrus

(do not use while sunning, as citrus oils can increase a sunburn)

Orange blossom water

20 drops Grapefruit essential oil

20 drops Lemongrass essential oil

15 drops Bergamot essential oil

5 drops Cypress essential oil

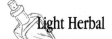
Light Herbal

Lavender floral water

20 drops Rosemary essential oil

20 drops Sandalwood essential oil

5 drops Eucalyptus essential oil

15 drops Juniper essential oil

If the unpleasant body odor is localized to the feet, then an aromatic footbath is very helpful. Use the bath salt recipe on page 299 . Mix 4 to 6 drops of Cypress essential oil in about 1 to 2 tablespoons of the bath salts and add to the basin. Soak feet for 15 to 20 minutes. Follow with the foot powder recipe given in this chapter, which aids in keeping the feet dry and odor-free. You can substitute any of the essential oils listed in this section in the foot powder recipe so it will be extra deodorizing for this problem.

Full aromatic baths can be taken several times weekly, to aid in naturally deodorizing the skin and killing odor-producing bacteria. Choose a total of 8 to 10 drops of essential oils and add to the bath water. I suggest you read over Chapter 11: The Aromatic Bath for more information on bath carrier choices, the use of water temperature, and other suggestions that will positively affect your skin's health, in addition to your mood.

Essential oils that are natural germ busters and show antiseptic properties are many. Almost all essential oils have anti-bacterial benefits; however, there are some essences that are stronger in this area than others. Keep in mind that only skin-friendly essential oils are recommended for application to the skin. Review Chapter 1: Common Sense Safety for those that are possible skin irritants, phototoxic, etc. Essential oils useful as antibacterial agents on the skin are bergamot, cypress, clary sage, eucalyptus, lavender, lemon, lemongrass, juniper, grapefruit, mandarin, neroli, patchouli, sandalwood, peppermint (in low dilution), petitgrain, pine, rosemary and tea tree. *Note:* Do not apply essential oils in the under-arm areas as the heat, moisture, and decreased ability of the oils to evaporate in this body area could cause skin irritation or sensitization.

Antiseptic herbs include basil leaves, lavender flowers, lemonbalm, marjoram, oregano, peppermint, garden sage and sweet thyme. These herbs can be made into an infusion (tea) and used as the floral water part in the Body Splash recipe. Additionally, these herbs can be incorporated into the daily diet.

Is There Anything for Scars?

First of all, if you use the appropriate essential oils in first aid treatments and post-surgical procedures, you can diminish or prevent scarring. Scars can be the result of trauma wounds, chemical and thermal burns, surgery, or stretchmarks. Scarring of the skin is the result of fibroblast cells having done their job of repairing a wound or skin inflammation. Because wounds undergo several stages of repair, including cleaning up the area and killing bacteria, the actual scarring does not take place until three to seven days later. It is then that the fibroblast cells do much of their work of forming collagen and elastin to close up the wound. However, in deep wounds, or those which have become infected, often fewer collagen and elastin fibers are present, giving the firmness and non-elastic characteristics to many scars.

Preventative aromatherapy application may involve using essential oils pre-operatively for several months to tone, strengthen, and nourish the skin prior to surgery. Using essential oils in compresses, local baths, and massage oils after surgery can further aid healing, prevent infection, and diminish scarring. The most impressive effects I have seen from therapeutic use of essential oils is on thermal burns and trauma wounds. In fact, Rene Gattefosse, a French chemist who was researching the cosmetic uses of essential oils back in the late 1920's, had burned himself in a laboratory fire, had used lavender essential oil as an immediate first-aid treatment and had continued to apply it daily. It is said that the wounds he had suffered in the accident did not become infected, healed in a very short time, and did not scar! It was shortly after this incident that Gattefosse dedicated his remaining years of research and study to the therapeutic applications of essential oils.

Curative aromatherapy applications involve using essential oils after the fact, when scars are present. These types of scars, as you might expect, will be more challenging to alter. Scars typically have a diminished blood supply and may be very firm. By using specific essential oils, along with heat and massage, circulation can be increased to the scarred tissue. Also long-term use of nourishing and moisturizing carrier oils, including Vitamin E, and essential oils can have a reducing effect on old scars.

Essential oils that aid healing, kill bacteria, and reduce inflammation are the oils to use to prevent scarring. As stated earlier, it is these stages that take place prior to scar formation, and can complicate and slow the healing process altogether. By using therapeutic essential oils promptly in wound healing, we are able to prevent infection and decrease inflammation and hasten the natural term of events. Ultimately, if a great deal of tissue has been lost, as in ulcers or trauma wounds, fibroblasts will need to fill in the area, and more often than not will involve fewer blood vessels and fewer elastin cells in that area.

Aromatherapy treatment of scars involves applying the oils three times daily, for three to six months, when a scar has been present for a long period of time. In preventing scar formation, as in thermal burns, apply two or three times daily until total healing has taken place, up to a few weeks. Once the wound has healed, begin applying the essential oils in a carrier and always include Vitamin E.

Lavender is one particular essential oil that can be applied directly to a wound or burn without needing to dilute it in another oil or carrier. It should be applied to any burn immediately to prevent infection and prevent scarring. Lavender can also be used in cool or warm compresses or sterile dressings.

An excellent all-around scar preventative oil is given below. You may choose to keep it in a first aid kit, or prepare it when needed. Immediately after a burn or wound, you can apply "neat" lavender essential oil, especially if it is a mild or small wound, or apply a dressing. A wound dressing (or compress) can be made by saturating a sterile gauze pad with aloe vera juice and several drops of lavender essential oil; leave this on the wound for 8 to 10 minutes or until it has dried. Do this three times per day.

After the wound has closed and healing has taken place, begin applying the oil blend given below to aid in scar prevention and to promote healing to underlying tissues in the dermis. It can be used post-surgery, on stretchmarks, trauma wounds, and on burns. It can also be used on older scars to help soften and reduce their appearance. Remember, the older the scar, the longer treatment will take: allow at least three to six months of treatment to see any change of old scar tissue. In this preparation greater amounts (more than twice the normal quantity) of wheat germ and Vitamin E are used to aid healing and to prevent scar tissue from forming. This is a potent preventative, so use it sparingly on scar tissue and the immediate surrounding skin. You can gently heat this oil, by placing it in a warm water bath, to increase absorption into the skin.

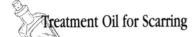

Treatment Oil for Scarring

to prevent and reduce scarring

1 tbls. Calendula infusion oil

1 tbls. Hazelnut or Olive oil

1 tsp. Wheat germ oil

1/4 tsp. Rose hip seed oil

1/4 tsp. Carrot seed oil

20 drops Lavender essential oil

5 drops Frankincense essential oil

800 IU's Vitamin E

In an amber glass bottle, add the calendula, hazelnut, and wheat germ oils. Add the carrot seed and rosehip seed oils, along with the vitamin E. Vitamin E gel capsules can be used by cutting one end and emptying contents into the bottle. Shake this mixture of oils well. Add the essential oils and shake gently to combine well. Label with instructions for use. To use apply three times daily to closed wounds and scars.

Other essential oils used in preventative or curative applications to scar tissue are bergamot, chamomile, frankincense, eucalyptus, geranium, hyssop, juniper, lavender, lemongrass, mandarin, neroli, patchouli, rosemary, and sandalwood.

Carrier options noted for their healing properties are hazelnut, calendula, carrot seed, comfrey, olive oil, wheatgerm, rosehip seed and vitamin E.

Relief for Rashes, Contact Dermatitis

A skin rash that appears following contact with a substance or irritant which causes a skin reaction is referred to as contact dermatitis. Symptoms include a red rash, intense itching, and skin inflammation. Thickening of the skin, scaling, raised red spots, or blisters may develop and break open, forming crusts or scabs. The most common substances which cause dermatitis are poison ivy, oak, and sumac (discussed in Chapter 8), industrial chemicals, metals, solvents, detergents, cosmetics, dyes, some textiles, and medicines. The most frequent cosmetic ingredients which are known to cause dermatitis are synthetic fragrance, preservatives, propylene glycol, formaldehyde, sunscreens, and deodorants. Also, there are several essential oils that can cause skin irritations and inflammation. Refer to Chapter 1 for review of the hazardous and skin-irritating essential oils.

> **Case History:**   *A young man experienced contact dermatitis around his neck following several days of wearing a new necklace made of leather which was dyed black. He had no history of allergic type reactions and was surprised to see the effects of dermatitis. When I saw him, it had been three days following the initial reaction. He had not put anything on it for treatment; however, he had washed the area in the shower. It appeared red, bumpy, and itched intensely. Aloe vera juice was immediately applied and lavender compresses were done twice per day. During the day, chamomile and lavender floral waters were misted on the neck to help with itching and decrease swelling. His healing was complicated by very hot weather and the need to wear tailored shirts during the day at work, which further irritated the rash.*

Immediate washing of the area is necessary when a rash appears from direct contact with skin irritants. However, in the case of poison ivy or oak, it is not advised to use soap as this will spread the irritant to other areas of the skin. Rinse with cold water to flush the substance from the skin and then apply hot water for a few seconds. Aloe vera juice or gel can be applied to the rash, in addition to floral waters of chamomile and lavender. Following this initial first aid, cool compresses, baths or oils can be used as a more intensive form of treatment.

Since itching and inflammation are very common in contact dermatitis cases, the use of cool compresses and tepid baths, particularly those which include baking soda, is most helpful. See Chapter 8 for aromatic baths which are very effective in this area. The cool compress recipe given below is for general use involving red, inflamed skin rashes. These compress treatments can be done three times per day. Depending on the size of the area that is affected, a washcloth, small flannel cloth, or large toweling can be used. If a large area is covered with the rash, the baths may be more appropriate. Vinegar and witch hazel are astringents that are effective for itching skin. One half cup of either can be used in the compress water, or a combination of both as shown here.

Cooling Relief for Dermatitis

an aromatic compress for swelling and itching

1/4 cup cider vinegar

1/4 cup witch hazel lotion

1 – 2 cups cold water

2 tsp. baking soda

4 drops Lavender essential oil

2 drops Chamomile essential oil

2 drops Bergamot essential oil

bowl or basin

washcloth or flannel cloth

ice pack (optional)

towel

In a bowl or basin (or sink if a larger area needs to be covered), add the vinegar, witch hazel, and water. To the baking soda, add the essential oils and mix well. This is used as the carrier for the oils and to help with itching. Add to the water and mix well by stirring. Soak the cloth and wring most of the water from it. Apply to the rash. Lay an ice pack over this and wrap with the towel. Leave on for a total of 20 minutes. Change the compress once it becomes body temperature or begins to dry. Apply the compresses three times per day as needed.

Essential oils which help relieve itching are bergamot, chamomile, cedarwood, jasmine, lemon, and peppermint (use 1% dilution or less). Anti-inflammatory essential oils are useful in dermatitis, as this is an inflammatory process involving the dermal layer of the skin. The essential oils effective in decreasing swelling are chamomile, clary sage, carrot seed, geranium, lavender, lemon, myrrh, patchouli, peppermint (1% or less), and rose. Rose has proven able to decrease histamine production, which is important in allergy-related conditions.

Anti-inflammatory herbs are elderflower, oats, chamomile, St. John's Wort, lavender, lemon juice, calendula, parsley, yarrow flowers and comfrey. These can be made into strong infusions and applied by compress or spray.

First Aid for Boils and Infected Pores

Blocked and infected pores are fairly superficial skin conditions, in comparison to boils which are located deeper in the skin and often involve hair follicles and surrounding tissue. Both are caused by infection, usually bacterial in origin. Symptoms include redness, swelling, heat, blisters or pus-filled lumps. Do not attempt to squeeze boils or infected pores, as this will encourage spread of the bacteria to surrounding areas and will injure the tissue, very possibly causing scarring. Very gentle treatment is necessary, keeping the infection localized and to a minimum.

If you find yourself continually developing boils or infected pores, it may be a sign of a weakened immune system, poor diet, inadequate hygiene, or diabetes. Repeated exposure to environmental pollutants may also be the cause. See a health care professional who is knowledgeable in natural alternative medicine to identify the underlying cause of this recurring ailment.

Essential oils are very effective for healing infected pores and boils because they are strongly anti-bacterial and anti-inflammatory agents which are safe and gentle to use on the skin. The aromatherapy method best suited for this ailment is the hot compress. By utilizing both moist heat and antiseptic essential oils, the blocked pore or boil is gently encouraged to come to a head and be released by the body. In traditional medicine and herbal folklore, poultices were made with parsley, chickweed, and comfrey to draw out the infection. Alternatively, onions were softly baked and cut in half and applied to the boil to draw and bring the infection to a head. Swimming in the salt water was also a remedy for relieving such skin infections.

Here is an aromatic compress made with hot salt water and Epsom salts, along with antibacterial and anti-inflammatory essential oils. The compress can be applied three times daily to encourage the infection to surface and be expelled from the body. Be careful to use proper water temperatures to prevent burns.

Hot Compress for Boils

to draw infection out and decrease swelling

2 cups hot water

2 tbls. sea salt

2 tbls. Epsom salt

4 drops Chamomile (or Lavender) essential oil

2 drops Tea Tree essential oil

2 drops Lemon essential oil

basin or bowl

small flannel cloth

plastic wrap

towel

In a glass bowl or basin, add the hot water (see hydrotherapy guidelines in Chapter 11). In a small dish, add the sea salt and Epsom salts. Add the essential oils to the salts and mix well with the back of a spoon. Add the aromatic salts to the hot water and stir. Soak a piece of flannel cloth in the water solution. Wring most of the water from the compress and apply over the boil or infected pore. Cover with plastic wrap and towel. Replace the compress with a fresh, hot one when it has become cool or dry. Leave on for a total of 20 minutes. Repeat three times daily until the infection comes to a head and is released.

Once the boil has opened, strict measures should be taken not to spread the bacterial infection to other parts of the body. *Staphylococcal aureus* is the typical bacteria present in these types of skin infections, and they spread very easily. Therefore, once the boil has opened, sterile dressings should be applied and showers taken, rather than baths. A few drops of lavender or tea tree essential oil can be applied to the dressing before covering the open wound. Change three times daily, as drainage from the wound will continue. Wear gloves, or use meticulous hand washing, following the handling of soiled dressings and wound care. Dispose of the bandaging appropriately to inhibit contamination.

Once the wound has healed and is completely closed (with no signs of infection), the Treatment Oil for Scarring on page 186 is recommended to prevent scarring, especially if the infection involved facial areas. Follow the instructions given there regarding scar prevention and healing.

Essential oils that are effective for treating boils and infected pores are those which possess strong anti-bacterial and anti-inflammatory properties. Those that are antibacterial (and gentle enough for use on the skin) are bergamot, chamomile, eucalyptus, lavender, lemon, clary sage, and tea tree. Those that are anti-inflammatory agents are chamomile, clary sage, geranium, lavender, lemon, myrrh, neroli, patchouli, carrot seed, and rose.

Herbs which are useful to take internally to fight infections are garlic, onion, echinacea and goldenseal. Those that can be used topically are aloe vera, parsley, chickweed, and comfrey. See information in Chapter 12 for first-aid treatments including herbal poultices.

Lifestyle and dietary recommendations include strengthening the immune system and general health by eating a healthy diet, adopting a stress-relief program, and avoiding environmental pollutants, if these are factors in recurrent skin infections. Eating more foods rich in Vitamins A, C, and E and zinc can be helpful. Avoid taking baths, once the boil has opened, to prevent the infection spreading to other areas. Both meticulous handwashing and good hygiene are crucial. Drink lots of pure water and herbal teas to help cleanse the body from the inside. (Use a combination of the herbs given above to make herbal teas.) Also drinking hot water with fresh lemon juice is helpful in aiding the body with elimination of toxins.

Quick 'n' Easy Remedy for Warts

Abnormal skin growths that can be flat, hard, soft, and varied in size, are called warts. They are typically flesh-colored and appear on the hands, knees, or face. Common warts, as they are often called, can be rough, raised, scaly papules. All warts are considered contagious, as they are viral-related; however, the way they are spread is relatively unknown. A break in the skin, with a lowered immunity could make a person more suscepti-ble. Children and young adults are the population most often afflicted.

Warts which are discolored or painful should be examined by a physician for correct diagnosis and treatment. Be sure to report any changes in a wart or mole to your doctor, as this could be a warning sign of something more serious.

To make an aromatherapy remedy for warts, mix equal parts of lemon, lavender, and tea tree essential oils in a small amber glass bottle. Purchase a box of small round bandages at your local pharmacy. Simply put one or two drops on the inside of the bandage and apply directly over the wart. Alternatively, you can use a cotton swab to apply this oil direct-ly onto the wart. Avoid getting the essential oils on the surrounding healthy tissue. Reapply either application discussed above, two or three times daily until the wart has disappeared.

Most useful for treating common warts are anti-viral essential oils such as bay laurel, black pepper, eucalyptus, geranium, lemon, tea tree, laven-der and cypress.

No More Dandruff

Dandruff, which is medically termed seborrheic dermatitis, is a condition that affects the skin of the scalp. Symptoms are a flaky scalp, dry or oily skin condition, loose scales with or without itching of the scalp. It may be caused by poor circulation, fungal infection, or overuse of high alkaline shampoo or hair products. Many dandruff treatments include salicylate con-stituents, which are closely related to aspirin or salicylic acid. Certain herbs and essential oils naturally contain this constituent, and can be used in aro-matherapy applications such as scalp treatment oils and rinses.

For dandruff control, daily vigorous brushing before shampooing is recommended to loosen any dead skin cells from the scalp and to increase scalp circulation. Wash with a natural baby shampoo or one specifically designed for dandruff, but of natural ingredients. If using a baby shampoo, or neutral base shampoo, you can add up to 80 drops of essential oils to an 8-ounce bottle, making your own dandruff shampoo.

Herbs and plants which contain salicylates are meadowsweet, birch, willow bark, wintergreen, poplar, and black haw. Of these, the only essen-tial oil I recommend for personal use is the birch essential oil. It should only be used in .2% (or less dilutions) for dandruff conditions. It is best used as part of a synergy blend, incorporating other beneficial essences in working together to remedy dry, flaky scalp conditions. The recipe given below reflects this recommendation, and is enough to add to 8 ounces of neutral or baby shampoo. Be sure to label the bottle to prevent others in the house from using it. Do not use this on babies or young children or if you are pregnant.

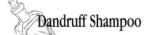

Dandruff Shampoo

add this blend to 8 ounces of shampoo:

40 drops Lavender essential oil

20 drops Rosemary essential oil

10 drops Birch essential oil

10 drops Cedarwood essential oil

Mix the essential oils together. Add to an eight-ounce bottle of shampoo and shake well to mix completely. Use daily or every other day, by using a small amount to massage into wet hair. Massage for 3 to 5 minutes before rinsing completely. Rinse several times, ending with a cold water application. This is an optional step, but helps close pores and stimulate scalp circulation. Follow with the vinegar rinse.

During the Victorian era, herbal vinegars were popular for hair and skin care. They were easy to make from herbs in the garden and countryside and were very effective for hair rinses, facial toners, and bath additions. Along the way, these herbal and floral vinegars lost popularity as store-bought and perfumed preparations became widely available. When it comes to dandruff control, herbal hair rinses that contain vinegar are one of the most beneficial after-shampoo rinses you can use. Vinegar, diluted in herbal infusions or floral waters, helps to normalize the scalp's delicate pH balance and aids in toning the skin. It also successfully removes oil and shampoo residue from the hair. Witch hazel lotion can also be used in this way. Mix up this recipe and store it in a plastic bottle with a squeeze top. Recycle one of your old shampoo or conditioner bottles.

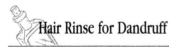

Hair Rinse for Dandruff

8 ounces floral water or herbal infusion

2 tbls. cider vinegar or herbal vinegar

Lavender floral water can be used, or you can make your own herbal infusion. Simply take fresh or dried flowers and herbs (from the list below) and pour hot water over them, about 2 or 3 tablespoons per cup, to make a strong infusion. Nettles and rosemary herb make a nice tea to add to this recipe.

Herbal and floral vinegars are easy to make. Obtain a good apple cider vinegar (organic preferably) and pour into a wide-mouthed glass jar. To one quart of vinegar, add one to two handfuls of fresh-picked flowers and herbs. Set in the sun for a few weeks, shaking daily. Or, if you are in a hurry, gently heat the vinegar and add to the herbs and allow to steep for several days. Strain and bottle. Label contents. This can be added to baths, hair rinses (as above) and diluted even further for use as a facial toner. For dandruff, use lavender, rosemary, and basil. This is great for adding to olive oil to make a very flavorful salad dressing too!

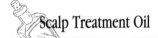

Scalp Treatment Oil

for dandruff control

2 tbls. Jojoba oil

1/2 tsp. carrot seed oil

10 drops Lavender essential oil

5 drops Rosemary essential oil

3 drops Cedarwood essential oil

2 drops Birch essential oil (optional)

Mix the jojoba and carrot seed oil in a small glass bottle. Add the essential oils and shake gently to mix well. Label. Apply at night after brushing the hair and scalp completely. Put several drops on your finger tips and massage into the scalp (not the hair). In the morning shampoo and rinse.

Essential oils which are useful for dandruff conditions are cedarwood, eucalyptus, lavender, lemon, patchouli, rosemary, clary sage, tea tree, lime, basil, birch, and cypress.

Carrier oils that are best for hair preparations are carrot seed, evening primrose, borage, jojoba, and sweet almond.

Traditional herbs used in scalp conditions such as dandruff are aloe vera, sage, rosemary, lavender, myrtle, witch hazel, borage, and nettles. These can be made into herbal vinegars for hair rinses.

Adding Lustre to Dull Hair

Dull, lifeless, brittle, and dry hair can be the result of overshampooing or chemical hair treatments, sun exposure, chlorinated swimming pools or hot tubs, certain medications, vitamin deficiencies, a poor diet, or even from just using the wrong shampoo or conditioner.

You can add specific essential oils to your natural or neutral shampoo to customize your own hair treatment shampoo. Use about 80 drops per 8 ounce bottle of shampoo.

For dry hair use cedarwood, sandalwood, or lavender.

For oily hair use rosemary, lemongrass, or ylang ylang.

For normal hair use lavender, geranium, or clary sage.

Herbs can also be used successfully to add highlights and shine to the hair. Strong herbal infusions can also be used as rinses to cover gray hair.

For dark hair use rosemary and sage herbs.

For light hair use chamomile herb and fresh lemon juice.

For red and auburn hair use calendula and madder root.

To cover graying hair use rosemary and sage herbs.

My friend has used strong infusions of rosemary to cover her gray for the last several years. It works so nicely, I never knew she had any gray hair until she told me! It tends to work best, I am told, with brunette and dark hair.

The herbs listed above can be made into herbal vinegars and diluted to make excellent hair rinses. Herbal and floral vinegars were used by Victorian women for ages. See the previous section which gives basic instruction on brewing your own herbal vinegars. Simply use the herbs best for your hair color and type.

Although I don't know of any women who brush their hair one hundred times every night, brushing can be good for your hair *if* you are using the correct hairbrush! Most hair brushes are made of synthetics, such as plastic and nylon, and can damage the hair by stretching and stripping it. These materials can be too stiff against the scalp as well. Natural boar bristles are still the best, as they give your hair a healthy glow and do not pull or stretch the hair shaft. Natural bristles can help clean your hair by removing excess oil and dirt. Boar bristles can also be safer to use for scalp exfoliation and stimulation.

In addition to finding a good natural bristle brush, the correct hairbrush designed for your hair type is also important to give you shiny and lustrous hair. The following styles of hair brushes can be found in specialty stores or beauty supply stores.

For long hair and for blow-dry styling use a Half Round Hairbrush.

For strong, thick, and shorter hair use a Club Hairbrush.

For delicate and thinning hair use a soft Club Hairbrush.

For long straight hair use an Oval Hairbrush.

For short or fine hair use a Professional Hairbrush.

An easy way to give shine to your hair, while softly fragrancing it at the same time, is to put a drop or two of lavender or rosemary essential oil on your hair brush before brushing your locks. You may find yourself brushing your hair every evening (like in the old movies) as this is an aromatic way to end the long day and naturally perfume your hair for bedtime. The lavender essential oil will even help you sleep!

Counteracting Hair Loss and Thinning

Hair loss and thinning ranks right up there with wrinkles and aging skin. Nobody wants to experience them! But when it happens to you, it can be devastating. What causes hair loss? Several causes have been linked to hair thinning or hair loss: vitamin deficiencies, thyroid or pituitary deficiencies, certain illnesses such as scarlet fever, the heredity factor, stress, overshampooing, swimming frequently in chlorinated pools, and as a side effect of cancer treatments such as chemotherapy and radiation of the head area.

Essential oils remedy hair thinning because they nourish deep in the dermal layers of the skin and in tiny blood vessels, where the hair follicle is located. See Cross Section of Skin page 16 and the physiology of the skin in the beginning of this chapter for visualization of these structures. Herbs, plant oils, and essential oils that can reduce hair loss are discussed in this section.

Of course, if your hair loss is caused from a deficiency, that must be addressed with the help of your health care practitioner. If the reason for your hair loss is from medications or cancer treatments, I'm afraid aromatherapy will not be of help to you. However, when treatment is completed, try using the aromatherapy blend given here to nourish and stimulate new hair growth. Many people experience a change in their hair texture and color following such treatments, so be prepared.

Stress is a major factor in many people experiencing hair loss. Adopting a good stress-release and stress prevention program will be very important, along with taking a good anti-stress vitamin. See Chapter 9 for in-depth discussion on stress and aromatherapy usefulness in this area.

This aromatic scalp treatment oil is effective when used over two to three months. This period of time will allow several hair growth cycles to take place and an improvement in hair growth will be visible. Use this oil several times weekly, after hair care, leaving it in to be absorbed into the scalp. It is called a scalp treatment because the hair itself is not the focus, rather the scalp, more specifically the hair follicle and microcirculatory system. Using warmed oil will increase the absorption of the oils considerably.

Scalp Treatment for Hair Loss

to reduce thinning and provide nourishment

1 tbls. Jojoba oil

1 tbls. Calendula infusion oil

1/2 tsp. Carrot seed oil

10 drops Lavender essential oil

6 drops Clary Sage essential oil

4 drops Cedarwood essential oil

4 drops Rosemary essential oil

In a small amber glass bottle, add the jojoba oil and carrot seed oil. Add the essential oils and shake to mix. Label. Warm the oil before application by placing it in a warm water bath. Apply by massaging a few drops into the scalp area. Leave in to be absorbed. Apply several times weekly.

Essential oils useful in counteracting hair loss are cedarwood, chamomile, clary sage, cypress, lavender, lemon, juniper, grapefruit, rosemary, patchouli, rose, and ylang ylang.

Carrier oils or infusion oils to use as part of your aromatic blend include carrot seed, calendula, jojoba, borage, evening primrose, castor oil, and St. John's Wort.

Lifestyle recommendations include avoiding hair chemical treatments, swimming in chlorinated pools (or wear a cap), and overshampooing, especially with harsh detergents and synthetic fragrances, etc. Use natural alternatives described in the previous sections. Use a natural bristle hairbrush specific for your hair type (described earlier in this chapter). Take action to alleviate stress in your life and use aromatherapy, meditation, exercise, and breathing exercises to develop a holistic program. Exercise and massage also help to increase circulation to the scalp. Bend over, hanging the head lower than your heart, and brush your hair and massage your scalp with your fingers. Better yet, ask a friend to give you a scalp massage which will be a stress-relieving treatment as well.

Dietary recommendations include vitamin supplementation of the B-Complex vitamins (stress vitamins); zinc helps keep the hair strong and niacin may help by improving circulation. Taking natural flax oil daily, in addition to eating more raw nuts and seeds, will benefit your hair and scalp condition. Drink plenty of pure water and eat a healthy diet based on fresh fruits and vegetables and whole grains.

CHAPTER 8

Aromatherapy Treatments for Children

Comforting the Young with Safe Alternatives

This chapter considers the gentle therapeutics for the young and sensitive smaller persons within our care. This population is deserving of a special chapter, as treatment of children involves more extreme care than adults would need, using highly diluted aromatherapy applications and weaker herbal infusions. Children typically respond very positively and require shorter recuperation and healing times. Children are very sensitive to their environment, both on a physical and emotional level. Promoting good health in children is of great importance, and includes basics such as eating good food, getting adequate exercise and enough sleep.

The child's developmental stage will often influence the type of accident or ailments that are likely to occur. Children, especially toddlers, are naturally curious, impulsive, and impatient. They have a strong desire and need to explore and experience their environment with all their senses, in particular the sense of touch. There needs to be a balance between providing safety for your child and allowing enough space for exploration. Although an estimated 90% of all accidents are preventable, prompt first-aid treatment and infection prevention are extremely important. This age group may experience a higher incidence of accidents as they explore the world around them. School-age children, on the other hand, are more susceptible to colds, flu, and other contagious illnesses as they enter daycare, public schools, and social groups.

It is important to keep in mind that children require safe and gentle alternatives when they become ill or require first-aid treatment. Personally, as a mother of three, I turn to these natural approaches first when my children need support in healing. However, if any of the medical emergency symptoms are present (on page 24 of Chapter 2), then immediate medical attention is necessary. Some of the common ailments that children frequently experience are covered in this section: chicken pox, poison ivy rashes, insect bites, sunburn, teething discomfort, first aid for minor skin abrasions, and treatment of diaper rash. Four alternative methods of herbal healing which have proven very effective in the treatment of children are flower essence therapy, homeopathy, herbal infusions, and aromatherapy. The latter two are discussed here.

Aromatherapy—the therapeutic use of essential oils in 1/2 to 1% dilutions (or less). Those most often used in children's ailments include anti-inflammatory and antiseptic essences. Children respond extremely favorably to aromatherapy. Methods include aromatic baths, lotions, and inhalation. For massage, children especially enjoy and react positively to foot and hand massage. A drop or two of essential oils on a pillow case can help with sleep disturbances or nasal congestion. Sleep pillows are also gentle sleep inducers and a recipe for my Sweet Dream pillows is given in Chapter 13, page 332. Humidifiers are another way you can utilize aromatherapy inhalation safely for children. Perform a skin patch test if using an essential oil for the first time on the skin. See directions on page 9 for skin testing.

Herbal infusions—the therapeutic use of specific herbs in the form of herbal tea is used with much success as a dilute tea, bath or compress. In preparing herbal infusions for children, use the following guidelines for safe and effective treatment:

Child less than 1 yr. = use 1 part tea to 4 parts water

1 to 3 yrs. = use 2 parts tea to 3 parts water

3 to 5 yrs. = use 3 parts tea to 2 parts water

5 to 10 yrs. = use 4 parts herbs to 1 part water.

Many skin problems can be avoided by using all-cotton underclothing and avoiding synthetic fabrics as much as possible. Avoid the use of talc and mineral-based skin care products or those with synthetic fragrances. As a general rule, creams, oils, and ointments are used for dry skin conditions. When the skin is moist, wet or oozing, liquids and lighter lotions are appropriate to use. As with all medicines (and cleaning supplies, chemicals, etc.), keep your oils out of reach of children.

A common symptom in children's ailments such as chicken pox, insect bites, and poison ivy reactions is "itching." Itching is actually considered a mild form of pain since the message is transmitted by nerve fibers in the same way that other pain signals travel. Scratching overstimulates this nerve path and causes the body's natural painkillers known as "endorphins" to be released. However, continuous scratching may cause an itch to worsen, impair the integrity of the skin, and possibly cause an infection.

How to Use Essential Oils to Relieve Itching and Promote Healing for Chicken Pox

Chicken pox is caused by the varicella-zoster virus. It is highly contagious via direct or indirect contact. The common age at which most children contract chicken pox is between 2 and 8 years of age. The incubation time is 14 to 21 days after exposure to the virus. The communicability period is from the onset of fever (usually one day before lesions appear) until the last vesicle has dried and scabbed over completely (5 to 7 days).

Symptoms include general malaise, fever for 24 hours or less, a rash of small red spots which turn into blisters, break open, and crust over to form scabs. Itching can be mild to severe, and scratching may cause scarring and infection. Typically, the rash appears on the trunk and head, and then appears on the limbs.

Caution: Chicken pox is a severe condition in pregnant women and is generally more severe for adults. Although uncommon, chicken pox can be complicated by secondary bacterial infections of the skin, pneumonia, and encephalitis.

Case History: *There are many case histories I could share with you, but I think my own family's story highlights just about every possibility you could experience with your own children. When my youngest boys were in first grade, one of them came home with a note from school and a mild fever. There was a chicken pox outbreak in the school and surrounding areas! Kristopher was the first one to develop it. One and a half weeks later, Ryan came down with it, and then to our surprise our eldest son got it for the second time! All in all, I was housebound with children for close to 6 weeks! The recipes given in this chapter were welcome relief for all the children. They healed quickly, had very little scarring and at most the itching was mild or moderate. My 15-year-old experienced a horrendous amount of pox all over, including his eyes, throat, and ears! He had had a mild case of chicken pox when he was in preschool so we thought he was done. When adults or teenagers get chicken pox, the symptoms and rash can be much more pronounced. The spray seemed to be the most helpful and easiest to use. He opted for the tepid shower in lieu of the aromatic bath, and misted with the chicken pox spray afterwards. A hairdryer was used to dry affected areas well before dressing.*

For local treatment of chicken pox, a spray can be made of essential oils that are astringent, relieve itching, promote healing, and guard against bacterial infection. This spray is a very convenient way to apply the herbal medicine, as swabbing the skin with cotton balls can prompt itching. Alternatively, an 8-ounce bottle of Calamine lotion can be used as the carrier, and the essential oils in the recipe given below can be added. Be sure to shake well to combine the oils completely in the lotion. Witch hazel is an astringent and will aid in drying the blisters that develop. Aloe vera is anti-inflammatory and helps to heal and prevent scarring of skin eruptions. Honey is used primarily as a carrier for the essential oils since they will not emulsify in the liquids on their own. However, honey is anti-bacterial and anti-inflammatory as well and certainly is beneficial for these reasons. The essential oils in this recipe both help with itching and inflamed conditions and aid healing and prevent secondary bacterial infections. Carrot seed oil is an essential oil, and is often used in 10% dilutions (or less) to aid in skin healing, prevent scarring, and as an antioxidant. It is optional in this recipe; however, if you are concerned with scarring, I strongly suggest you include it. Remember to do a skin patch test on the child to check for skin sensitivity before applying this (or any new essential oil) to a large area. (See Chapter 1, Common Sense Safety, for details.)

A Healing Spray for Chicken Pox

to relieve itching, promote healing of vesicles

1/2 cup distilled Witch Hazel lotion

1/2 cup aloe vera gel (or concentrated spray)

40 drops Lavender essential oil

15 drops Lemon essential oil

15 drops Bergamot essential oil

5 drops Peppermint essential oil

1 tsp. carrot seed oil (optional)

1 tbls. Honey

You will need a spray bottle or mister, with a relatively fine spray nozzle. In a measuring cup or glass, mix very well the essential oils and carrot seed oil in the honey. Add the aloe vera gel and mix completely. Then add the witch hazel and combine well. Pour into the spray bottle and label. Spray onto affected body areas, avoiding the eye area. Use as needed several times per day to relieve itching and help heal blisters.

The aromatic bath is another very effective treatment providing cooling relief for itching and to promote healing. Baking soda is very effective in easing the itching caused by chicken pox. Tepid water is indicated for inflammatory conditions and will also help to relieve hot spots and itching. Lavender essential oil is the ideal essence to use since it is anti-infective, anti-inflammatory, and calming to the nervous system. Tea Tree essential oil is included for its healing and antibacterial properties. Chamomile essential oil is anti-inflammatory and is extremely helpful in conditions where itching is a major symptom. Most young children love baths and can be entertained (or distracted from itching) for quite a while with water toys.

Aromatic Bath for Chicken Pox

1 cup baking soda

2 drops Lavender essential oil

1 drop Chamomile essential oil

1 drop Tea Tree essential oil

Fill the bath with tepid water. See Chapter 11: The Aromatic Bath for hydrotherapy guidelines and water temperatures. To 1 cup of baking soda, add the essential oils and mix well with the back of a spoon. Add to the bath and stir until dissolved. Allow the child to soak for up to 30 minutes, depending on comfort level.

Herbs can be made into strong infusions to be added to the bath water or used as topical compresses, poultices, or lotions. Useful herbs include chickweed, calendula, comfrey, lavender, witch hazel, and St. John's Wort. Lotions are recommended for moist blister-type vesicles, rather than an ointment. Herbal tea can also be made to be taken internally to aid the healing process. Herbs traditionally used are chamomile, lemonbalm, echinacea, elderflower, and burdock. Be sure to follow the guidelines given in the beginning of this chapter for safe dosing according to the child's age.

Lifestyle recommendations include keeping nails short to prevent infections from scratching. Keep the child isolated until all lesions have crusted and completely scabbed over (at least 5 to 7 days). Encourage rest and sleep. Spray the air with Pure for Sure antiseptic blend on page 335 or use pure eucalyptus essential oil for disinfection.

Dietary suggestions include drinking plenty of liquids, including diluted herbal teas and juices (especially carrot juice), and plenty of water. Garlic and onion soup will aid healing and prevent infection. (Recipe given on page 97.)

How to Use Essential Oils to Relieve Itching and Promote Healing for Sunburn

Burns are caused by excess exposure to the sun or other heat source. This chapter will address superficial second degree burns only. First degree burns involve only a portion of the outer skin layer, the epidermis. (See Physiology of Skin on page 16.) Symptoms include redness and pain with slight swelling and inflammation. Typically the epidermal layer peels within 5 days, becomes itchy and pink, and is well on its way to total healing in about one week. There is usually no resulting scar from a first degree burn.

A superficial second degree burn also involves partial thickness of the skin, but the dermis as well as the epidermis layer. Symptoms are pink or red discoloration of the skin, blister formation, edema (swelling and inflammation) with superficial layers of the skin damaged. The wound is moist and painful. This type of injury takes about ten to 14 days to completely heal and is prone to infection. First or second degree burns can result from either the sun or a heat source. For the sake of simplicity I will refer to "sunburns" in this chapter but the information applies to thermal burns as well.

Prolonged UV ray exposure causes severe sunburns which can affect deeper cells in the skin, and lead to skin cancer many years later. More than 50% of the skin damage resulting from overexposure to the sun occurs before the age of 18 years. It is crucial that we protect our children by preventing sunburns.

UVA are the longer sun rays which can penetrate clouds, car and home windows. These rays are strongly linked to the formation of wrinkles and, more important, malignant melanoma, a fatal form of skin cancer. As a cancer nurse working in Seattle, I saw many fishermen, avid golfers, and construction workers who had developed skin cancers on unprotected areas of their body such as the neck, back of the hands, and ears. You probably wouldn't think that Seattleites could get skin cancer since they don't see the sun for months at a time! Even clouds don't protect us from the harmful UVA rays.

UVB rays, on the other hand, are the shorter wavelength sun rays. They are responsible for rapid sunburns, wrinkles, age lines, and cataracts of the eye.

Be aware that certain medications, such as diuretics and antibiotics, can increase sun sensitivity, making you more susceptible to sunburn. Also, some essential oils and many perfume oils are phototoxic and should be avoided when in direct sunlight. Refer to Chapter 1: Common Sense Safety for more detailed information on this subject.

Aloe vera, which is anti-inflammatory and healing, has been used for centuries to heal burns. Lavender and tea tree essential oils can be added to this to make a first-aid treatment for sunburn as described above, or use in the form of a gel or spray. It can be added to the aromatic bath, compresses, and lotions. Research studies show that using aloe vera before sunning protects the immune system from the deleterious effects of UV ray exposure. Therefore, it is not uncommon to find aloe vera in sunscreen products marketed today.

There are several good carriers that can be used for the aromatic sunburn bath. Many of the recipes given in Chapter 11 are very effective, and include honey, milk or cream, and aloe vera. The ultimate answer to treating your sunburned skin is to soak in a bath with an abundance of healing herbs, soothing essential oils, and aloe vera. This recipe is a bit more complicated than the others, since you have to prepare a strong infusion (tea) of the herbs; however, if your body is screaming for it, you best make it! It will be worth the extra effort. Lavender and peppermint are the perfect pair to take to the bath for sunburns. Lavender is calming to the skin and nervous system, while peppermint (in small doses) is cooling. For small children or to save time, this recipe can be made without the herbal infusion.

Aromatic After-Sun Bath

to treat sunburn

1/4 cup of the following herbs: calendula, comfrey,
    raspberry leaf, slippery elm

1 qt. boiling water

1/2 cup baking soda

1/2 cup apple cider vinegar or Witch hazel lotion

1/2 cup Aloe vera gel or juice

2 tbls. honey

2 drops Lavender essential oil

1 drop Peppermint essential oil

Note: Adults can use twice the amount given for essential oils. Make a strong infusion of the herbs listed by pouring boiling water over them in a bowl or pot and allowing it to steep for 20 to 30 minutes. Strain and set aside. Fill the bath with tepid water. Add the herb tea mixture to the bath, along with the baking soda, vinegar, and aloe. Mix the essential oils with the honey to combine well and add to the bath water by stirring well with your hands. Soak for 20 minutes or longer. Pat dry gently. Follow with After-Sun Healing Spray if desired.

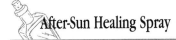

After-Sun Healing Spray

to heal sunburned skin

1/2 cup distilled water

1/4 cup Witch hazel lotion

1/4 cup Aloe vera gel or juice

8 drops Lavender essential oil

2 drops Chamomile essential oil

1 drop Geranium essential oil

1 tsp. honey

In an 8-ounce (or larger) spray bottle, add the water, witch hazel, and aloe. Combine the essential oils and honey, and mix very well with the end of a spoon. Add the aromatic honey to the water mixture. Shake well to completely mix. Label contents with directions for use. Shake well before applying to the skin. Avoid the eye area. Apply freely several times per day.

Olive oil is an excellent oil to heal burns and scalds, and has traditionally been used in this way for centuries. The extra virgin (first pressing) is high in vitamins and minerals. Calendula oil is another ingredient I recommend to add for any healing skin preparation. Refer to Chapter 15 for directions on how to make your own calendula infusion oil. Wheat germ oil is an anti-oxidant and is useful for burns and damaged skin. The following body oil recipe includes all three of these fine healing oils, in addition to essential oils.

For adult usage, double the amounts of essential oils listed, as this blend is designed for children, and reflects a much lower dilution.

Aromatic Body Oil for Sunburns

for children

5 tbls. Extra virgin Olive oil

2 tbls. Calendula infusion oil

1 tbls. Wheat Germ oil

16 drops Lavender essential oil

2 drops Neroli essential oil

1 drop Chamomile essential oil

In a 4-ounce amber bottle, add the essential oils. Add the olive, calendula, and wheat germ oils and shake gently to mix. Label contents. This oil goes on easily when the skin is moist. Spray the body with Lavender flower water, or don't completely dry after bathing. Spread this oil on in a thin layer. It will help to seal in the moisture on the skin and glide on easily when applied in this way. Note: Apply this oil after the skin has cooled for several hours or overnight.

Preparing a Lavender mist, or using authentic lavender floral water as a body mist, is simple yet very refreshing and soothing for sunburned, hot, and dehydrated skin. Turn to Chapter 12 for directions on how to prepare your own facial or body spray. Take it to the beach and keep it in the cooler for a refreshing skin-loving treat. It encourages relaxation too!

Heatstroke or sunstroke is a systemic reaction to excessive exposure to heat or sunlight. Taking a tepid aromatic bath and drinking cool peppermint tea will have a mild cooling effect on the whole body. Get plenty of rest and drink lots of fluids. A cool compress to the forehead, or a cool foot bath would also help. Choose one of the essential oils useful in treating sunburn for any one of these methods. Refer to Chapters 11: The Aromatic Bath, and 12: First Aid Treatments for directions on preparing these.

Honey can be used as a healing agent for dressings because it is antibacterial and anti-inflammatory. When essential oils are combined with it, you multiply its effects. I recommend you use Lavender or Chamomile essential oil, along with one drop of Tea Tree for dressings. Mix the essential oils in the honey first, then apply a thin layer to the gauze dressing and apply to the burn. Aloe vera gel, or the fresh juice from the plant, can be used in the same way.

Essential oils useful in treating sunburns and thermal burns are lavender, chamomile, eucalyptus, geranium, tea tree, and neroli.

Lifestyle recommendations involve education and prevention. Use of broad-spectrum sunscreens which block both UVA and UVB rays are best, with as SPF of 15. Reapply after swimming or water play, according to product labeling. Be sure you protect your little ones with shade, adequate clothing, sun hats, sunglasses, and sunscreen.

How to Use Essential Oils to Relieve Itching and Promote Healing for Insect Bites

Insects such as mosquitoes and horse flies cause bites, while bees, yellowjackets, hornets, and wasps inject poison which causes a sting. It is helpful if the stinger, if present, can be scraped off the skin before applying treatment. Other than for this step, the treatment for insect bites and bee stings is relatively the same. There is local inflammation, itching, or pain present.

Allergy Alert: If a bite or sting causes swelling of the face and lips, difficulty breathing, severe itching, abdominal cramps, or diarrhea seek immediate medical attention.

Lavender essential oil can be applied directly to the bite (or sting) by applying one drop "neat," which means undiluted. Lavender and Tea Tree essential oils are the only essential oils that can safely be used this way; all others must be diluted. Alternatively, a cotton swab can be moistened with fresh lemon juice, apple cider vinegar, or witch hazel and one or two drops of essential oil applied to it and dabbed onto the skin.

Essential oils that help relieve the pain, itch, and swelling of bites and stings are basil, bergamot, chamomile, eucalyptus, lavender, lemon, lemongrass, patchouli, pine, and tea tree.

A paste made from baking soda, meat tenderizer, or clay powder can be used as well to relieve the discomfort of a bite or sting. To this paste you can add one or two drops of the listed essential oils helpful for these conditions. Poultices made from one of the following herbs (calendula, garlic, onion, plantain, marshmallow root, and St. John's Wort) have been used in traditional herbal medicine for external application. Rubbing an ice cube over the area that has been stung is also helpful in relieving immediate swelling and pain.

Lifestyle recommendations include prevention and awareness that camp sites, hiking trails, and picnic rest areas are common areas for stinging insects. Yellowjackets nest on the ground, and are often stepped upon by unwary persons who may be barefoot. Therefore, you should wear shoes or sandals while at such places. Also be aware that bees are attracted to bright clothing, sweet smells, and perfumes.

Natural Alternatives for Insect Repellants

Insects have an extremely sensitive olfactory system (sense of smell). It is what guides them to specific plants and other insects in what is a complex interrelationship. Certain plants emit aromatic molecules (essential oils) to attract particular insects to them to aid in self-preservation via pollination, while others can emit specific aromatic molecules to ward off or deter specific insects for self-protection.

Most commercial products on the market used as bug repellants are harmful and contain irritating chemicals that should not come into contact with the skin, eyes, or mucous membranes (or be inhaled, for that matter). On the other hand, several herbs and essential oils are very useful to repel insects and are relatively safe and natural alternatives if used properly. Pennyroyal herb has been used for centuries in this way, and the essential oil made from that plant is used extensively in many preparations.

However, this oil can be very dangerous, especially for pregnant women, if used improperly and is not recommended for personal use, although making an infusion (herbal tea) is fine. See Hazardous Essential Oil list on page 18.

Citronella is another well known active ingredient in bug repellants, and is frequently found in outdoor candles. It is the scent familiar in many products, including Ivory soap and Avon's Skin-So-Soft lotion. The latter is a product helpful with deterring bugs, simply because it contains citronella oil. Citronella has a very strong odor intensity and can be quite overpowering if used in too high a dilution.

The following essential oils have been found to have moderate to high effectiveness in keeping various insects away from you:

To repel mosquitoes: Basil, cedarwood, citronella, geranium, juniper, and rosemary.

To repel house flies: Citronella, geranium, and juniper.

To repel fleas: Cajeput, lemon, and pine.

To repel ants: All mints.

Essential oils useful as insect repellants are basil, cajeput, cedarwood, citronella, eucalyptus, geranium, juniper, lavender, lemongrass, patchouli, peppermint, pine, rosemary, and tea tree.

Herbs useful as insect repellants are garlic, lavender, lemonbalm, all types of mint, pennyroyal, southernwood, wormwood and tansy.

To make an insect repellant to apply to the skin, you can make the following tea spray or a vegetable oil-based aromatherapy blend. Or you can forgo the skin application completely, and put a few drops of essential oil on your clothes, sleeping bag, hat, and tent. It doesn't have to be on your skin to keep the bugs away! Remember they have a very keen sense of smell. Here is the recipe for a bug repellant oil to apply to your skin.

Bug Off Skin Oil

to apply to the skin; avoid the eyes

2 tbls. vegetable oil

5 drops Cedarwood essential oil

4 drops Lemon essential oil

2 drops Geranium essential oil

1 drop Citronella essential oil

In a plastic squeeze bottle (which is convenient for camping), add the essential oils. Omit the lemon essential oil if you plan on being in the direct sunlight, as lemon oil is phototoxic and can cause a sunburn if put on immediately prior to sunning. Lemongrass, rosemary, or eucalyptus can be substituted for the lemon oil. Add the 2 tablespoons of vegetable oil and shake well. Label contents with directions for use.

A tea spray can be made from various herbs to be used as a room mist or to apply on clothing and the skin. Reminder: This is made into a tea from the fresh or dried herbs, not the essential oil!

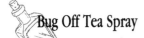 ## Bug Off Tea Spray

to repel most bugs and insects

2 tbls. each of the following herbs:

Lavender, Pennyroyal, Southernwood, Tansy, and Wormwood

1 cup boiling water

Pour a cup of boiling water over the above herbs and allow to steep for 15 minutes or longer. Cool, strain, and pour into a small spray bottle. Label contents with directions for use.

My teenager likes to camp a lot, and uses a blend of geranium and citronella essential oils in a vegetable oil base to soak strips of cloth with the solution. He ties the cloth strips around trees surrounding his camp, to successfully keep the mosquitoes away.

Treatment for Ringworm

Ringworm is a superficial fungal infection of the skin and is not a worm at all. It has a peculiar "ring" growth formation, which is how it got its name. It grows outward from the center, leaving an inactive middle portion, and developing the red ring appearance on the skin. The medical name for ringworm of the scalp is Tinea Capitis. It is most common on the scalp and appears in rings of vesicles which can be very itchy and can cause hair loss in patches. It is also contagious; infected pets, soil contamination, and person-to-person are the most common sources of infection. Common use of hair brushes, combs, and hats can easily spread this from child to child.

Ringworm can also appear on the body in a single ring patch or multiple patches and is called Tinea Corporis or Circinata. Typical locations where it may grow are the exposed areas of the arms, hands, and feet. It can also extend into areas of the scalp, hair, and nails.

Topical antifungal agents are necessary to treat ringworm infections. This skin condition can be stubborn to treat, so you must be patient and consistent with aromatherapy treatment and hygiene. Most ringworm conditions need at least 10–14 consecutive days of treatment to complete the regime. In some stubborn cases, a month may be necessary to totally rid the child of this fungal growth. The important thing to remember is to apply this treatment two to three times per day, for 10 or more consecutive days. This is a challenge, but must be done to be successful.

Case history: *A 6-year-old boy had ringworm on his thigh and one arm. It did not itch, but did appear in ring formation of about 1/4-inch diameter when first observed by his mother. I presume the child got the infection from his pet dog or from playing in the woods and soil. By the time I was consulted, the rings had grown to approximately 3/4- to 1/2-inch and multiplied to several areas on the arm and thigh. The young boy claimed it itched only slightly and he was not bothered by it. The mother applied the ringworm treatment oil twice per day, and gave him several baths weekly. The infection completely disappeared within 11 days. It has been over 1 year and he has not been re-infected since.*

The following aromatherapy treatment oil is very concentrated and is designed for local areas only. This is a 10% dilution preparation, which is much higher than the normal dosage for all-over body treatment or for regular massage concentrates. Because fungal infections can be resistant to treatment and they are usually treated with local application, a stronger blend is warranted. Some experts suggest you use specific essential oils "neat" or straight on the skin. I find the oil base encourages slower evaporation of the essences and is very effective. However, since this is a fungal infection, a light oil is recommended rather than a heavy ointment, as fungi thrive in moist, dark, and warm conditions.

Ringworm Treatment Oil

a fungal treatment

2 tbls. vegetable oil (sesame or soy)

25 drops Tea Tree essential oil

15 drops Lavender essential oil

5 drops Geranium essential oil

5 drops Peppermint essential oil

400 IU Vitamin E

In a one-ounce amber glass bottle, add the essential oils and vitamin E. You can use vitamin E gel caps by cutting one end and squeezing the contents into the bottle. Add the vegetable oil. Shake the bottle to mix. Use a Q-tip to apply the oil to the affected skin areas. Be sure to cover the entire patch. Apply this treatment oil three times per day for at least 10 consecutive days.

Sea salt baths and soaking in the ocean have been a form of treatment for a host of skin conditions, including fungal-type infections. An aromatic bath which contains sea salt is especially useful in treating widespread fungal infections, while compresses and foot baths are effective if this condition is localized.

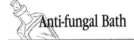 ## Anti-fungal Bath

for ringworm and other fungal infections of the skin

1 to 2 cups sea salt

4 drops Lavender essential oil

1 drop Geranium essential oil

1 drop Tea Tree essential oil

Fill the bath with warm water. Add the essential oils to the sea salt and mix. Add to the bath water and stir well with your hands. Soak for 20 minutes or longer if comfortable. Dry the skin well. A blow dryer can be used on a low setting to dry affected areas of infection. Apply ringworm treatment oil.

Essential oils that show anti-fungal properties are chamomile, cedarwood, eucalyptus, fennel, geranium, lavender, myrrh, patchouli, sandalwood, and tea tree. Of these, the safest for children are lavender, tea tree, and geranium. Remember to use caution with peppermint essential oil by diluting it highly before use.

Lifestyle modifications are extremely important whenever you are dealing with a contagious ailment such as ringworm. Excellent hygiene, including using clean towels daily, wearing clean cotton clothing, and completely drying the skin after bathing are crucial to preventing spread to other areas, or to other members of the family. Putting clothes through two drying cycles in the dryer guarantees they will not harbor fungi. Keeping children's nails short may be helpful in preventing scratching and spread of ringworm. Use an anti-fungal or natural vegetable-based soap which contains anti-fungal essential oils. A diet rich in fish and flax (seed) will also be of benefit.

Natural Prescriptions for Diaper Rash

First of all, you are not a terrible mother if your child gets a diaper rash! I will share several helpful and practical tips for preventing diaper rash and give you some wonderful all-natural recipes for treating it. Diaper dermatitis is a rash appearing on the buttocks which is red and may or may not have eruptions. It causes discomfort for the baby, especially when the diapers are soiled and wet or when cleansing the buttock area during a diaper change.

Washing the buttocks and perineum thoroughly and drying well before reapplying the diapers are very important. Change diapers as soon as they become soiled or wet. Avoid powders which can cake to the skin, and mineral oil which can clog pores and prevent adequate drying of the skin. Avoid plastic pants and disposable diapers which discourage air circulation and retain body heat and moisture. Washing cloth diapers with vinegar or borax will neutralize the ammonia that is produced from urination. All cotton diapers are best to use most of the time, and disposable diapers can be used when traveling or for convenience on occassion. Dry the diaper area thoroughly following bathing and diaper changes by using a hair dryer or allowing your baby to air dry for a few minutes in the sunlight when possible.

A solution of white distilled vinegar and water (1 to 4 ratio) can be used to wash the diaper area. This will neutralize the concentrated urine and ammonia present and balance the skin's pH. *Note:* It also discourages yeast, a common cause of rash. Cotton cosmetic pads or towelettes can be soaked in this solution and stored in a zip-lock plastic bag for travel use.

This oil blend will prevent diaper rash and treat mild cases of skin irritation. Use sparingly to protect the skin and provide a natural and gentle barrier. For extremely dry skin an ointment can be made by following the directions on page 319 in Chapter 12 and then adding the essential oils given in this recipe.

Aromatic Oil for Baby

to prevent and treat diaper rash

4 tbls. Calendula infusion oil

10 drops Lavender essential oil

1 drop Chamomile essential oil

In a 2-ounce amber glass bottle, add the essential oils. All lavender essential oil can be used in lieu of the chamomile. Add the calendula oil. Shake to mix well. Label with directions for use. Apply on dry skin, in small amounts.

Lifestyle recommendations are to cut down on dairy products and sweets (including juices). Use cloth diapers and avoid baby skin products (soap, powder, lotions, and bubble bath).

Safe and Easy First Aid for Minor Cuts, Wounds, and Abrasions

There are many conditions which fall into this category of minor cuts and abrasions, such as paper cuts, slivers, scrapes, and so forth. When the body's immune system is strong, and skin integrity is otherwise excellent, a minor cut does not pose very much danger. However, cleaning the wound with soap and water or an antiseptic vinegar is necessary, in addition to applying first-aid treatment. Depending upon the wound, compresses, ointments, bandages, or more elaborate dressings may be needed. Essential oils are very helpful in first-aid treatment as they possess antibacterial, anti-inflammatory properties which aid healing and prevent infection.

Warning: Tetanus, or lockjaw, is a disease caused by an anaerobic bacteria (clostridium tetani) which is found in the soil and animal fecal matter and can be introduced into the body by any break in the skin. The major symptom of tetanus is stiffening of the muscles, including the jaw. Seek medical attention immediately if these symptoms are present. It is recommended that everyone receive a tetanus booster every ten years for protection.

An antiseptic vinegar can be made and kept in the first-aid kit for washing minor wounds. It helps itching conditions and provides local washing in addition to killing germs.

Antiseptic Vinegar

an aromatic first-aid wash

1/2 cup distilled water

1/2 cup apple cider vinegar

1 tsp. honey

6 drops Lavender essential oil

2 drops Tea Tree essential oil

1 drop Chamomile essential oil

1 drop Lemon essential oil

You will need an 8-ounce amber glass bottle. Mix the essential oils with the honey. In a glass measuring cup or bowl, combine the aromatic honey with the water and vinegar. Stir well and pour into bottle. Shake well to mix. Label contents with directions for use. To use, simply soak a cotton ball with the solution and clean the wound.

To make an antiseptic ointment with all-natural ingredients use the recipe given on page 318 in Chapter 12 and add the following essential oils to kill germs and aid healing.

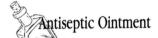

Antiseptic Ointment

to apply to minor wounds

Heavy-duty Ointment

40 drops Lavender essential oil

20 drops Tea Tree essential oil

10 drops Chamomile essential oil

10 drops Lemon essential oil

Prepare the heavy-duty ointment according to the directions given on page 318. Before pouring the mixture into the clean storage jar, add the essential oils while still in a liquid state. These essential oils are the best antiseptic essences for general first-aid usage. Apply a small amount of this ointment to the cleaned wound. May cover with bandaging if necessary or leave open to air.

Essential oils that are useful in first-aid treatment of minor cuts and wounds are bergamot, chamomile, eucalyptus, fir, frankincense, geranium, hyssop, juniper, lavender, lemon, lemongrass, myrrh, patchouli, pine, rosemary, and tea tree.

Traditional herbal medicine has employed herbs in the form of fresh poultices and unguents for ages with great success. Some of the popular herbs for first-aid treatment are aloe vera, calendula, comfrey, echinacea, goldenseal, St. John's Wort, and slippery elm.

Aromatic Bedtime Secrets to Encourage Slumber

After a long day, I know of no greater challenge than trying to get a child to sleep against his or her will. Although there have been times in my life when I wished to sedate my children, I have found other gentler approaches to promote sleep, which include encouraging a positive bedtime routine.

Children love routines. Structure makes them feel safe and cared for. Taking the time to prepare your child for bed by following a routine can save hours of restless and sleepless nights for both of you!

This routine has worked for our family (and many others) for encouraging children to go to sleep.

The 4-B's (B-4) Before Bedtime

1. a warm aromatic *Bath*—children relax and get clean while playing with bath toys.
2. read a *Book*—when they get older, they can read to you.
3. go to the *Bathroom*—so they don't wake to void during the night.
4. a *Bear hug* and *Butterfly kiss*—a big hug and a delicate butterfly kiss (brushing your eyelashes by blinking against the child's cheek).

Kids love the great big bear hug followed by the gentleness of the butterfly kiss. By the time they soak in a warm bath of relaxing and calming essences, get a book read to them and receive nurturing, they will be ready to go to bed. However, as a parent you must set structure also, in letting them know that you need quiet time too. Another bedtime secret is to tuck a sleep pillow inside the child's pillowcase to encourage sleep. I have given you my recipe for a sleep pillow I make for my family called "Sweet Dreams." The directions are on page 332 and include many sleep-inducing herbs such as lavender, hops, and sweet woodruff. A drop or two of lavender essential oil on the pillowcase will support slumber too!

Before you ever get to the bath stage, you can offer your child a cup of diluted chamomile herbal tea, made according to the guidelines stated in the beginning of this section under "herbal infusions for children." Also, warm milk with a sprinkle of nutmeg works well in relaxing a child before bedtime.

Children are great fans of foot or hand massages. Favorite scents include lavender and mandarin essences. When they get into bed, massage their feet or hands with a little aromatic massage oil to promote relaxation and deep sleep. When the feet are warmed by local massage it seems to be especially comforting. The following recipe is very basic and simple to prepare. It is also useful during the day or early evening when children tend to be overactive or overtired.

Aromatic Massage Oil for Children

a relaxing hand or foot massage blend

2 tbls. warm vegetable oil

5–10 drops essential oil of Lavender or Mandarin

Mix the child's favorite essential oil (or combination of the two essences) in the warm vegetable oil. This can be made ahead and kept in an amber glass bottle or prepared in a shallow dish in half the amounts given. Massage the feet, working toward the heart. Use gentle but firm pressure.

The aromatic bath recipe given on page 302 called *Child's Play* is recommended, in addition to using any of the listed oils for relaxation. A bath using pure lavender essential oil is particularly satisfying.

Essential oils useful for insomnia are those which promote deep relaxation and are soothing to the nervous system. It is important that you use essential oils in normal doses, which for children are half the adult dose. See guidelines given in the front of this chapter and review Chapter 1: Common-Sense Safety for dosing children. Using too much essential oil can produce overstimulation, rather than relaxation. This pertains to adults as well. Of all the essential oils about to be listed, lavender, chamomile, and mandarin are the safest and most pleasant for children.

Essential oils useful for relaxation are basil, bergamot, cedarwood, chamomile, clary sage, cypress, frankincense, geranium, hyssop, jasmine, lavender, mandarin, marjoram, myrrh, neroli, nutmeg, orange, patchouli, sandalwood, tangerine, rose, and ylang ylang.

We have already discussed many lifestyle recommendations, which include developing a bedtime routine. Avoid caffeinated beverages such as cola and hot chocolate. Give the children chamomile tea or warm milk instead. And remind them to visit the bathroom afterwards.

Calming the Overactive Child with Aromatherapy

The overactive child isn't necessarily "hyperactive" or overly active all the time. Sometimes children are overactive only at certain times of the day, or after eating certain foods, or reacting to their environment. Overactive doesn't mean abnormal or that something is wrong. However, by visiting a health care practitioner who specializes in natural medicine, you may be able to identify the cause of your child's hyperactivity. Its main sources in children are: intolerance to milk, wheat, sugar, chocolate, oranges, yeast, antibiotics, and food additives. They also may have deficiencies in zinc or magnesium, or may be suffering from low blood sugar (hypoglycemia), allergy, or a yeast infection. However, treatment of hyperactivity will not be the focus of this section; rather a discussion of over-activity in children is addressed, specifically how this state of overstimulation and excitement can benefit from relaxation and sedative essential oils. These oils can also help ease tantrums, anxiety attacks, and overtiredness, in addition to overactivity. Aromatherapy works on a subtle level, and is very unlike regular drugs which tend to take over the body's normal rhythm. Relaxation oils are natural plant derivatives which aid the body in relaxing, slowing the respiration and heart rate, and soothing an overstimulated nervous system. Reviewing the section on how essential oils are absorbed via the olfactory system would be useful to help understand how psycho-aromatherapy affects the nervous system.

There are several essential oils that can help to relax a child by affecting the nervous system. The most effective methods utilizing aromatherapy are those which can cross the blood-brain barrier by inhalation and direct olfactory and brain stimulation. Less direct, yet very effective, is the massage method whereby the sense of touch is combined with aromatherapy to benefit the entire body. When using therapeutic essential oils for relaxation, or for any other psycho-emotional outcomes, you must make sure that the essences are used within normal dosages, and not overused. If too much essential oil is used, or abused, the opposite effect of overwhelming the nervous system (and other systems involved) will result. Review the beginning of this chapter's discussion of treating children with aromatherapy and Chapter 1: Common-Sense Safety.

Case history: *A friend of mine complained that her teenage daughter would come home from middle school every afternoon acting very "hyper," loud, obnoxious and "testy." It began to bother her mother so much that she asked me for aromatherapy suggestions. I gave her a recipe for a room mist and a synergy blend for use in her diffuser. Massage was not a viable option that her teenage daughter would be open to, so I focused on inhalation methods to introduce the oils. Her mother diffused the essential oils in the kitchen and family room right before she came home from school. The room mist was used in her bedroom and sprayed on the phone! Her mother was very pleased with the calming effects of the oils, in addition to their nice scent. It was well received by the daughter as well, as she said she was able to concentrate better on her homework and felt less hurried. She looked forward to the relaxation of being home after a hectic day at school. She called the room spray "Mellow-mist" as this was the effect it had on her. Months later, my friend used the same recipes for her husband, who was experiencing a lot of stress at work. It helped him too!*

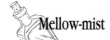 **Mellow-mist**

a room spray to relax

1 cup distilled water

20 drops Mandarin essential oil

10 drops Lavender essential oil

5 drops Marjoram essential oil

5 drops Sandalwood essential oil

a spray bottle with a fine mist nozzle

Fill a spray bottle with 1 cup of distilled water. Add the essential oils. Shake well before each use, as the essential oils float to the top of the water and are not soluble in water on their own. Use this aromatic water to mist a room, furniture, pillowcase or the telephone.

Aromatic baths can be very relaxing and calming for the overactive child. One of the single essential oils listed below can be used, or one of the recipes given in Chapter 11: The Aromatic Bath, specifically Serenity, Glad to Be Home, and Child's Play. Be sure to use half the adult dose for children, as many of these (except Child's Play) are given in amounts for adults. All these recipes include essential oils that are known to be relaxing and regulating. Also, footbaths are another nice way to enjoy the benefits of aromatherapy.

A diffuser, an electric nebulizer that emits pure essential oils into the air, is a most effective way to use aromatherapy for this purpose. With every breath, essences are having a direct effect on the nervous system. Chapter 13 is dedicated to all the various inhalation methods, including diffusers and room mists. Look ahead to that chapter for more ideas after reading this section if you wish. The Slow Down and Relax synergy blend, or the one below, is good recipe for calming the overactive person.

Slow Motion

a synergy blend for overactivity

4 parts Lavender essential oil

1 part Clary sage essential oil

1 part Cedarwood essential oil

1 part Sandalwood essential oil

This blend is meant to be used for inhalation purposes only. If a diffuser is to be used, then larger portions will be needed. Use one eye dropper to equal one part, or one teaspoon to make larger amounts. Diffuse 10 or 15 minutes prior to child coming home from school, or use as needed for overactivity. Diffuse for 15 minutes at a time. The essences will last several hours in the room air. May be diffused up to three times per day. Do not overuse!

Essential oils that can help the overactive child are chamomile, cedarwood, clary sage, lavender, mandarin, marjoram, neroli, orange, sandalwood, and tangerine.

Review the previous ailment section on promoting sleep. Many of the suggestions there will be appropriate for relaxation during the day, such as the aromatic massage oil, reading a book, and hugs!

Easing Teething Discomfort Safely

Most children can experience some discomfort with teething. Sometimes teething is very obvious: their cheeks become flushed, their gums are red and swollen, and they are more irritable than usual. Or you may be total-ly surprised when it happens, and the only indication is a runny nose, mild fever or drooling. All these symptoms are from the teeth erupting through the gums.

Thankfully nature has provided us with the chamomile plant, which is one of the most powerful anti-inflammatory essences known. A weak herbal infusion (tea) can be made from German chamomile (Matricaria chamomilla), also known as blue or Hungarian chamomile. This diluted herbal preparation can be sweetened with honey, and is generally well liked by children. Refer to the beginning of this chapter for herbal infusion dosing for children. And, of course, there is essential oil of Roman chamomile (Anthemis nobilis), also known as true chamomile or sweet chamomile. It is very effective as an analgesic when mixed with a vegetable oil and applied to sore and irritated gums. The following recipe is very effective and safe for babies experiencing teething discomfort.

Teething Oil

1 tbls. Olive oil

1 drop of Chamomile essential oil

Add the essential oil to the olive oil. Rub a small amount onto the affected gum line. Store in a small amber glass bottle with an eyedropper and label. Keep it in the refrigerator for future use, as the cool oil will provide addi-tional relief. Take it out a few minutes before applying, as the olive oil will thicken.

Lifestyle recommendations include offering cold teething rings, meant to be refrigerated, or natural teething biscuits such as those below made with natural ingredients.

Tasty Teething Biscuits

1 egg - beaten

3 tbls. honey

1 tbls. vegetable oil

1/4 cup condensed milk

1 tbls. wheatgerm

1 tbls. ground fennel seed

1 cup flour (whole wheat preferably)

Combine the wet ingredients in a bowl. Add the dry ingredients and mix until the dough is well combined and stiff. Roll out to about 1/4-inch thickness, and cut into rounds with a cookie cutter or open end of a glass. Place on an ungreased cookie sheet. (Let stand overnight for extra-hard biscuits). Bake at 350 degrees for 15 minutes or until lightly browned. Cool and store in an airtight container.

First Aid For Fevers

A rise in normal body temperature (above 98.4° F) is considered a fever. Besides measurement of temperature, symptoms may include shivering, coldness, heat, sweating, and delirium, depending upon the extent of temperature rise. A fever is a natural response by the body, for an increase in body temperature can kill germs and therefore protect the organism. If a fever rises above 103° F degrees, call your physician. The aromatherapy applications discussed here relate to mild to moderate fevers. Interfering with the body's attempt to protect itself is necessary when the fever gets too high, or causes discomfort. I would give the fever a chance to do what it is meant to do for at least three to four hours before initiating the first-aid recommendations.

Warning: Do not give aspirin for fever conditions, as this has been linked to Reye's Syndrome, which can lead to liver and brain damage.

Simple Compress for Fever

1 cup ice cold water

3 drops Lavender essential oil

1 drop Eucalyptus essential oil

washcloth

bowl

In a bowl add about 1 cup of ice-cold water. Add the essential oils and swish to disperse in the water. Soak the washcloth and then wring out most of the moisture so it is not dripping wet. Apply to the forehead. After it dries, or warms to body temperature, reapply a fresh compress. Check the temperature every 30 minutes. Do not use this on children younger than three years old without advice from your health care practitioner.

Folk medicine and grandmothers alike have used the sponging technique for high fevers. Tepid or cool water was used, and the feverish person was sponged down in an attempt to cool the body. A larger body surface was treated in this way. You can easily add essential oils known to have febrifuge (fever relieving) properties to decrease the body temperature. When a larger body surface is treated, as in sponging, a smaller amount of essential oil is needed. Also, tepid water is used, not ice-cold temperatures which would be too extreme for a whole-body treatment.

Aromatic Sponging

first aid for fever

basin of tepid water
2 drops Chamomile essential oil
washcloth or natural sea sponge

Fill a large basin half full with tepid water and add the essential oils. Swish the water to disperse as much as possible. Soak the sponge or cloth in the water. The feverish person should be lying on a bath towel. It is not necessary to remove all the clothing; just the upper chest, back area, and legs need to be exposed. Gently squeeze out the sponge, leaving it wet enough to cool the body. Starting from the neck down, sponge the body. Resoak the sponge as needed. Then do the same for the back side. Do not allow the person to chill, as this will cause heating of the body.

Essential oils capable of lowering body temperature (fevers) are basil, bergamot, chamomile, eucalyptus, ginger, hyssop, juniper, lavender, lemon, lemongrass, rosemary, tea tree and peppermint. Those that are antibacterial and antiseptic are listed on page 324 and would be appropriate to use as room mists or in a diffuser to prevent others from getting sick.

Bedrest is in order, along with drinking plenty of fluids. Taking extra Vitamin C is a prudent measure as well. The Old-Fashioned Onion and Garlic soup on page 97 can be made to help fight cold and flu symptoms.

CHAPTER 9

Aromatherapy Treatments for the Emotions, Moods, and Memory —Psycho-Aromatherapy

A Look at Psycho-Aromatherapy...

There is an old proverb that says "Food nourishes the body, but flowers heal the soul." Actually, I think the two—the mind and body—are inseparable. However, for the sake of understanding and study, they are often separated into two entirely different subjects. Science likes to compartmentalize to make such subjects manageable, although there are no systems within the body that work in isolation. John Madden, Ph.D, explains the body and mind connection as "when the mind thinks, the body listens." Many of the teachings and writings by Deepak Chopra, MD, have reflected similar perspectives on understanding the mind/body connection, which he calls "quantum" healing.

My aim is not to attempt to explain such complex issues, but to acknowledge the very real connection of the mind and body, and present aromatherapy applications that affect mood, emotions, and memory. Well known for its benefit as an aid to stress reduction and relaxation enhancement, aromatherapy is now beginning to be applied to other areas of emotional ailments and mental health challenges. For centuries, natural plant essences were used in the form of perfume and incense for aphrodisia, communing with the divine, prayer and meditation, and to ward off evil spirits. Today, the use of essential oils is being explored in the areas of memory recall, hypnosis, child-birthing, pain control, insomnia, meditation, and for various aspects of environmental fragrancing.

"The brain is the organ of longevity," says George Allan Sacher. It is also where the olfactory system directly integrates with the limbic portion of the brain, as reviewed in Chapter 1. It is 10,000 times more sensitive than any other sensory organ the body possesses. Because the limbic, or old brain, is where emotions, moods, memories, sexual desires, and various physiological functions originate, inhalation is the easiest and most direct route to affect these areas. In fact, essential oils are one of the few chemical constituents that are able to cross the blood-brain barrier. More study is needed; however, this may be an area of great potential in terms of immune strengthening, fertility problems, as well as psychological applications.

The brain physically consists of blood and nerve tissue. Somewhere between the physical and the non-biological lies the mind or spirit. There is an interrelationship between these aspects of the human physiology and the mind. Evidence is mounting connecting the thoughts and emotions to the general health of a person, and even linking certain emotions to specific ailments. For example, Dr. Dean Ornish's work has found a correlation between unexpressed emotion, namely anger, and heart disease. Emotional stress causes physical changes in the body which, over a lifetime, may result in a disease process. Stress causes a great deal of wear and tear on the nervous system and affects numerous other systems within the body. The endocrine, cardiovascular, respiratory, digestive, and immune systems are also negatively affected, particularly by chronic stress.

The brain is responsible for several functions. It regulates the endocrine system, muscles, heart rate, respiration, and all thought processes. It is recognized as the seat of consciousness and intelligence. It is where visualization, beliefs, reasoning, and memory originate. The brain is responsible for all conscious action and emotional responses. Its primary cellular unit is the neuron, which secretes an electrical neuro-chemical. In the healthy brain, there are healthy neurotransmitters in adequate number, making it possible to think clearly, recall memories, and the like.

The three basic neurotransmitter chemicals are acetylcholine, serotonin, and dopamine. Each has its own specific responsibilities. Serotonin is a sedative-like neuro-chemical manufactured by the brain to produce a feeling of well-being, relaxation, and deep sleep. Dopamine, on the other hand, produces a state of alertness and aggression. Acetylcholine is responsible for motor activity, action, and coordination. The use of therapeutic essential oils, such as chamomile and lavender, can affect serotonin levels by stimulating the portions of the brain responsible for its production. Other essential oils which stimulate alertness or have invigorating qualities, act similarly upon the brain via the olfactory and brain connection.

The brain is very much affected by our diet, since the neuro-chemical and electrical pathways must be supplied with adequate essential fatty acids, vitamins and minerals to work properly and stay in communication with each other. The brain is also affected by fragrance. With every breath, the aromatic molecules present in the air are inhaled and messages to the brain are sent. Unless the scent is detectable, only the unconscious brain is registering the information. However, physiological as well as psychological effects are taking place without your awareness. I strongly recommend that you read *An Open Invitation—Two Ways Essential Oils Enter the Body* (Chapter 1), inhalation specifically. That section will help you understand the olfactory system and brain connection and its importance in the relationship between the limbic brain and scent associations.

The use of essential oils in psycho-aromatherapy, or psycho-aromacology, is very exciting, although caution and discernment are required. Aromatherapy must always be utilized safely and in moderation. A subtle, pleasing aroma is most beneficial for obtaining mood, emotional, or psychological effects, but if the olfactory senses are overwhelmed by overuse of aromatics, the body can react negatively. For example, erogenous scents can be alluring and very pleasurable in minute amounts; however, if the scent is too concentrated, the risk of having an effect opposite from the one intended is highly possible (if not predictable), producing a repulsive rather than aphrodisiac aroma.

Scientists suggest any aromatic molecule, whether natural or synthetic, will have a psychological effect. But aromatherapists, or aroma-practitioners, strongly believe that only the natural essential oils and aromatics will have a therapeutic effect on the person because the use of synthetic scents risks sensitivities and non-productive results. More and more people are experiencing for themselves the effect aromatherapy has on their moods and emotions. Certainly, as studies show brain wave changes with particular aromas, and science can "measure" the effects, aromatherapy is becoming increasingly accepted among the general population.

Are You Stressed?

Of course you're stressed. Everyone experiences stress. Stress can be any factor that causes physical or mental tension, and can be experienced in varying degrees. Babies experience stress when they are hungry or get startled. Older children experience stress at school in the form of peer pressure or when taking exams. Adults, more than anyone, can experience the greatest amount of stress from work, family responsibilities, health, finances, and marital relationships. The fact is, you cannot always change outside stressors, those factors in the environment which cause anxiety. But you can learn to change how you will react. This is the key to coping with stress. It isn't about control; rather it is about identifying stress and finding better ways to handle it.

Some of the symptoms of stress are listed here, but realize there are many more which would likely take up several pages. Some of the more familiar include fatigue, headache, neck and back pain, palpitations, indigestion, stomach pain, loose bowels, depression, irritability, aggression, difficulty concentrating, and recurrent infections, such as colds.

There are several major health conditions strongly associated with chronic physical and emotional stress: angina, asthma, cardiovascular disease, depression, headaches, hypertension, immune depression, colds, PMS, and ulcers. And this is only a partial list.

Some unhealthy reactions to stress include irritability, inclination to argue, overeating, crying spells, loud and fast talk, overwork, aggressive behavior, isolation, drinking alcohol, or excessive sleeping. These reactions can certainly affect your enjoyment, your appreciation of life, and your state of health, as well as relationships.

One of the hardest things to do when you are under stress is also the most helpful: set aside time for yourself. Do things for yourself. Walk along the ocean or in the park. Water is very soothing. Take a cold shower or hot aromatic bath. Right after work seems to be the most frequent time for people to feel the greatest amount of stress. Set an electric diffuser to go on shortly before you arrive home from work. Put on some relaxing music or nature sounds, or better yet, take a walk. Exercise helps immensely with stress. While in your car commuting home, play tapes or do breathing exercises.

Nature in itself is a stress reducer. Billboards in Japan are painted with nature scenes to promote relaxation for their overcrowded, stress-prone inhabitants. The Japanese also catch cat naps on the subways, which are jam-packed with people. It is not surprising that one of the most densely populated countries in the world utilizes aromatherapy in its workplaces. In fact, Japan is very active in research in the psychological effects of fragrance, notably natural essences.

Identify your stressors by taking this "at home" test. Look at your coping options listed in part on the *50 Fun Coping Strategies*, and the aromatherapy recommendations and recipes given here. As I have said before, prevention is the best key to maintaining good health, which certainly applies to dealing with stress.

Do Any of These Stressors "Hit Home"?

Day-to-day life has countless stressors. Identifying even the smallest irritant, as well as major life stressors, assists us in recognizing the amount of stress we actually encounter . . . and the value of coping skills.

Stressors have a cumulative effect and can have unhealthy consequences relating to personal health, relationships, and all other life areas.

Check (✓) below the stressors you've experienced in the last few months.

❑ Your alarm clock not going off.
❑ Your favorite sports team losing.
❑ A recent illness.
❑ Dealing with bureaucracy/red tape.
❑ A divorce.
❑ Losing a friend's long-distance phone number.
❑ Working with incompetent people.
❑ Not being able to find a Kleenex . . . and needing it!
❑ Birth of a child.
❑ Being late on a deadline.
❑ Hearing disparaging comments about a minority.
❑ In-law problems.
❑ Spouse being under stress.
❑ Recent death of someone close to you.
❑ Having difficulty motivating yourself.
❑ Losing a game.
❑ Wanting to eat, but on a diet.
❑ Having only cold water for a bath.
❑ Spouse late coming home.
❑ Not being able to find the car keys.
❑ Anxiously awaiting a phone call.
❑ Late paying a bill.
❑ Someone telling you what to do.
❑ Moving to a new city.
❑ Not enough time for yourself.
❑ Having an empty gas tank and being in a rush.
❑ Sexual problems.
❑ Threat of war.
❑ Planning a large event.
❑ Being in trouble with the law.

❑ Anniversary of a beloved's death.
❑ Not having enough money to pay the bills.
❑ Parents treating you like a child.
❑ A new job.
❑ Someone telling you how to feel.
❑ Inability to conceive a child.
❑ Having no money and not wanting to borrow.
❑ Arguing with a good friend or relative.
❑ Out-of-town relatives staying with you.
❑ Spouse being too dependent on you.
❑ Seeing signs of aging in the mirror.
❑ Unwanted pregnancy.
❑ Not feeling well and not knowing why.
❑ Best friend asking to borrow money.
❑ An appliance/machine not working.
❑ Too much to do, not enough time.
❑ Someone canceling plans one-half hour before.
❑ Moving to a new house or apartment.
❑ Good friend feeling depressed.
❑ Someone telling you how to drive.
❑ Job interview.
❑ Boss putting pressure on you.
❑ Saying "yes" to too many things.
❑ Waiting in a long line.
❑ Being charged too much money.
❑ Electricity going out.
❑ Children not taking responsibility for themselves.
❑ _____
❑ _____

These stressors may not change; however, your ability to "cope" with them *can* change!

From *Life Management Skills* ©1991 Wellness Reproductions Inc. (800) 669-9208.

A Gallup poll taken in July 1994 showed job stress and money problems were the two most frequent causes of stress for adults. Family responsibilities and stress was third on the list. Housework and health problems were fourth and fifth, with stress caused from child care following.

Chronic stress is perhaps more damaging than the acute form, which causes a "flight or fight" response. In chronic or prolonged forms a cycle can develop whereby physical tension is experienced, which affects the immune system by weakening it, resulting in decreased energy, mental tension, compromised health, and disturbed sleep. Likewise, mental stress can cause the same stress cycle. The goal is to prevent stress, and next to be able to cope with it once it is experienced.

The relaxation response interferes with the stress cycle by breaking the chain of events. All of the coping strategies discussed here are capable of promoting a relaxed state. Essential oils used in aromatic baths, massage application, and inhalation methods have the potential to enhance physical and mental relaxation, thereby increasing energy and strengthening the immune system. Relaxation promotes better quality sleep and clear thinking and alertness. More energy means an active lifestyle and better health. So you can see how incorporating relaxation and a good stress-relief program can prevent chronic stress from taking a strong hold in your life by interrupting this cycle of events.

Effective Tools and Treatment for Alleviating and Coping with Stress

Relaxation is a skill which can be learned. Its positive effects last throughout the day. When relaxation is experienced on a regular basis, pain is decreased, illness is less likely and stress is lowered. Balance is key in a good stress-reduction program, as well as prevention. Refer to the holistic health wheel illustration on page 23 to review what areas in your life may be unbalanced. Make a list of what brings you joy and health, and another list of what you spend your time doing, including responsibilities, work, etc. Compare the lists. Which one is longer? See what items you can let go of and cross off the list. See where you might be able to organize or delegate some things to others. There is more to life than work. The old saying "stop along the way to smell the roses" is about just this very topic. If you work too hard, you are bound to lose sight of what is really important in life, like your health and your family.

During the day take breaks to go outside for a quick stroll, or spend the time in a quiet place and practice the breathing exercises, or simply close your eyes and "be" for 5 to 10 minutes. In the long run you will have more energy and work more efficiently when fatigue is prevented. Hook up a diffuser in your work area to combat stress and purify the air. Inhalation of essential oils during the day is one of the most effective and easiest ways to enjoy the benefits of aromatherapy. Room sprays are another simple method to encourage relaxation in the office. I suggest you read Chapter 13: Breathe Easy for a complete discussion on inhalation methods and excellent synergy blends to prevent stress. Recipes such as *Slow Down and Relax, I Love My Job,* and *Tropical Oasis* are a few good choices that offer anti-stress benefits. I am including several more options here, that can also be used in the home, office, psychotherapy setting for hypnosis, medical treatment exam rooms or hospitals, and other places where stressful conditions are present. Since these recipes are made of pure essential oils, without a carrier, they are to be used in a diffuser, aroma lamp, or simply inhaled from a tissue to which you have applied a few drops. For diffuser use, you will need to make a substantial amount to run through the machine. Alternatively, only a few drops are needed for the aroma lamp or handkerchief methods. Please refer to Chapter 13 for more options.

Anti-Stress Synergy

4 parts Lavender essential oil

2 parts Bergamot essential oil

1 part Ylang ylang essential oil

Deep Relaxation Blend

6 parts Lavender essential oil

2 parts Marjoram essential oil

1 part Mandarin essential oil

Lavender Fields

6 parts Lavender essential oil

1 part Sandalwood essential oil

In addition to making the list suggested above, there are many other helpful stress reducers. Organizing your time better is one of them. Creating a personal space of comfort which promotes relaxation and peace and quiet is crucial. Practice "being" and not "doing." If you are a busy type, try knitting or crocheting; this can be relaxing for some. Regular exercise in the form of walking, yoga, and dancing are ways to alleviate stress and prevent it. The breathing exercises given on page 102 of Chapter 4 are very effective in stress reduction and can be done almost anywhere.

Massage, especially aromatherapy massage, is a wonderful way to reduce stress. Ask for a massage or give yourself a mini-version of one. Progressive muscle relaxation exercises are very relaxing and increase your body awareness to differentiate when the muscles are tense or in a relaxed state. The massage oil blend below is designed for a full body massage (2% dilution). Take this with you to the massage therapist or use it at home. The oil should be warmed prior to applying it to the skin. See Chapter 12 for aromatherapy massage tips. Take turns with your mate once a week or more, giving each other a simple aromatherapy massage using this easy recipe for calming the mind and body. Don't be fooled by its simplicity. It's wonderful!

Massage Oil for Stress

2 tbls. sweet almond (or vegetable oil)

10 drops Lavender essential oil

2 drops Neroli or *Rose essential oil*

In a shallow dish or bottle, add the essential oils. Add two tablespoons of warm vegetable oil or sweet almond oil. Mix well. Apply to the skin with slow rhythmic hand strokes, working towards the heart. Be sure to pay special attention to the hands, feet, and neck.

Prayer, meditation, hypnosis, singing, gardening, walking along the beach, and flying a kite are all very different ways people can choose to relax. The list of *50 "Fun" Coping Strategies* is interesting because it presents many different ways to handle stress and to unwind. Some you may find appropriate for you and others you will not be interested in at all. Find the things that sound good to you. Practice, put forth the time and energy it will take to learn these skills. You will live with a fuller appreciation of life and live longer!

50 "Fun" Coping Strategies

Feed the ducks
Skip rocks on a lake
Read a good book
Build a puzzle
Keep a journal
Take a walk with a friend
Watch an old classic movie
Do a relaxing aromatic foot bath
Ask for an aromatherapy foot or back massage
Play with bubbles
Have a pillow fight
Simplify your life

Go kite flying on a windy day

Ask a friend for a hug

Give three compliments today

Give yourself affirmations

Listen to your favorite music

Take a long, warm, aromatic bath

Play with bath toys in the tub

Visit a botanical garden or park

Learn how to Rollerblade

Make a snowman

Watch a funny movie

Eat by candlelight

Roast marshmallows over a fire

Take a bike ride with a friend

Go canoeing

Pet a dog or cat

Suck on a lollipop

Listen to the ocean in a shell

Browse in a book store

Grow some herbs in a window box

Drink warm milk with nutmeg

Play hand shadows on the wall

Write to an old friend

Finger paint

Visit a museum

Go bird watching

Tell stories

Climb a tree

Start a new hobby

Visit a new park and explore

Treat yourself to a three-day weekend

Look at the stars

Go horseback riding

Build a sand castle

Go on a picnic

Skip rope

Hoolahoop

Sit under a tree and daydream . . .

How do you know if these coping strategies are working? Your mind will be quiet. You will feel more peaceful and your body will feel calm and relaxed. The effects of a good stress-release program will last throughout the day. You will experience less illness, less pain, and experience fewer unhealthy reactions to stress in the future.

Aromatic baths are one of my favorite ways to unwind and pamper myself. They are especially helpful in relieving stress and aiding relaxation at the end of a long day. The warmth of the water, in addition to the relaxing benefits of the essential oils, melts away muscle tension and helps to quiet the mind. There are many recipes and a entire chapter dedicated to *The Aromatic Bath* in this book. I suggest you read Chapter 11 next if this method of relaxation appeals to you. Some good anti-stress recipes there are the *TGIF Blend, Serenity Blend, Undress-De-Stress* and *Glad To Be Home* blends. I am including several recipes here that also aid in relaxation and stress-reduction, using aromatic baths and inhalation, along with an herb tea you can make. Bath salts, honey, milk and other carriers can be used to transport the essential oils into the bath water. Recipes for these are in Chapter 11. Concentrate on your breathing while soaking. Breath by inhaling deeply and slowly. Visualize being in your favorite place; it may be an herb garden, flower garden, or at the ocean. Exhale through your nose, pushing out all the day's stress and negative energy. Repeat this several times if you wish, until you find yourself in a peaceful and restful place.

For stress, the aim naturally is to relax and unwind the mind and body and a very warm bath will be most effective to this end. However, staying in a hot bath too long can have a draining effect and should be avoided. See hydrotherapy guidelines for bath temperatures in Chapter 11. Take a warm bath right after work or before retiring. Darken the room and light a few candles which can facilitate relaxation. Close the bathroom door, and hang a "Do Not Disturb" sign on the door to discourage interruption. You will get the most amount of benefit from the essences if they are contained in the room. If you have a tension headache, rub a few drops of lavender on your temples before soaking in the bath water. See "tension headaches" in this chapter for more on that topic.

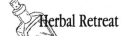

Herbal Retreat

Bath Salts (or other carrier)

7 drops Lavender essential oil

2 drops Lemongrass essential oil

1 drop Basil essential oil

Add the essential oils to the carrier and add to a full bath. Warm to hot water temperature is suggested. Soak for 20 to 30 minutes.

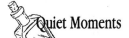

Quiet Moments

2 tbls. Honey (or other carrier)

6 drops Sandalwood essential oil

2 drops Bergamot essential oil

2 drops Ylang ylang essential oil

In a small dish, add the honey. Mix in the essential oils and combine well by stirring. Add to a full warm bath. Soak for 20 to 30 minutes.

Stress-Release Soak

1/4 – 1/2 cup heavy cream (or other carrier)

6 drops Lavender essential oil

2 drops Mandarin essential oil

1 drop Bergamot essential oil

1 drop Clary sage essential oil

In a cup add the cream. Add the essential oils and mix well to combine. Dry powdered milk can be used as an alternative to the cream. Simply make a thick paste with water and add the essential oils to it. Add the aromatic cream to a full warm bath and stir with your hands. Soak for 20 to 30 minutes.

If you haven't the time for a full aromatic bath, do a foot bath by using half the amount of essential oils (4–5 drops per foot bath). See directions for "Quick 'n' Easy Shortcuts" in Chapter 11. Bath salts and Castile lotion are your best options for foot bath carriers. Brew a cup of *No Worries* herb tea to sip while soaking for additional benefit.

This herbal tea blend is very soothing to the nervous system. It can be consumed several times per day or taken an hour before bedtime to encourage a restful sleep. Use 1 to 2 teaspoons per cup of hot water and allow to steep for 5 minutes. This can be made in a larger quantity and kept in the refrigerator. It doesn't have to be hot to drink; it makes a nice iced beverage blended with fruit juices or sparkling mineral water. You do not have to wait to be under stress to enjoy it either! Use dried herbs and flowers to prepare this mixture and store in a glass jar.

No Worries Herb Tea

relaxing blend for stress

2 parts Chamomile flowers

2 parts Lemonbalm herb

1 part Catnip herb

1 part Lavender flowers

1 part Peppermint leaf

1 part Rose petals

1 part Lemongrass (optional)

A pinch of nutmeg to taste

Vanilla Honey (optional, recipe on page 295)

Combine the dried herbs, flowers, and spices in a glass jar. Label. To prepare one cup of herbal tea, use 1 to 2 teaspoons per cup of hot water. Steep for 5 minutes.

Essential oils useful for stress reduction and promoting relaxation are basil, bergamot, chamomile, clary sage, geranium, juniper, lavender, lemongrass, marjoram, neroli, rose, sandalwood, and ylang ylang.

Dietary recommendations include avoiding caffeine, sugar, salt, and nicotine. By adopting a healthy diet which includes raw nuts and seeds, flax oil, whole grains, fresh fruits and vegetables, pure water, and herbal tea, you will be building the body, not draining it of energy. Bananas, rice, milk, and pasta contain tryptophan, an amino acid that encourages relaxation. Eat more of these. Bring healthy snacks to the office or have them handy during the day. Lowfat granola, dried fruit, fruit and vegetable juices, yogurt, raw vegetables, rice cakes, popcorn, and whole grain crackers are some excellent choices that will provide you with energy and fight fatigue.

Recovery from Nervous Exhaustion

Nervous exhaustion or mental exhaustion is a "burn out" state of fatigue most often caused by a combination of factors such as overworking, high levels of chronic stress, and not receiving enough positive feedback. Often perfectionism underlies the exhaustion—the belief that you must do it all, and do it perfectly. Clearly a good stress reduction program was not in place or was not being practiced if you get to this point of extreme weariness. At this time realize that you are very prone to catching colds and infections, as the immune system, as well as the nervous system, has been overwhelmed.

Case history: *A 42-year-old business manager of a software company talked to me about his feeling "burdened" and "burned out." He had neglected his family, his personal needs, and much of the household responsibilities. He was working 50 to 60 hours per week at a very stressful job. He traveled frequently and ate poorly, as he wasn't home most evenings in time for dinner. He was a prime example of nervous and mental exhaustion. Fatigue was evident. He knew he needed to take action to remedy the state he was in. In general his health was good. His major complaint was feeling "tightly wound up like a rubber band" and having very little energy. To make a long story a little shorter, he made his lists and crossed out much of what he could delegate to others at work. He used the aromatherapy recommendations in the sauna at the exercise club, took baths at home (sometimes with his wife), and purchased a diffuser for his office. He did the deep breathing exercises regularly and started running again in the morning before work. He started eating healthier and brought snacks to work and on his business travels. Within a week or more he began feeling more in control of his life, more positive, and seemed to have more free time.*

Re-Charge Synergy Blend

for nervous tension

6 parts Lavender essential oil
3 parts Basil essential oil
2 parts Pine essential oil
1 part Nutmeg essential oil

Mix the essential oils in an amber glass bottle. Use a few drops in an aroma lamp or inhale from a tissue. Ideally, this blend is nice to use in a diffuser to disperse the essential oils into the room air two or three times per day. See Chapter 13 for inhalation methods and directions.

Re-Fuel

an aromatic bath to relieve nervous tension

Bath salts (or other carrier)
5 drops Patchouli essential oil
3 drops Clary sage essential oil
2 drops Eucalyptus essential oil

Choose a carrier to transport your essential oils into the bath water. Bath salts contain Epsom and sea salt and make a good choice. Add the essential oils to the carrier and mix well. Pour the bath preparation into a full warm bath and stir with your hand. Soak for 20 to 30 minutes.

Essential oils that are helpful in conditions of mental and nervous exhaustion are those which affect the nervous system and aid in regulating and relaxing. Those used most often are basil, clary sage, eucalyptus, geranium, ginger, grapefruit, hyssop, jasmine, lavender, lemongrass, marjoram, neroli, nutmeg, patchouli, petitgrain, rosemary, ylang ylang, and pine.

Lifestyle and dietary changes are crucial to prevent fatigue and to build the body's defenses and nourish the nervous system. Taking a midday catnap for 20 minutes can bring added energy. Exercise is recommended on a regular basis, to help with stress and encourage better sleep. Start slow and at a level comfortable for you. Walking is a great form of exercise, especially when it's done outdoors in nature. Stretching exercises are also good as is yoga. The Sun Salutation yoga asanas are particularly effective for both stretching all the major muscle groups and for vitality. Developing a regular sleep pattern by going to bed and rising at the same time can be helpful. Take time to relax during the day, and listen to nature sounds or relaxing music. And have more fun—humor is good medicine for you!

Also, prioritize your day, performing major tasks in the morning and fewer in the afternoon when you may be less energetic. Confront your perfectionism by allowing yourself to be human. Be realistic in your expectations of yourself and others. And, by all means, ask for help either by finding a good friend to listen to you or by delegating tasks.

Dietary recommendations include avoiding unhealthy foods in general, and eating small frequent healthy snacks during the day to prevent fatigue. See the previous section on stress and the recommendations given there. All of them apply to you. Take the stress test and see where you can prevent future stress and adopt a good prevention program.

How to Use Aromatherapy to Relieve Anxiety

Anxiety is caused by stress. It is a general feeling of apprehension. Fear may be the underlying feeling that has not been outwardly expressed. Behaviors that may be part of anxiety are negative thinking, uncontrollable and recurring thoughts, mild disorientation, nervous tension, and irritability. Procrastination is another behavior seen in anxious people, and is the flip side to perfectionism. Symptoms can include tight breathing, palpitations, and increased perspiration. Chapter 5 discusses palpitations due to anxiety and gives information that may prove useful to you as well.

Use the *Slow Down and Relax* inhalation blend in Chapter 13 or use *A Peaceful Pace*, which is another inhalation blend given in Chapter 5 on page 121. The latter was specifically designed for anxiety and is highly recommended to use three times daily in a diffuser or aroma lamp. The most effective methods to incorporate aromatherapy for anxiety are inhalation, aromatic baths, and massage. A lifestyle that includes these methods, in addition to herbal teas and dietary changes, will provide the best outcome and prevention program.

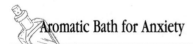 ### Aromatic Bath for Anxiety

Bath salts (or other carrier)

5 drops Lavender essential oil

3 drops Ylang ylang essential oil

2 drops Bergamot essential oil

Add the essential oils to the carrier. Add the bath preparation to a full warm bath. Soak for 20 to 30 minutes.

This massage oil can be applied to the back or used as a foot or hand massage preparation. It is concentrated, and not designed for whole body application. Adjust if necessary by using the User-Friendly Blending Chart in Chapter 15 for dilution change. A back massage is very rewarding and relaxing for the receiver, especially one experiencing anxiety. Take your time giving this massage and prepare the environment using some of the suggestions given in the helpful hints in Chapter 12.

Anti-Anxiety Massage Oil

apply to the back area

2 tbls. vegetable oil

12 drops Lavender essential oil

6 drops Ylang ylang essential oil

4 drops Frankincense essential oil

3 drops Clary sage essential oil

In an amber glass bottle, add the essential oils and vegetable oil. Shake gently to mix well. Label. To use, warm the oil by placing in a hot water bath. Apply to the back area in light and gentle strokes.

Essential oils useful in anxiety are basil, bergamot, chamomile, clary sage, frankincense, hyssop, jasmine, juniper, geranium, lavender, lemon, neroli, orange, petitgrain, rose, ylang ylang, and sandalwood.

Lifestyle recommendations include relaxation exercises such as deep breathing exercises (page 102), and concentrating on your breath. These decrease stress and aid in relaxation by blocking out external stimuli. Changing negative thinking patterns is not easy but can be done .

Confronting any recurring fears or fearful thoughts may be necessary to face the apprehension that is sometimes experienced. It is human to feel fear, but it should not predominate in your thoughts. Moving through the fear, taking action, and finding someone to listen to you may all be of help. Take the stress test and see which areas of your life cause you the greatest stress and worry.

Dietary recommendations include avoiding stimulants such as caffeine, alcohol, and cola drinks. Supplement your diet with vitamin-rich foods, especially Vitamins B and C, and the anti-oxidants. Refer to the section on stress for more dietary suggestions. Drink the herbal tea recipe given there called *No Worries*; it will benefit you in relieving feelings of tension.

Potent Remedies for Tension Headaches

Tension headaches are typically slow to develop and are a result of stress. They can be frontal (forehead area) or temporal (in the temple region on either side of the head) or in the back of the head at the base of the neck. Headaches range in intensity from mild to severe and, if ignored, can be quite debilitating. Overstimulation, such as loud noise or straining the eyes, can result in a tension headache. Long hours of unrelieved working and also emotional tension can cause this stress-related condition; prevention is important in any treatment.

There are several types of headaches, including migraines, which can have a wide variety of causes, such as hormonal imbalances, medications, water weight gain and bloating, and food allergies. Here we are addressing stress headaches caused by nervous tension or muscular tension. People who have experienced whiplash or other neck injuries often complain that the neck area is their weak spot as a result. If they do not pay attention to their stress levels and their body's reaction to stress, they can find themselves with a tension headache.

> **Case history:** *A woman in her early thirties who was late to a class I was teaching came hurrying in looking very stressed. After sharing her mishaps and events that she had just experienced, she sat down and asked what I had for a headache, as her head was throbbing painfully. I warmed some headache oil in my hands and applied it to her temples, massaging very gently and with light pressure. I suggested she concentrate on her breathing and slow it down. I allowed her to inhale the essences from my cupped hands by placing them over her nose and mouth area. Within a few minutes her headache was gone. She was very pleased with the quick results and the rest of the class was amazed.*

There are many different ways to handle tension and the headaches that are caused by it. Review the section in this chapter which discusses stress and the various ways to cope with it. Below is a recipe for a headache oil which is extremely effective for headaches caused by stress. It is a massage oil concentrate and should be used in small amounts on the temples and hairline. Plain lavender or peppermint essential oil both work singly, but I choose to use them together in this blend. Lavender is known for its soothing properties on the nervous system, while peppermint is a mild analgesic and anti-inflammatory agent. They work synergistically to remedy a headache.

Headache Oil

massage oil for tension headaches

1 tbls. vegetable oil
10 drops Lavender essential oil
5 drops Peppermint essential oil
200 IU's Vitamin E (optional)

In an amber glass bottle, add the essential oils and vegetable oil. Add the vitamin E. If using the gel capsule form of Vitamin E, cut off one end and squeeze the contents into the oils. Shake well to mix completely. Label with directions for use. To use, warm a few drops of the concentrated oil and apply to the temples of the head and just beyond the hairline. Typically this area is sore to the touch if the headache is severe. Gently massage this area with a light pressure. Inhale the essences from cupped hands following the massage. Breathe slowly and concentrate on the breath.

Another excellent remedy for headaches is the cold footbath with essential oils. I know it sounds strange, but by soaking your feet in cold water you draw blood from the head, which brings immediate relief for headaches. Also, there are reflexology points of the hands and feet that can be used for this ailment. Read the section on footbaths in Chapter 11: The Aromatic Bath for more information on this method of applying aromatherapy.

Aromatic Footbath for Headache Relief

2 tbls. Castile lotion (or other carrier)
4 drops Lavender essential oil
2 drops Peppermint essential oil
A basin or tub
cold water
a towel

Fill a tub or basin (large enough to hold both feet comfortably) half full with cold water. See hydrotherapy guidelines in Chapter 11 for water temperature uses. To the castile lotion soap, or other carrier that you have chosen, add the essential oils and mix well. Add to the water and stir with your hands. Soak both feet in the cold aromatic water for 15 to 20 minutes. Sit comfortably while doing the footbath. Concentrate on breathing slowly and deeply. Relax.

Cool or warm aromatic compresses can be used for effective headache relief as well. If you have a frontal headache, a cool compress can be made with lavender essential oil. For headaches which involve the base of the neck and head area, a warm compress will aid blood flow and give relief. Please refer to Chaper 12 for directions on how to prepare compresses.

Other headache remedies include meditation, visualization, breathing exercises (page 102), yoga, listening to relaxation tapes and reflexology. For mild eyestrain and headache you may want to try an eye pillow made with lavender flowers. It offers relief for mild symptoms and can be kept by the bedside or in an office drawer. My recipe for eye pillows can be found on page 332 of Chapter 13: Breathe Easy. Also, an idea similar to the eye pillow is to warm your hands by rubbing them together briskly and cupping them over your eyes for gentle relief. If eye strain is a probable cause, review that topic in Chapter 3. If your headaches are a result of hormonal fluctuations as in PMS or menopause, turn to those ailments for further recommendations regarding aromatherapy applications.

Lifestyle recommendations include avoiding stress and finding ways to cope with it in order to prevent these headaches. The recommendations given in the Stress section will be very helpful. Keep the headache oil or eye pillow handy at the office or at home. Remember to listen to your body and take care of your headache promptly, rather than waiting until it is severe.

Dietary suggestions include looking at your diet to see if there are particular foods which cause the headaches. Salty foods can cause water retention and be a factor in some headaches; avoidance may help. Refer to the beginning of Chapter 2 on the digestive system for information regarding expansive versus contractive food properties. This subject of using food as medicine may be useful in some cases.

What Is Depression and Can Aromatherapy Really Help?

Depression has many symptoms which can range from mild to severe. A depressed mood can include feeling down, powerlessness, boredom, weight loss or gain, sleep problems, agitation, fatigue, loss of interest in activities, difficulty in concentrating, and indecisiveness.

Causes of depression are still debated and theorized in many respects. There can be a genetic factor, or possibly a neuro-chemical imbalance of the brain. It can come from stress, negative thinking, and poor coping styles. Inadequate social and family support is another factor to consider in depression, as well as unexpressed anger or loss. It is most common in women, and may be related to hormonal factors and body image perceptions. Depression experienced following childbirth is not uncommon, and is discussed in Chapter 10: Aromatherapy Treatments for Women Only. Depression appears among teenagers and adults, and especially among the helping professions, such as nurses. It also occurs frequently among people of poor health and those who are experiencing grief over the loss of a loved one. Also see Anosmia in Chapter 3 for the link between a decreased or absent sense of smell and depression.

People who have Seasonal Affective Disorder (SAD) experience depression when they are deprived of sufficient light. Sunlight sends signals to the brain via the optic nerve to stimulate the hypothalamus. This portion of the brain is responsible for regulating moods, sleep, and hunger. Therefore some of the symptoms of SAD are decreased energy, difficulty concentrating, sleepiness, cravings for sweets, and depression. Use of essential oils for regulation and balance by stimulating the hypothalamus can help in this area: frankincense, bergamot, and geranium, and the citrus oils can have a generally uplifting and "sunny" effect. Light therapy is now being explored for people experiencing this disorder.

The word "depression" means to "push down." Periods of stress or loss may cause one to feel "blue" or "down in the dumps." Aromatherapy can help in mild forms of depression, and is the topic of this section. However, if you, or someone you know, is severely depressed, additional support and therapy are necessary because it is unrealistic to think aromatherapy will affect a deeply depressed person. Depression is sometimes a complex condition involving many facets of a person's life. There is no simple answer or one individual remedy, although aromatherapy can be very helpful in complementing other forms of therapy.

Some treatments useful for depression are cognitive behavior therapy, which looks at changing the belief system and unhealthy behaviors of a person experiencing difficulty functioning. Anti-depressant drugs are widely prescribed in the United States for treatment; group therapy support is considered helpful as well. Exercise, flower essence therapy and light therapy are additional ways to counteract depression.

Case history: *A 55-year-old psychotherapist consulted with me for depression. She had just experienced several losses in her life over the past six months, and was also experiencing anxiety. She had used anti-depressant drugs in the past and wanted to avoid taking them if she could. We worked together to implement an aromatherapy plan that would benefit her lifestyle and emotional needs. She followed the dietary recommendations made to her as well as taking daily walks outside on her lunch break. More important, she began using essential oils in her bath, in massage preparations, and in a diffuser which she used in her office between client appointments and in her bedroom at home. She also used a blend of oils for a hand and chest massage. Working* *with this woman and seeing the positive results take place prompted me to incorporate the anger and sadness oils in depression blends. She did not need to go on any medications, and seemed to be completely over her depressed feelings within about two weeks. Prior to this, her experience with depression had lasted for several months before she "came out of it," and that was with the aid of anti-depressant drugs.*

Inhalation, aromatic baths, and full body massage are the ideal methods of applying essential oils to those experiencing feelings of hopelessness, boredom and loss of interest. The goals for overcoming this health challenge are to diminish the feeling of depression, to enhance a feeling of well-being and to prevent physical illness.

You will notice that many of the essential oils used for depression are from flowers and fruit. These essences tend to be light and ethereal in nature, with an uplifting effect on the mind and emotions. Pure Bulgarian rose oil is one of the most employed essences for use in depression, grief, bereavement, sadness, and low self-esteem. Unfortunately, it is also one of the most expensive essential oils you can buy, and with good reason. It takes several thousand pounds of hand-picked rose petals to make one pound of its precious aromatic oil. Although it is used primarily in the perfume industry (fine European perfumes) and in high-end aromatherapy skin care preparations, it is highly recommended as an anti-depressant. Regarded by many aroma practitioners as the strongest anti-depressant known, rose oil is well worth its costly price tag which, for 1/16th of an ounce, can be somewhere between $30 and $60 dollars. This amount, however, used for inhalation purposes only, can last about six months when used twice daily. Bulgaria produces the finest rose oil in the world, and is the essence of choice for psycho-aromatherapy.

This particular blend for depression is by far my favorite and generally the most popular, because it works well for many people and has a heavenly scent that is extremely pleasurable to use. The clary sage is euphoric and anti-depressant. Ylang ylang is useful in states of anger and is anti-depressant. Geranium is regulating and balancing, while the basil is helpful in clearing the mind, is anti-depressant and useful for mental fatigue. Sandalwood is the base note essence in this blend which eases nervous tension and concentration difficulty. This blend is made entirely of essential oils (no carrier oil), and is designed for diffuser use. It can also be used in an aroma lamp, potpourri burner, or a few drops on a tissue. This is an inhalation synergy blend that should be used three to four times daily. If using an electric diffuser, allow it to run for 15 minutes at a time. Read Chapter 13: Breathe Easy for alternate inhalation methods.

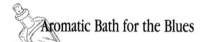

Nature's Answer

an inhalation blend for mild depression

4 parts Clary sage essential oil

4 parts Ylang ylang essential oil

3 parts Geranium essential oil

2 parts Basil essential oil

1 part Sandalwood essential oil

Mix the above essential oils in an amber glass bottle. Label. To use in a diffuser, simply add to the bottle or reservoir for the apparatus. If using this blend in an aroma lamp or simmering pot, add 4 to 6 drops and allow to diffuse into the room.

Besides the daily inhalation blend, taking an aromatic bath two to three times per week is especially helpful. Sometimes the aromatic baths are effective enough on their own as a remedy for mild bouts of depression or feeling blue. Draw a warm bath and soak for as long as you are comfortable.

Aromatic Bath for the Blues

for mild bouts of depression

1/4 cup Honey (or other carrier)

3 drops Lavender essential oil

3 drops Ylang ylang essential oil

2 drops Basil essential oil

2 drops Geranium essential oil

1 drop Grapefruit essential oil

Mix the essential oils in the honey. For other carrier options refer to Chapter 11: The Aromatic Bath. Fill the bathtub with warm water and then add the aromatic honey mixture. Stir well using your hands. Soak for 20 to 30 minutes. Play your favorite music and light a candle or two. Sip on a cup of *Feel Good* herb tea (recipe given later in this section) while in the tub.

Last but not least, an aromatherapy massage oil to use if you are feeling down. Getting a full-body massage is one of the best ways you can treat yourself. It is pampering and nurturing, in addition to very satisfying, as touch is a basic need. Massage and aromatherapy go hand in hand in treating nervous system ailments such as depression. This blend can be diluted further to make a whole-body massage oil that you can bring to the massage therapist with you. See the User-Friendly Blending Chart in the back of this book for easy blending directions. Otherwise, if you will be applying this oil, a concentrated version can be made for use on smaller body areas. This is a concentrated massage oil blend, designed for application to the back of the hands, and upper chest (between the breasts and lower neck region).

Elation Formulation

a concentrated massage oil for mild depression

2 tbls. sweet almond oil (or vegetable oil)

1 tsp. Wheat germ oil

8 drops Lavender essential oil

8 drops Ylang ylang essential oil

2 drops Basil essential oil

2 drops Geranium essential oil

2 drops Bergamot essential oil

In an amber glass bottle, add the essential oils. Add the sweet almond oil and wheat germ oil. Shake gently to mix well. Label. To use apply a small amount onto the back of the hands and chest area. Inhale the essences from your hands after application to the skin. During the day, inhale from the back of the hands. The oils will also be absorbed through the skin. Apply two or three times daily.

Feel Good Herb Tea

to encourage a feeling of well-being

3 parts lemonbalm herb

1 part Lavender flowers

1 part Rose petals

1 part Spearmint leaf

1 part St. John's Wort

1 part marjoram

Vanilla honey to taste (recipe page 295)

Mix the above herbs and flowers in a bowl. Store in a glass jar and label. To prepare use 1 to 2 teaspoons of herb per cup. Pour hot water over herbs and allow to steep for 5 to 10 minutes. Flavor with honey or lemon if desired. Drink up to three cups per day.

Essential oils used for depression are basil, bergamot, cedarwood, clary sage, frankincense, geranium, grapefruit, lavender, lemon, jasmine, myrrh, neroli, rose, sandalwood, spruce, orange, and ylang ylang. Essential oils that can have a positive influence on feelings of anger, which are associated with depression, can be useful as well and include rose, chamomile, ylang ylang, and rosemary. If the depression is associated with a loss, then essential oils helpful for grief and bereavement, such as lavender, rose, frankincense, neroli, hyssop, and marjoram, should be included.

Traditional herbs that may help depression are basil, thyme, lemonbalm, St. John's Wort, lavender, spearmint, peppermint, rose petals, gingko, marjoram, lemon verbena, and ginseng.

Lifestyle recommendations involve being in the company of others and avoiding isolation. Set your day's tasks by prioritizing, and be realistic in your goal setting. Exercise is extremely beneficial as it produces "feel good" hormones and boosts circulation. Exercise will also keep your body trim and strengthen the immune system. Take daily walks, preferably in the park or along the sea shore, to connect with nature and appreciate the beauty it offers. Fresh air and deep breathing exercises are both good in aiding relaxation and promoting good oxygenation of the entire body. Give yourself a "treat" or special activity occasionally, such as fresh flowers, but avoid using food as a reward if this is an issue for you. Volunteering and helping others is another way to focus on someone other than yourself and your own problems. Ask for support from friends, family, or church members. Replace negative thinking with positive affirmations.

Dietary suggestions include avoiding caffeine, black tea, and alcohol. Use the herbs listed above in cooking, fresh in salads, and as spices. Eat more wheatgerm, which is an energizer. Pears, apples, and nuts contain bromine which assists the nervous system in functioning properly.

Best Insomnia Blends

There are approximately 40 million Americans who suffer from chronic sleep disorders, while another 20 to 30 million experience occasional bouts of sleep disturbance. Insomnia is a symptom, not an ailment, that is associated with poor-quality or disturbed sleep. It doesn't necessarily equate to the number of hours you sleep, but rather to how you feel when you awaken the next day. Insomniacs may have trouble getting to sleep or getting back to sleep once they have awakened during the night or early morning hours. People who suffer from insomnia will feel fatigued and possibly irritable when they start a new day, rather than feeling refreshed. Sleep is vital to good health. Without good quality sleep, energy is not restored and rejuvenation is impossible. If insomnia is experienced for long stretches of time, it will affect the person's general health as the immune and nervous systems are compromised. It has been shown in recent studies that natural killer cell activity (immune defenses) is lowered in persons who have been deprived of sleep, and who are, therefore, more prone to colds.

There is no single answer to sleeping better. Aromatherapy and a few lifestyle recommendations can greatly affect your sleep in a positive way; however the underlying cause must be identified.

It is not uncommon to be bothered by occasional bouts of insomnia; after all, there are many factors that can cause this symptom. The average number of hours a person sleeps is about 7 to 9 hours per night. Perhaps the most frequent causative factor known to disturb sleep is stress. Nervous tension, mental exhaustion, environmental stress, worry, anxiety, depression, relationship problems, are all stress-related conditions capable of causing you to lose a full night's sleep. Developing coping strategies to deal with stress on a day-to-day basis is crucial in preventing sleep disturbances and other stress-related symptoms. I recommend you next read the section on stress if it is the reason for your insomnia.

Other factors that have been linked to sleep difficulties are consuming heavy meals or large amounts of liquid right before bedtime. Indigestion or the need to get up and urinate is almost guaranteed if you choose to follow this kind of pattern. Drinking coffee or smoking cigarettes can interfere with sleep, as they are stimulants. Another factor is a high body temperature. Normally, the body temperature becomes cooler as metabolism and digestion slow down. A cooler body temperature is associated with deep sleep. Some water beds which do not have the ability to naturally adjust (lower) during the night can affect a person's sleep, and possibly inhibit a deep state of sleep. People who exercise right before they retire for the evening may have the same problem as their body temperature is warmer and will take hours to decrease. Background noises or interruptions from the external environment are yet another reason why you may find yourself tossing in bed during the night. Women are more prone to sleep disturbances, especially during menses, PMS, pregnancy, or menopause.

Children often have trouble sleeping and will benefit from a bedtime routine that encourages relaxation and special "together" time. This subject as it relates to children is covered in Chapter 8: Aromatherapy Treatments for Children.

Case history: *A 28-year-old woman who had insomnia and woke up almost every night at 2:30 a.m. wanted to use aromatherapy for sleep induction as she was dissatisfied with her present program. She had tried various over-the-counter sleeping pills, in addition to prescriptions from her medical doctor. She purchased an electric diffuser and put it in her bedroom. A blend was designed for her to use nightly one-half hour before she retired, and again at 2:00 a.m. It took a few weeks before she could discontinue the sleeping medication, but by that time she was off all drugs and sleeping well during the entire night with the aromatherapy nebulizer only. We have adjusted the aromatherapy blend to fit her needs as it has been well over two years since her insomnia problems.*

Essential oils are used extensively in hospitals in the United Kingdom to assist patients in falling asleep. Rather than dispense sleeping pills routinely, nurses will sprinkle a few drops of Lavender essential oil on the bed sheets or offer aromatic baths. Lavender was also found to increase analgesia in lessening pain that was associated with tension. Which reminds me that pain is certainly a factor in sleep disturbances. If this is one of the main reasons why you may be experiencing sleep loss, I suggest you review the chapter on musculo-skeletal ailments, as this chapter discusses pain relief.

A surprisingly easy remedy for promoting sleep is to spray your legs with cold water and Lavender essential oil. This is especially welcoming during hot, humid summer evenings, but can be just as effective during the drier winter months. Store this spray in the refrigerator to stay cold and bring it to your bedside at night.

Aromatic Leg Spray

to promote sleep for the restless

1 cup cold water

12 to 16 drops of Lavender essential oil

spray bottle with a fine mister

To a plastic spray bottle, add the water and essential oil. Label. This preparation does not contain a carrier to disperse the essential oils into the water, so it is necessary to shake this well before each use (application). Spray the lower legs. I suggest you sit at the bedside and spray your legs over the floor rather than above the sheets, to prevent the bedding from getting damp.

Inhalation of essential oils prior to going to bed, and diffusing the oils again while you sleep, can be extremely effective in preventing you from waking during the night. Bedrooms are a convenient place in which to use diffusers because they are small areas and you spend a lot of time there. It only makes sense that this is where aromatherapy should take place for insomnia problems.

This inhalation blend is designed for general use, meaning it aids in relaxation and promoting sleep by calming the nervous system. An aromatic diffuser is the most effective method to use with essential oils for inhalation; they run by electricity and can be connected to automatic timers to go on while you are asleep. Alternatively, a few drops of essential oils can be sprinkled on the bed linens, or a room mister can be made. See Chapter 13: Breathe Easy for detailed discussion on these and other inhalation methods. Not recommended for persons with extremely low blood pressure because of the marjoram essential oil. See Essential Oil Reference Guide for Marjoram.

Peaceful Sleep

to encourage sleep

7 parts Lavender essential oil

2 parts Marjoram essential oil

1 part Clary sage essential oil

Mix the essential oils in an amber glass bottle. Use a few drops to apply to the bed linen, pillow, etc. Or prepare a large amount to run through a diffuser. Alternatively, add 20 drops (or double this recipe if using drops as a measurement) and add to 4 ounces of water to make a room mister. Shake before each use.

Essential oils that are commonly used for insomnia because they have relaxing and sedative characteristics are chamomile, clary sage, frankincense, lavender, marjoram, neroli, petitgrain, rose, sandalwood, and ylang ylang. Many of these essential oils work by stimulating serotonin production. Lavender is by far the most popular essential oil for relaxation and encouraging sleep. Please review the essential oil reference information prior to using any of these oils on a regular or consistent basis. Some, such as marjoram, have contraindications that may or may not apply to you.

Traditional herbs that have sedative qualities are chamomile, lemonbalm, hops, skullcap, passionflower, and valerian. These herbs can be taken in the form of herbal infusion, herbal capsules, or tincture form. There are numerous other herbs and flowers which have relaxing properties as well. I have included a recipe for sleep pillows in Chapter 13; you may be interested in making and keeping this small pillow sachet inside your pillowcase to encourage sleep and peaceful dreams. The recipe for Sweet Dreams sleep pillow contains a multitude of these herbs and flowers.

Other ways people have overcome their sleeplessness is by the old remedy of having a cup of warm milk before you go to bed. I suggest you sprinkle a little nutmeg in the cup and then add the warm milk. It is very comforting and will help ease muscle tension as well. Regular exercise (during the day) is helpful for people who are restless at night. But remember not to exercise at least one hour or more before retiring as this raises body temperature. Use of bright lights during the day can also be of benefit to reset the body's internal rhythm—when to be awake and asleep. Others suggest you don't go to bed unless you're ready to sleep. Also relaxation and breathing exercises, as well as listening to a relaxation tape before bed, can be helpful.

How Essences Can Help You Focus, Meditate, and Study More Effectively

The brain remains a mystery in many ways. Scientists are still puzzled about the multitude of functions and capabilities the human brain possesses, and the mind and body connection is just beginning to be accepted by Western cultures. Considering only a very small percentage of the brain is actually utilized, there is much left to ascertain through research. What is known about the brain is that every detail of our lives is recorded in this astonishing "computer." You do not even have to be consciously aware of or remember these events for the memory to be stored. Because there is an intimate relationship between the limbic brain that is responsible for memory, as well as certain regulatory functions, and the olfactory system (sensory organ), it stands to reason that scent can trigger memories, help one stay focused, and aid in memorization and studying.

Memories can be triggered by any of the senses, but the strongest association is made through the sense of smell. The scent of baking bread or warm oatmeal cookies may trigger a memory of your mother working in the kitchen when you came home from school as a child. Or an old boyfriend may be suddenly remembered when you smell the after-shave or cologne he used to wear. Memory can also be triggered visually, by a familiar landscape or a person's facial expression. Music and sounds can also trigger memories and specific times in a person's life, such as a special song and your first school dance. Studies show that a memory linked with a scent is recalled more easily. This is due to the fact that the limbic or "old" brain is so closely associated with the sense of smell, and to some degree conditioning has taken place.

A Japanese study involving keypunch operators found that when lemon scent was piped into the ventilation system, errors were decreased by 53%. Lemon is an uplifting scent that is used for memory stimulation and mental alertness. High-stress hormone levels have been linked to decreased memory. A diet based heavily on meat and high sodium foods has been associated with poor memory recall, as has inactivity and high blood pressure.

The hormone pregnenolone may help brain cells to communicate better, thereby increasing memory and learning ability. It is being investigated for its possible usefulness in Alzheimer's disease. It is normally produced in the brain and adrenal glands. If this theory proves accurate, adrenal gland-stimulating essential oils may be helpful. Essential oils known to work by stimulating the adrenals are cedarwood, citronella, geranium, and clary sage. However, much more information is needed for this to be conclusive.

Memory loss has been linked to low estrogen levels in several studies. Women are more likely to contract Alzheimer's disease than men. Symptoms of this disease range from simple memory loss to severe dementia. Essential oils that mimic estrogen may prove useful, especially in postmenopausal women. Refer to the beginning of Chapter 10 for a listing of essential oils that possess hormone-like properties. Interestingly, many of the essential oils known to help with memory and mental concentration include these essential oils as well. Clary sage, cypress, and basil essential oils are three essences that appear on both lists (hormone-like essential oils and known memory stimulants).

To study for a major exam, I recommend you use basil and lemon essential oil while you study for the test, and inhale the essences again just prior to and during the examination to trigger the memory recall associations made while studying. Scent has also been used to help children and adults with learning disabilities. All in all, the use of aromatics necessitates additional research in these areas. I wish I had had this synergy blend around when I had to take state boards and certification tests! This is an inhalation blend which can be used by placing a few drops on a tissue and inhaling while studying, and again before the test and during the exam. A diffuser can be utilized very easily in the room where the studying takes place and on a regular basis during the school year to help with concentration, alertness, and memorization. Refer to Chapter 13: Breathe Easy for additional recommendations and uses for inhalation. You will find other recipes there including *Mint Conditioning* which is another synergy designed for inhalation to sharpen alertness and mental acuity.

Memory Recall Synergy

a study aid

5 parts Lemon essential oil

3 parts Basil essential oil

2 parts Rosemary essential oil

Make an ample amount by using dropper-full measurements to use for a diffuser. If only a few drops will be needed for a potpourri burner, aroma lamp or tissue, then count the essential oils by drops.

Essential oils that increase alertness and aid one to concentrate are basil, cypress, eucalyptus, ginger, juniper, lemon, lemongrass, pine, peppermint, and rosemary. The essential oils for meditation are a little different as their focal point is in breathing, deep relaxation, and centering. These essential oils can be very helpful in prayer, meditation and yoga exercises, and were often the essential oils used for ceremonial rituals in ancient (and present) times. The essential oils useful in relaxation and breathing are clary sage, cedarwood, eucalyptus, frankincense, lavender, myrrh, neroli, patchouli, sandalwood, pine, rose, and ylang ylang.

Traditional herbs useful for stimulating and fortifying the brain are peppermint, spearmint, gingko, ginseng, gotu cola, licorice, lemon grass, ginger, and rosemary.

Herbal Tonic for the Brain

a stimulating and fortifying tea

2 parts Spearmint or Peppermint herb

2 parts Lemonbalm herb

2 parts Gotu cola nut

1 part Rosemary herb

1 part Gingko biloba

1 part Siberian Ginseng root

1 part Licorice root

Ginger honey to taste (optional)

Mix the above herbs and ground root into a jar and label. To prepare bring 2 cups of water to a boil and add 2 to 3 teaspoons of herbal tonic mix. Reduce heat to simmer the tea gently for 5 minutes. Remove from heat and allow to steep for another 5 minutes. Strain and drink. Two or three cups per day can be taken.

Dietary recommendations include adopting a diet based on fresh fruits and vegetables and whole grains. Vitamin B's aid in stress and the anti-oxidant supplements are useful for fighting free radical damage. Eating raw nuts and seeds and taking flax oil and wheat germ may help brain cells communicate better and therefore increase memory and mental functioning. Incorporating the herbs used for fortifying the brain is suggested, by making the herbal tea given in this section, or by taking them in capsule or tincture form. Follow the directions stated on the product label for dietary recommendations on the latter herbal forms. A recent analysis done by Jorg Grunwald, Ph.D. (Berlin, Germany), showing the *European Phytomedicines Market* figures and trends reflected Gingko biloba and Ginseng as the two leading European plant products purchased. In Europe, where up to 30% to 40% of the cost of all herbal remedies is reimbursed, phytomedicines (which include herbal and essential oil preparations) have long been accepted throughout history as safe medical alternatives in health maintenance. These are primarily used by the aging population for circulatory and brain functioning aids.

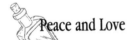

Peace and Love

a meditation oil

18 parts Frankincense essential oil

10 drops Lavender essential oil

10 drops Sandalwood essential oil

5 drops Cedarwood essential oil

5 drops Ylang ylang essential oil

Mix the essential oils in a small amber glass bottle. Label. This recipe can be added to 2 ounces of vegetable oil and 1 teaspoon of wheat germ or jojoba oil to make an anointment oil, or leave as is (without a carrier) to be used for inhalation. A few drops in a potpourri burner or aroma lamp are convenient for meditation purposes. See Chapter 13 for more inhalation options.

Stimulating Scents for Invigoration

This is an exciting topic, as essential oils can display their effectiveness in mental stimulation, alertness, and general invigoration rather quickly. Inhalation of the essential oils immediately affects the mood and mental state. Several conditions and circumstances may require the use of stimulating essential oils: boredom, lethargy, mental exhaustion, lack of motivation, a need to stay awake and alert, such as when driving and working the night shift. Many of the essential oils utilized in this area are also useful in stimulating the immune system.

I was part of a small study investigating the stimulating properties of black spruce essential oil. Following a long hot day of notetaking, lectures, and discussion, many of us were lethargic, to say the least. Some people were even napping! A naturopathic physician went around the room applying the essential oil of black spruce to each individual. Within moments, many of the test subjects experienced feelings of invigoration and mental alertness. I can speak only for myself when I say that the essence had an immediate effect on my feeling of sleepiness. I was alert within what seemed like seconds!

Studies were also done on truck drivers, testing the usefulness of eucalyptus essential oil for increasing alertness and preventing lethargy. The drivers were asked to inhale the eucalyptus oil periodically and whenever they felt tired. It was shown more effective than caffeine and other stimulants without their side effects. My husband and I have used essential oils while traveling to help keep us awake and invigorated while driving on long car trips. Very effective in increasing alertness, aromatherapy provides a pleasant side benefit in the natural aromatic environment it provides to confines of an automobile.

It is interesting to note how many of the stimulating essential oils are derived from tree sources. Could this be why we feel so alive when we visit forests that are abundant with these trees? Eucalyptus, pine, cypress, cedarwood, fir, spruce, and juniper all possess stimulating, mentally invigorating properties. Every Christmas, when we sit around the decorated evergreen tree, I am reminded of how excited and happy I feel being in the presence of these scents.

Stimulating scents are handy when, at the end of the day, you find yourself tired and worn out. Unfortunately, that very same night you are expected to meet friends out for dinner and dancing—essential oils to the rescue! A foot bath is the best thing you can do for yourself to give life and energy to a weary and fatigued body and soul. The following recipe is tried and true to invigorate you.

Energize Me

a stimulating foot bath

2 drops Pine essential oil

2 drops Rosemary essential oil

1 drop Clary sage essential oil

1 drop Peppermint essential oil

2 tbls. bath salts (recipe on page 299 or other carrier)

basin of cold water

a towel

Mix the essential oils in the bath salts. Add the aromatic salts to the basin of cold water and stir with your hands. Sit comfortably in a chair, allowing your feet to soak in the foot bath for 20 minutes. Sit quietly while doing some deep breathing exercises (on page 102 in Chapter 4).

The aromatic bath recipes in Chapter 11 are other wonderful treatments you can do to increase alertness. Some good choices are *TGIF Blend, Reviver Blend,* or the *Footbath for Tired, Aching Feet.*

An inhalation synergy for mental alertness can be found in Chapter 13 called *Mint Conditioning.* I am including another recipe for inhalation here that can be used anytime you need to stay awake, alert, and mentally stimulated. It is very useful for people who must read, study, or work numeral figures all day, to aid in preventing mental exhaustion. It is also very well suited for inhalation during exercise workouts, as it is very stimulating and refreshing. This may help you to stay motivated while performing stationary exercise such as rowing, cycling, and stair-stepping. Put on a nature video and diffuse this blend for the next best thing to being outdoors in the fresh air. It is a blend of fruit, spice, and tree essential oils. Very stimulating indeed!

Invigoration

a synergy blend for inhalation

2 parts Eucalyptus essential oil

2 parts Juniper essential oil

2 parts Grapefruit essential oil

1 part Clary sage essential oil

1 part Ginger essential oil

Combine the essential oils in an amber glass bottle. Use in a variety of ways for inhalation, such as diffuser, humidifier, aroma lamp, or tissue. See Chapter 13 for more inhalation method options.

Drinking an herbal tea can give you an additional lift too. This is a simple blend of some stimulating herbs that can be taken anytime you need a gentle nudge to take action. It makes a nice cool beverage on a hot summer day. Garnish with fresh lemon peel and mint leaves for a festive drink.

Refreshing Herb Tea

4 parts Lemonbalm herb
4 parts Peppermint herb
1 part ground fennel seed
1 part fresh or ground ginger root
cinnamon to taste
fresh lemon peel
Ginger honey to taste

Mix the dried ingredients in a jar and label. To prepare bring 2 cups of water to a boil. Add 2 to 3 teaspoons of the herb tea, grated ginger, and fresh lemon peel and simmer gently for 3 minutes. Remove from heat and strain. Add ginger honey (recipe on page 38) to taste. Drink hot or cold.

Essential oils that have stimulating qualities are basil, cypress, cedarwood, eucalyptus, fir, ginger, juniper, lemon, lemongrass, peppermint, pine, rosemary, and spruce. The essential oils that can produce a feeling of euphoria are also included for their benefits in invigoration, and include clary sage, jasmine, grapefruit, ylang ylang, and rose.

What Are Aphrodisiacs and Do They Really Have an Effect on Us?

Aphrodisiacs are substances that are capable of enhancing sexual pleasure or sexual desire. Actually, they have been around a long, long time. Throughout history food was used as an aphrodisiac. It was used to energize the physical body and affect circulation, often producing a positive effect on the entire body, including the sexual organs and emotions. Traditional herbs have been used for centuries to stimulate circulation and aid in conditions of impotence.

Also introduced in the form of perfume, aphrodisiacs were used to affect the emotions directly and as a personal scent to attract romance and love. Perfume is still used today for similar reasons, although it should be worn to make the wearer feel good, rather than to try to attract someone. Aromatherapy is more than perfume. Essential oils have the potential to affect the circulatory, hormonal, and nervous systems, all of which are involved in this subject. Essential oils are mood-enhancing substances that are capable of creating many different moods or feelings such as warmth, femininity, euphoria, romance, or spirituality. Aphrodisiacs can be used to enhance feelings of self confidence, joy and a general feeling of well-being. They become therapeutic when they affect the emotions and the nervous system. Aromatherapy, more than any other form of complementary system, has unlimited potential in this area. The olfactory system and its direct association with the limbic system is real and powerful. Pleasure, reproductive cycles, sex drive, memory, and emotions are seated in the limbic brain. The therapeutic application of essential oils can ease stress and promote relaxation, which can aid with "performance" issues. Letting go of the worries of the world and becoming more aware of your body are other issues that must be addressed. Patchouli, ginger, and myrrh can be useful for this.

Before you become convinced that you have any kind of problem with your sex life, be aware that most Americans have sex only once per week. That isn't what the magazines, movies, and romance novels lead us to believe. More often than not, both stress and not making it a priority are the underlying issues. In fact, it has been said that good health means good sexual health as well. However, there are some conditions that can affect sexual desire and sexual performance; some can be serious and need to be evaluated and ruled out by a health care practitioner. Here are some of the common conditions, all associated with sexual difficulties, that may be getting in the way of your full enjoyment of your sexuality.

Sexually Transmitted Diseases

Cancer

Diabetes

Arteriosclerosis

Overweight

Prostatitis

Pelvic Inflammatory Disease

Endometriosis

Ovarian Cysts

Fibroids

Medications

Hormonal changes

Cystitis

Depression

Stress

The last four ailments on this list are covered in this book; therefore you should start there to remedy your situation before expecting this chapter to be effective. Experts claim that male impotence is caused by several factors, including problems within the vascular, neurological or cardiovascular systems, infection, alcohol-related, or due to medication side effects. In women, estrogen levels and insufficient foreplay may be factors in the decreased interest in sexual activity.

The importance of the olfactory system and its role in sexuality is plain to see. It is known that anosmia or hyposmia (an absent or decreased ability to smell) has been associated with a decreased interest in sex. As we discussed previously about smell and aphrodisia, our sense of smell is very important in our lives, especially in the sexual arena. In fact, as many as 25% of the people who experience smell disorders also lose interest in sex. Therefore, keeping your sinuses healthy could be the hidden key in creating a healthy sex life. Turn to Chapter 3 following this section to review anosmia's symptoms, causative factors, and remedies.

The pituitary, also known as the master gland of the endocrine system, is responsible for controlling hormone production of other glands. There is an association between an underactive pituitary gland and a decreased interest in sex as well. Essential oils have the ability to stimulate the pituitary gland, and interestingly are comprised of many of the essences known to be aphrodisiac. They are clary sage, jasmine, patchouli, and ylang ylang.

Whether you are aware of it or not, the color of your skin (skin type) and the color of your hair play an important role in sexual attraction. Different skin types and hair colors produce different individual smells. Every person has his or her own "personal scent," much like a set of fingerprints, with no two being exactly alike. Newborn babies are able to identify their mothers by smell, as can couples. Of course, much of what we perceive is subconscious, or below a level of conscious awareness. Sexual attraction and arousal are unconscious, as well as visual and physical (conscious). It is on the subtle and subliminal level that scent plays a major role. Kissing is still one of the best ways to intimately "smell" each other. In fact, the word "kiss" means "to smell" in several languages. The face is one of the places where there are ample sweat glands, which play a key role in producing a person's characteristic smell. Other regions of the body with a large number of sweat glands and hair are considered erogenous (arousing sexual feelings) body zones. It is primarily these areas, and the odors produced there, that make up the smell characteristic to each and every person.

Care should be taken when associating scent with lovemaking, as it needs to be subtle. By incorporating essential oils into the experience you can escape into a different state of mind. You can use aromatherapy to create a romantic retreat away from the rest of the world, without ever leaving the bedroom! It is an easy way to discover new experiences. The best aphrodisiac will make use of the brain, because this is where the sexual center is located, in addition to memories and hormone regulatory functions.

However, minute and diluted forms of scents must always be created with sensitivity and a delicate hand. If the blend is too concentrated it will be unpleasant or repulsive, rather than erotic, and is called anaphrodisiac. The aim is to create a subtle body odor, together with other pleasurable scents that will delight and arouse. A blend of the erogenous, stimulating or calming, and euphoric essential oils would make a well-rounded aphrodisiac synergy.

Jasmine absolute (which means it was solvent extracted due to its low essential oil content) is the most sought after fragrance in the perfume industry because it has a very erogenous effect on humans. Ambrette seed (Hibiscus abelmoschus, L.) and angelica are two essential oils not mentioned previously in the book. Their useful application is primarily in the perfume and aphrodisiac area as well, as they are essential oils which resemble the musk scent. Musk was originally obtained from the sexual glands of specific animals, such as the civet cat and the musk deer. Aromatic substances known as pheromones are produced by an individual (or animal) which affect the sexual physiology of another. They are excreted by the sweat glands in the armpit, face, chest, genital, and anal regions of the body. These aromatic molecules are not present until after puberty, and are the reason why children's sweat has very little odor. Only recently have scientists acknowledged that not only animals, but humans too, produce and react to these aromatic substances called pheromones.

Therefore, after all this discussion I hope you see the need to consider many things in creating an aphrodisiac blend. Skin, hair color, personal body odors, past experiences, personal preferences, olfactory condition, pituitary health, and other factors discussed in these pages all come into play. Aromatherapy applications can be very effective for setting a mood, affecting the emotions, and stimulating the brain to achieve aphrodisia. Aromatic baths, massage oils, and inhalation make the most sense as they also encourage intimacy and touch. Essential oils can also be used in the Jacuzzi, sauna, or shower. Sprinkling a few drops onto the bed sheets and using candles, diffusers, and room sprays are other ideas to experiment with. Several bath recipes that have aphrodisiac qualities are given in

Chapter 11. They are called *Woodstock* and the *Lover's Bath*. At the end of Chapter 13, a very special inhalation recipe is given, called *Love in a Mist*.

Here is a very sensual massage oil designed for the whole body (2% dilution). I suggest warming the oil in a hot water bath prior to application to increase absorption. There is enough here for two bodies, so decide who will go first. Review the helpful tips for aromatherapy massage in Chapter 12 if you need additional information . Notice the alternate oils for dark and light skin types. If this oil appears strongly scented, simply add more vegetable oil to dilute further.

 Love Oil

---

4 tbls. Sweet almond or Safflower oil

1/2 tsp. Evening Primrose oil (optional)

1/2 tsp. carrot seed oil (optional)

12 drops Sandalwood essential oil

6 drops Ylang ylang essential oil

4 drops Clary Sage essential oil

2 drops Rose oil (for dark hair and skin) OR

2 drops Neroli oil (for light hair and skin)

Mix the essential oils with warm safflower or sweet almond oil in a shallow dish. Apply to the body in small amounts using a comfortable pressure and working toward the heart. Avoid the face and genital area.

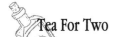 **Tea For Two**

---

an herbal tea for romance

2 tsp. Rose petals

1 tsp. Spearmint herb

1 tsp. Licorice root (ground)

1 tsp. Hawthorn herb

a pinch of the following:

coriander, cinnamon, and nutmeg

Vanilla or Ginger honey to taste (see recipes on pages 295 and 38)

Bring 3 cups of water to a boil. Place the herbs listed above in the hot water and simmer on low for 3 minutes. Remove from the heat and allow to steep for 5 minutes. Strain and drink.

Essential oils that have been referenced as having aphrodisiac properties are carrot seed, clary sage, black pepper, ginger, fennel, frankincense, geranium, hyssop, jasmine, juniper, myrrh, neroli, patchouli, pine, rose, rosemary, sandalwood, and ylang. ylang.

Lifestyle recommendations and suggestions include knowing your body and openly communicating desires, likes, and dislikes to your mate. Discuss your feelings and ask for what pleases you. You may not get it, but don't rely on "hoping" the other person guesses or figures it out. Spend more time alone with your mate and focus on each other. Make a commitment to each other that your relationship is a priority in your lives. Make eye contact and listen attentively. To be a good listener doesn't mean you have to "do" anything but hear what the other person is saying.

Dietary recommendations include eating foods rich in fatty acids, such as Vitamin E, niacin, evening primrose oil, and safflower oil. Nutrients that may be helpful are phosphorus and zinc. Some foods said to have aphrodisiac qualities are oysters, chocolate, raspberries, and elderberries. It was sometimes thought if a particular food looked like a sex organ, it would have aphrodisiac properties, merely by the suggestion made. But I think that only works for the highly visual person—I'll take chocolate and aromatherapy any day!

CHAPTER 10
Aromatherapy Treatments for "Women Only"

Brief Overview of Hormone Health

This chapter highlights challenges that are specific to women. Ailments unique to women are frequently related to the delicate balance of hormones. The two most important hormones are estrogen and progesterone. These hormones are produced in the ovaries from puberty until the menopausal period. Estrogen is responsible for the development and maintenance of the female sexual organs and the physical appearance unique to a woman's body. Progesterone's prime responsibility is to prepare the uterus for pregnancy. The cycles a woman experiences every month, from puberty to menopause, are a direct result of the levels of these two key female hormones.

PMS is frequently experienced up to two weeks prior to menstruation. The symptoms range from mild to severe and more than one-third of premenopausal women experience some form of PMS. Hormones are typically responsible for premenstrual symptoms. A dramatic decline in the levels of estrogen heralds the transition into menopause. Hormone fluctuations are natural and these challenges are unique to women. Our social culture strongly influences our perception of a woman experiencing these changes.

Aromatherapy can ease many of the symptoms caused by hormone fluctuations. Therapeutic essential oils, phyto-hormones, are used for their hormone-like properties which provide balance and relief from symptoms such as mood swings, depression, nervous tension, and water retention (bloating). Diet and lifestyle also plays an important role in alleviating many women's health problems. Diets low in caffeine, red meats, dairy, alcohol, and sugar, and high in fiber, vegetables, soy, and whole grains will be extremely helpful in a wide variety of female health challenges.

Considerations must be made when using aromatherapy for pregnant women and when employing the hormone-like essences for PMS or menopausal symptoms. Durign pregnancy, you must avoid certain essential oils completely, use some with caution and in low dilutions, and use only the safe essences that are very welcomed at this time. Research to identify how many essential oil constituents are absorbed by the fetus have not been conducted. However, we know that essential oils are absorbed via the olfactory system, crossing the blood-brain barrier, and are absorbed via the skin into the microcirculatory system; this suggests that aromatics may possibly enter the fetal blood stream. Also, if a pregnant woman uses a toxic essential oil or even a safe one in an excessive dose, she may cause harm to herself and her baby. This is a very fragile time of development for the baby and physically stressful for the mother. It is crucial that conservative and safe methods are utilized during pregnancy, both in regard to allopathic medicine and natural therapeutics such as aromatherapy and herbal therapy.

There are inherent dangers while using the hormone-like essential oils. Anise, star anise, and fennel essential oils may closely resemble female hormones in their physiologic activity. It is prudent to avoid such oils if you have a history of hormone-stimulated cancer. Uterine, ovarian cancer, and some breast cancers may be influenced by these essences since they are so closely related to how our own hormones act in the body. Although much of this work is theoretical, as a cancer nurse I strongly believe the correlation should be taken into consideration when applying these oils on a woman with a history of any of the above. Pre-pubescent girls should not be using these phyto-hormones on a regular basis as they may possibly stimulate hormone activity.

Another important area in women's health in which aromatherapy has much to offer is in using essential oils to nurture ourselves and help with stress relief. Women are nurturers by nature. As mothers, wives, and community activists, we give a lot of energy to others. It is important that we learn to take care of ourselves, and make our health a priority. When we fill our own cup, it will overflow and be shared with those in our lives. I am reminded of how adults are instructed to put on their own oxygen masks if an emergency arises on an airplane, before putting one on the child. This is for a very good reason, as caregivers must take care of their own needs before caring for others successfully. Aromatherapy will bring more pleasure and encourage self-nurturance into your lifestyle, in addition to supporting excellent health.

In addition to good nutrition and stress reduction, regular exercise and knowing (and listening to) our body is also important. Because you are a woman, and all women are at risk, you need to learn how to do breast self-exams. Breast cancer causes more deaths in women than any form of cancer other than lung cancer. However, more important is the fact that breast cancer may be curable, if found early. If you are over 50 years of age and have a family history of breast cancer, you are at greatest risk. According to the American Cancer Society, all women over the age of 20 should check their breasts for lumps, thickness, or other abnormal changes. It only takes a few minutes to do, and can be easily performed in the shower. Do the self-exam every month. The best time for menstruating women is immediately following their period.

Essential Oils That May Demonstrate Hormone-like Activity

Aniseed

Basil

Chamomile (Roman)

Clary sage

Cypress

Fennel

Geranium

Nutmeg

Star Anise

Reported Abortifacient Essential Oils (May Induce Abortion)

Do Not Use During Pregnancy.

Davana

Champaca bark

Boldo leaf

Ho wood

Mugwort

Pennyroyal
  (European, N. American)

Parsley seed

Rue

Savin

Sassafras

Red cedarwood

Santolina

Tarragon

Thuja

Tansy

Wormwood

Wormseed

Essential Oils to Be Used with Caution During Pregnancy

Caraway

Cedarwood

Chamomile

Clary sage

Cypress

Jasmine

Juniper

Lavender

Marjoram

Nutmeg

Peppermint

Rose

Rosemary

Essential Oils Regarded as Safe to Use During Pregnancy

in low dilutions and as directed

Bergamot	Orange
Geranium	Patchouli
Lavender (Angustofolia)	Sandalwood
Lemon	Tea Tree
Mandarin	Ylang ylang
Neroli	

Easing the Symptoms of Premenstrual Tension

Premenstrual syndrome, premenstrual tension, and PMS are some of the names given to a condition that presents recurring symptoms about one to two weeks before menstruation begins. Primarily caused by the increase in the level of estrogen and decrease in progesterone, many woman may experience a wide variety of unpleasant and uncomfortable symptoms. Symptoms can range from mild to severe. An estimated 30 to 40% of women experience some form of PMS. There are more than 150 symptoms associated with PMS. Some of the symptoms include:

bloating	cramping
nausea	headaches
breast soreness	breast swelling
constipation	diarrhea
acne	backache
weight gain	insomnia
swelling (hands, feet)	compulsive eating
food cravings	depression
fatigue	nervous tension
irritability	aggression
anger	decreased libido
tearfulness	

Most of the symptoms listed above are directly related to water retention and an increase in estrogen; however, a poor diet and other lifestyle conditions will intensify these symptoms. Essential oils can help to balance a woman's physical and emotional sensitivities at this time. Aromatic baths, massage oils and lotions, and inhalation of essential oils are the most beneficial methods used for this health challenge. When incorporating aromatherapy into your lifestyle, be sure to allow two to three months time before expecting dramatic results. Aromatherapy is a gentle and supportive form of natural healing when used as constitutional therapy. I suggest you start keeping a journal to record any symptoms you experience during the next several months, so you will be better able to evaluate your progress.

Case history: *A 38-year-old woman experiencing moderate to severe PMS symptoms two weeks prior to her next menses came to me for aromatherapy recommendations. She had dramatic mood swings with depression, bloating, carbohydrate cravings, and mild headaches. She was otherwise very healthy, ate a balanced, mostly vegetarian, diet and exercised regularly. Her irritability was beginning to affect her boyfriend and coworkers. She had tried many of the over-the-counter medicines suggested for PMS symptoms, but had not experienced much improvement. She was feeling desperate and confused. She made some changes in her lifestyle and diet, and began to take aromatic baths and apply massage oils. She also purchased a diffuser to use in her apartment. She began to feel a big difference about the sixth week, and by her second month she had very few symptoms. In the past she would know two weeks ahead of time when her period was coming because of all the PMS symptoms she would experience. By the second month, she said she had only one day of symptoms before her period came! The aromatherapy had helped balance her system, and she no longer had to suffer two weeks of misery. As part of her dietary change, she began taking aloe vera concentrate and herbal tea to nourish her system and help diminish water retention. It has been a few years since her PMS problems, and she says when she starts menopause she will certainly turn to aromatherapy to help her!*

The essential oils chosen for this recipe aid in bloating and water retention and help with depression, nervous tension, and irritability. The essences are regulating and balancing for the female reproductive system and generally relaxing and euphoric. This bath is best when taken three times per week, about two weeks prior to your menses. Other aromatic baths that will be beneficial for this time are the *Glad to be Home* and *Tune-Up* bath recipes given in Chapter 11: The Aromatic Bath. These help with fluid retention and balancing the body. For trouble sleeping soak in the *Serenity Bath* given in that chapter as well.

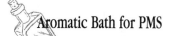 ## Aromatic Bath for PMS

carrier of your choice

5 drops Lavender essential oil

2 drops Geranium essential oil

2 drops Grapefruit essential oil

1 drop Clary sage essential oil

Choose a carrier such as honey or epsom salts for your essential oils. These will help with the water retention and muscular cramps and aches. Add the essential oils to your carrier and mix well. After the bath has filled, add the mixture to the water and stir with your hands. Close the bathroom door for the full inhalation effect. Hang a Do Not Disturb sign on the bathroom door if you feel you might be interrupted. Soak for 20 to 30 minutes in this warm to hot aromatic bath treatment.

A massage oil is very helpful in easing bloating, backache, and cramping, as it is a local treatment. When you are not using the aromatic baths, it can be very effective for the discomforts of premenstrual tension if used daily. Then a heating pad will give additional relief, or use the hot compress method for aromatherapy application. I find the mild to moderate cases of PMS respond quite well to massage oils alone, while the more severe PMS symptoms need the additional heat application for the greatest benefit. Compress instructions are given on page 319 in Chapter 12: First Aid to the Rescue. Turn there for additional information if you need to. The recipe below includes infusion oils of arnica or St. John's Wort (hypericum) to help with muscular cramping and general inflammation. Borage or evening primrose oil are known to increase prostaglandin levels, which decrease inflammation, and are of great benefit for PMS-related symptoms. This is a massage concentrate and should only be applied to local areas of the body, such as the lower abdomen and back. Do not use as a whole-body massage oil, as this preparation is too concentrated.

A Potent Premenstrual Potion

a massage oil for PMS symptoms

2 tbls. vegetable oil

2 tbls. Arnica or St. John's Wort infusion oil

2 tsp. evening primrose or borage oil

20 drops Lavender essential oil

10 drops Rosemary essential oil

6 drops Clary sage essential oil

6 drops Juniper essential oil

6 drops Lemon essential oil

To an amber glass bottle, add the essential oils. Then add the infusion and vegetable oils. Shake gently to mix well. Label contents with directions for use. To apply, massage a small amount of the oil to the lower abdominal region and low back area. Apply the aromatic oil with gentle hand pressure, working towards the heart to encourage blood return and increase lymphatic drainage. Inhale essences from the hands after application. Apply daily during episodes of PMS symptoms, up to two weeks prior to menses.

To benefit from inhalation of relaxation and uplifting essential oils, I recommend a diffuser as the most therapeutic way to absorb essential oils via the olfactory and respiratory system. Inhalation is the most effective method for aromatherapy benefits on the emotions. Since there is such a wide variety of emotional states that can be experienced by each individual woman during premenstrual syndrome, I have listed specific essential oils that can have a positive effect on the most common of these. That way you may be able to customize your very own blend that will be best for you. A few drops can be used in an aroma lamp or potpourri burner or a diffuser. Refer to Chapter 13: Breathe Easy for all the different methods for aromatherapy inhalation.

Irritability/aggression	*Depression/tearfulness*
(nervous tension, anxiety)	(including decreased libido)
Basil	Basil
Bergamot	Grapefruit
Frankincense	Sandalwood
Chamomile	Bergamot
Clary sage	Clary sage
Jasmine	Jasmine
Lavender	Lavender
Mandarin	Lemon
Marjoram	Mandarin
Rose	Neroli
Sandalwood	Rose
Hyssop	Sandalwood
Ylang ylang	Ylang ylang

Fatigue/lack of energy	*Regulating/balancing emotions*
Basil	Frankincense
Cypress	Bergamot
Ginger	Clary sage
Juniper	Geranium
Lemon	Lemongrass
Rosemary	
Eucalyptus	
Grapefruit	
Hyssop	
Peppermint	
Pine	

Other essential oils helpful in the treatment of PMS symptoms are those which demonstrate hormone-like activity similar to the female hormones. These include anise, basil, fennel, and nutmeg and are listed in the beginning of this chapter. Essential oils that help to alleviate stress in general are employed for this ailment and can be found in the chapter addressing stress relief.

The following herbal tea helps to nourish the female reproductive system during times of PMS or menopause.

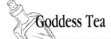 ## Goddess Tea

an herbal infusion for women

6 parts Raspberry leaves

4 parts Chamomile flowers

2 parts Rose petals

1 part Ginger root (fresh or dried)

1 part Licorice root (ground)

1 part Rosemary herb

Honey to taste (try ginger honey, recipe on page 38)

Combine all the dry ingredients in a clean glass jar and label. If using fresh ginger root, cut a 1/4-inch slice for each cup of tea. When using dried or dehydrated ginger, use 1/4 teaspoon (or to taste). If using ginger honey, you may omit it if you wish. Pour boiling water over 2 teaspoons of herb per cup. Allow to steep for 5 to 10 minutes. Drink hot or cold. Drink 1 cup daily.

Lifestyle and dietary recommendations include avoiding food additives, refined carbohydrates and sugar, caffeine, alcohol, salt, dairy, and meat. Eat lots of fresh fruits and vegetables, and plenty of whole grains. Be sure to drink plenty of fluids such as pure water and herbal tea. Drinking a cup of hot water and fresh lemon juice in the morning helps with cleansing the entire system and decreases water weight gain, as it is a natural diuretic. Taking a concentrated form of aloe vera has proven very beneficial for inflammatory conditions and constipation, two symptoms that are a problem for many women.

Unbelievably Simple Relief for Menstrual Cramps

Menstrual cramps can range in severity. Painful periods, also called dysmenorrhea, are most often caused by an underlying condition such as endometriosis, pelvic inflammatory disease, or fibroids. Extremely painful periods are not normal and should be checked by a health practitioner, to be dealt with holistically. Mild to moderate menstrual cramps are the topic of discussion here, and can be adequately treated with aromatic baths, compresses, and massage oils. Diet is very important, as many foods can aggravate cramping, muscle tension, and overall toxification of the body. In general, a healthy diet based on fresh fruits, vegetables, and whole grains will promote the body's ability to cleanse and detoxify.

A very effective massage oil can ease most cramps and aches caused by menstruation. This blend is made with the analgesic, anti-spasmodic and anti-inflammatory essential oils. Borage or arnica oils are used as a base for their benefit in prostaglandin production. Massage yourself with this oil twice per day to relieve discomfort in the pelvic region and lower back. Use the recipe *A Potent Premenstrual Potion* on page 264 in the previous section for PMS.

This bath recipe is so helpful! I use my homemade bath salts as the carrier, as Epsom and sea salt are useful for muscular aches and cramping. Or if you feel like being pampered, make the Botanical Bath recipe on page 298 for the ultimate bath concoction.

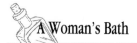

A Woman's Bath

an aromatic bath for menstrual cramping

carrier of choice (try the bath salt recipe page 299)

5 drops Lavender essential oil

2 drops Cypress essential oil

2 drops Nutmeg essential oil

2 drops Peppermint essential oil

Add the essential oils to a carrier, such as bath salts or honey. See recipes for carrier options in Chapter 11. Add the carrier and essential oil mixture to a full hot bath. Soak for 20 minutes. Do not stay in longer than 30 minutes, as it can have a draining effect on you. Wrap yourself in a warm terry bathrobe or towel, and rest for 20 minutes or so by lying on a bed and elevating your legs and feet (above heart level). This is very relaxing and takes the burden off the lower back and encourages good blood flow.

Essential oils useful in easing menstrual cramps are chamomile, cypress, basil, carrot seed, frankincense, clary sage, juniper, jasmine, lavender, marjoram, nutmeg, peppermint, and rosemary.

An herbal tea can be made with a combination of several herbs and taken once or twice per day. See the Goddess herbal tea recipe in the previous section which eases menstrual discomforts, including cramping.

How to Correct Cystitis

Cystitis is an inflammation of the bladder, typically caused by a bacterial infection or local irritation caused by having sex. Symptoms include painful and burning sensations when voiding (urinating). It is often characterized by frequent trips to the bathroom to pass only small amounts of urine. There may be a low-grade fever present and, depending on the duration and severity of the infection, fatigue may be a symptom.

Essential oils that contain antibacterial and anti-inflammatory properties are the aromatics chosen for this ailment; however, they must also be gentle enough to be used on delicate tissues such as the perineum. Sandalwood essential oil is both a gentle astringent and disinfectant and is included in most of my blends for urinary tract ailments. The most appropriate method of application of therapeutic essential oils is the "sitz" bath, which literally means "to sit." It is a local bath treatment which delivers the medicament directly to the area in need of healing and together with essential oils and warm water, provides a very effective and soothing remedy. A shallow bath at hip level in a regular tub with a few inches of water, or a large basin (bidet) in which you can sit comfortably, will suffice.

Sitz Bath for Cystitis

for bladder infections

3 drops Sandalwood essential oil

2 drops Tea Tree essential oil

1 drop Chamomile essential oil

1 – 2 tbls. Honey

2 tbls. Apple cider vinegar

Fill a large basin with warm to tepid water, or use the bathtub and fill only to hip level. If there is severe burning and local irritation, then use tepid water to relieve these symptoms. Otherwise, use warm water. In a small dish, combine the essential oils and honey. Mix well to blend. Add the cider vinegar to the bath water, and then the aromatic honey. Soak by sitting in the bath (with knees out of the water) for at least 15 to 20 minutes. Sip on herbal tea while in the tub if you wish.

After voiding, many may find the use of bathroom tissue too abrasive. A pleasant option for washing this area is an aromatic periwash made of distilled water, cider vinegar, and a few drops of essential oil, after every trip to the bathroom (which is often!). A plastic squirt bottle is handy to use as a peri bottle, or a plastic water bottle with the pull-out drinking spout.

In lieu of the toilet paper, rinse the perineal area with this soothing antibacterial solution. It provides cooling and healing relief without causing irritation. Blot dry with a clean towel.

Aromatic Periwash

to cleanse the perineum

7 ounces distilled warm water

1 ounce (2 tbls.) cider vinegar

1 drop Lavender essential oil

1 drop Sandalwood essential oil

In a clean plastic bottle, add the essential oils and vinegar. Shake well. Add the water and shake again to mix. Before using this solution, you must shake it well, as the essential oils separate from the water. Alternatively, by mixing the essential oils in honey beforehand, they will become emulsified in the water, but it makes this simple periwash a little more complicated. Rinse with this immediately after voiding. Pat dry with a clean, soft cotton towel.

A massage oil concentrate can be used for treatment of bladder infections as well. You can concentrate treatment by using essential oils in a massage oil or lotion base, and massaging them into the lower abdominal (pelvic) region over the bladder and lower back. If you are experiencing any back discomfort, then it is possible that the infection has moved into the kidneys. Seek medical care if symptoms of kidney infection appear.

The infusion oils listed in this recipe are optional, as well as the carrot seed oil; however, they have anti-inflammatory and healing properties and add to the efficacy of this blend. Refer to Chapter 15 for carrier oil information and recipes for making your own infusion oils.

Massage Blend for Cystitis

for local application

1 tbls. vegetable oil

1 tbls. Mullein or Calendula infusion oil

1/4 tsp. carrot seed oil (optional)

10 drops Lavender essential oil

6 drops Sandalwood essential oil

5 drops Cedarwood essential oil

4 drops Bergamot essential oil

>6>6>6>>>>t>6

In an amber glass bottle, add the essential oils and carrot seed oil. Pour in the vegetable oil and infusion oil. Shake gently to combine well. Label contents. Apply a small amount to the lower abdomen, above the bladder area, in addition to the lower back. Apply this treatment oil twice per day, morning and before retiring.

Essential oils known to be useful in bladder inflammation and infections are bergamot, cedarwood, chamomile, cypress, eucalyptus, frankincense, fennel, hyssop, juniper, lavender, marjoram, pine, rosemary, and sandalwood. Peppermint essential oil is not recommended as it is prone to cause irritation on sensitive skin.

Lifestyle recommendations include drinking plenty of fluids, at least 8 glasses per day. Extra fluids will encourage dilution of local bacteria and aid in flushing them from the system. Get more rest and avoid stimulants like caffeine, alcohol, and black tea. Drink herbal tea, and hot lemon water instead. Avoid sweets or juices.

How to Make an Easy Transition—Menopause

Menopause is a transition from the stage of childbearing to a state of greater maturity. This change is directly related to the decline of hormone levels causing the ovaries to cease producing eggs. Actually, as women, we are born with all of our eggs! You may have heard menopause referred to as "the change of life" or "the change." Menopause can trigger a host of symptoms and "changes" in your body, emotions, and outlook on life. As "baby boomer" women enter the middle or transitional years, mainstream America isn't far behind. Finally women's health challenges are visible. With public demand comes greater social understanding and an increased medical awareness and study. This is a positive and necessary turning point in support of better health care for women.

The average age at which a woman enters menopause is between 49 and 51 years. Some women may experience menopause much earlier at about age 40, while others do not start menopause until their late 50's. The perimenopausal period, which is the actual period between normal cycles and the cessation of menstruation, may last several months to several years. There are some women who appear to have more intense and frequent perimenopausal symptoms. Women who are in denial regarding their age and youthfulness seem to be more susceptible to the aging process in general, which includes menopause. Another group of women who may find themselves having a difficult time are those who have dedicated their entire lives to rearing children. Their personal "identity" became focused on child rearing and childbearing and it may be difficult for them to refocus. A positive outlook is very helpful in dealing with this challenging phase of a woman's life. Many women enjoy this new phase, focusing on studies or projects they were unable to tackle when their children were small. I am reminded of the question posed of perception, "Is the cup half full or half empty?" How do you perceive your reality? Do you view menopause as a sort of death sentence or a new beginning? Research and poll studies say that your outlook and belief system makes a difference.

The most common complaints are weight gain, sleep problems (night sweats), hot flashes, fatigue, and psycho-emotional changes. Weight gain can possibly be caused by a decreased metabolic rate rather than a decrease in hormone levels. This may be directly related to the lack of sleep caused by hot flashes and night sweats. Other complaints include a decreased interest in sex, forgetfulness, mood swings, water retention, palpitations, vaginal dryness (and inflammation and pain during intercourse), anxiety, depression, and headaches. Headaches may result from water retention.

There is a strong correlation between stress levels and the degree of severity of menopausal symptoms. Exercise helps in several ways: it increases metabolism, aids with stress relief, helps to lift depression and relieves the sleep disturbances. Daily exercise lasting at least 30 to 45 minutes and maintaining sexual activity will increase circulation to the pelvis and stimulate vaginal secretion.

There are many essential oils that can ease the symptoms of menopause and help in preventing them. Those that contain hormone-like chemicals can be used to "feed" the body, while other essences can be used to relieve water retention, flushing and sweats, emotional changes, etc. You will want to give aromatherapy, and other natural alternatives, time to take effect and make a difference. This may be one or several months of consistent aromatherapy applications. I suggest you keep a journal to record all of your symptoms and complaints so you will be better able to evaluate your progress. Make notes of which aromatherapy baths, oils, and inhalations you prefer and seemed to work best for you. As all women are different, so too must their treatment plan be. I have outlined common symptoms relating to menopause and the respective aromatherapy treatment for those complaints.

To ease symptoms of night sweats and encourage a peaceful sleep, essential oils which affect the nervous and circulatory systems are most effective: basil, chamomile, lavender, mandarin and marjoram, neroli, petitgrain, rose, sandalwood, and ylang ylang. To ease night sweats and as an aid in preventing them, essential oils of cypress, lemongrass, petitgrain, grapefruit, and lime are useful. The following recipes can be used before bedtime (body oil, aromatic bath) or during the night as an inhalation blend.

Peaceful Sleep Bath

to ease night sweats and promote sleep

4 drops Lavender essential oil

3 drops Marjoram essential oil

3 drops Lime essential oil

carrier of choice

(try Milk Maid's Bath or Honey Bath page 298)

To your carrier, add the essential oils and mix completely. Milk is great for dry skin, while honey is soothing; both recipes are given in Chapter 11: The Aromatic Bath. After the bath has filled, add the aromatic mixture and stir with your hands. Soak for 20 to 30 minutes. This bath is great before retiring, as it is relaxing. The lime essential oil is refreshing.

Inhalation is another method through which a direct effect on the limbic brain can be achieved. The best method of utilizing inhalation, especially during the night while you sleep, is the electric diffuser which can be connected to an automatic timer. If you awake at a certain time each evening, set the diffuser to go on 1/2 hour before that time. Ideally, the diffuser should go on every three to four hours for a ten-minute duration. The essential oils will last several hours in the room air, and you will be inhaling them while you sleep. Take care to use the recommended amounts and times (dose), as too much can waken you or have the opposite effect. The goal is to have a subtle background scent, not one that is overbearing. Alternatively, you can use an aroma lamp or potpourri burner, although these methods require a lit candle. For a simpler method of inhalation, place a few drops on your pillowcase. However, the diffuser is the most therapeutic method to utilize for inhalation purposes, such as for night sweats and sleeping disturbances.

Peaceful Sleep Inhalation Blend

to diffuse during the night

3 parts Lavender essential oil

2 parts Marjoram essential oil

2 parts Lime essential oil

1 part Mandarin essential oil

To make a large amount, enough to use in a diffuser: Measure each part with an eye dropper or teaspoon.

To make a small amount, to be used with an aroma lamp, light ring, etc.: Measure each part by drops. See Chapter 13: Breathe Easy for inhalation options.

The body oil recipe given below consists of a vegetable oil base with either borage or evening primrose oil. These oils are beneficial to feed the skin (and body) as they are high in GLA and promote production of prostaglandins. Vitamin E can also be added. See Chapter 15 for carrier oil choices and their properties.

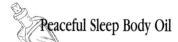 ## Peaceful Sleep Body Oil

to ease night sweats and promote sleep

4 tbls. vegetable oil

1 tsp. Borage or Evening Primrose Oil

10 drops Lavender essential oil

6 drops Grapefruit essential oil

5 drops Marjoram essential oil

4 drops Cypress essential oil

In an amber glass bottle, add the essential oils. Add 1 tsp. of borage or evening primrose oil (or combination). Add the vegetable oil and shake well. Label contents. Apply nightly on chest and neck areas. This is a body oil and can be used freely on the body.

Bloating and headaches are symptoms caused by water retention. Diuretic essential oils may be helpful for these conditions, in addition to avoiding sodium in your diet. Those oils to consider for these complaints are cypress, fennel, geranium, grapefruit, juniper, lavender, lemon, mandarin, orange, and rosemary. Include these oils in your aromatherapy oils, lotions, or aromatic baths. The *Cellulite Bath* and the *Menopause Bath* are good choices and include some of these essential oils. You can find the recipes at the end of Chapter 11: The Aromatic Bath.

For depression caused by menopause, use the essential oils of basil, bergamot, clary sage, grapefruit, jasmine, lavender, neroli, rose, sandalwood, and ylang ylang. Review the section on depression in Chapter 9 for wonderful, nurturing, and anti-depressant oil blends. The irritability and mood swings can be triggered by disturbed sleep, and may subside once a better night's sleep is experienced. Refer to Chapter 9: Psycho-Aromatherapy for stress relief essential oils and essences to ease anxiety. Also, in Chapter 13 inhalation and emotional effects of specific essential oils are discussed that may apply to your particular needs.

For a decreased interest in sex, the aphrodisiac essential oils discussed in Chapter 9 will be very effective. Try the *Lover's Bath* or the *Woodstock* blend given in Chapter 11. In addition to the aphrodisia information, I recommend you use a natural vaginal salve or cream on a regular basis to aid in replenishing the vaginal wall lining which is thinning at this time. Daily application of this salve will minimize inflammation and discomfort caused by intercourse. Exercise, including sexual activity, encourages circulation to the pelvis, and helps women who are experiencing changes in this area. You may already be using a vaginal cream or perhaps you will want to make your own. The replenishing salve recipe below is effective and relatively easy to make. It has all-natural ingredients and it is unlikely that you will be able to find a better vaginal preparation. After reading the information in Chapter 9 on aphrodisiacs, you probably will want to start the "exercise" recommendations!

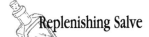 **Replenishing Salve**

for vaginal dryness

2 oz. natural vaginal cream OR
heavy duty ointment (recipe on page 319)
5 drops Frankincense essential oil
5 drops Sandalwood essential oil
5 drops Myrrh essential oil
800 IU Vitamin E

If making your own ointment, you may want to use less bees wax to make a cream consistency. Also, instead of using all olive oil for the base, I highly recommend using a combination of calendula, comfrey and St. John's Wort infusion oils. These oils will nourish and protect the delicate vaginal tissues. Follow the directions for making an ointment on page 319 and store in an amber glass jar. Apply a small amount daily. If using an already made product, such as a naturally-based vaginal cream that you have purchased, make sure you have a 2-ounce amount for this recipe. If the cream comes in a tube, you will need to empty the contents into a clean amber glass jar, and mix with the above essential oils and vitamin E. Please note that only 15 drops (total) of essential oils are needed for this preparation. That is about 1 1/2% dilution ratio, which is adequate for vaginal application.

Hot flashes (Power Surges!), sudden heat rushes that create havoc in public and at the oddest times, are bothersome to say the least! An easy and effective remedy is to inhale essential oil of peppermint. Many women choose to carry this in their purse, just in case! It has a cooling and refreshing effect on the nervous system. Try putting a drop or two of essential oil on a small folding fan for personal use.

There are many over-the-counter vaginal creams, doctor-prescribed pills, patches, creams, implants, and suppositories to replace hormones synthetically. Risks are involved with taking these products, so be sure to discuss all their inherent side effects with your health team, as well as other natural options available to you.

This herbal tea contains many traditional herbs helpful in relieving the common symptoms of menopause. Some are relaxing, diuretic, and tonifying. They may ease hot flashes and night sweats if taken regularly.

Menopause Support Tea

2 parts chamomile flowers

1 part ginseng root

1 part dandelion root and leaf

1 part licorice root (ground)

1 part valerian

1 part garden sage

honey to taste

Mix the dry herbs in a jar with a tight fitting lid. To make 1 cup of herb tea, place 1 teaspoon of herb in 1 1/2 cups of boiling water and simmer gently for 10 minutes. Strain. Drink one cup per day. If bloating is a complaint, add fresh lemon juice as it is a mild diuretic.

Lifestyle recommendations include those already mentioned in the context of this section, as well as actively seeking support for yourself while experiencing this transitional phase of your life. Communicate with your spouse. Talk with your friends. There are even newsletters and menopause support groups you can join. Also important is finding practitioners to be part of your health team that are knowledgeable in natural alternatives. Nutrition (including vitamin and mineral therapy), herbal medicine, homeopathy, and aromatherapy are example of complementary therapies that can be utilized for health support at this time.

Dietary recommendations include a low-fat, mostly vegetarian diet. Eating more soy products such as tofu, soy milk and cheese, in addition to yams, may decrease menopausal symptoms due to their phytochemical content which is similar to our own naturally occurring hormones lowered during menopause. Lowering your salt intake will diminish water retention and weight gain. Avoid alcohol and caffeine as these stimulants put additional stress on the body. It's also a good idea to increase your daily intake of foods rich in calcium and vitamin D to prevent osteoporosis.

The Challenges Specific to Childbearing

It is very important that you have already read Chapter 1, in particular the Common-Sense Safety information. Unless directed by a health care professional, follow the safety recommendations discussed in this book.When using aromatherapy during pregnancy, always be sure to double check that the essential oil you wish to use is appropriate and safe for application. Review the lists given in the front of this chapter to make certain; also cross reference the Essential Oil Reference Guide in Chapter 14. As you have read in other parts of this book, it is crucial that low dilutions be used when preparing therapeutic essential oil blends. one percent or less is recommended during pregnancy by most midwives and aromatherapists. Pay careful attention as you count the drops of essential oils. Use exact amounts or less, never more, than what is suggested in the recipe, especially when using aromatherapy in pregnancy. I lean toward being more conservative and preventative by making safety of utmost importance. You may find that you will personally want to use less than is recommended since your sense of smell is highly sensitive at this time.

Tips for Relieving Morning Sickness

One of the less pleasant effects of pregnancy is morning sickness. The feeling of nausea, with or without episodes of vomiting, is often experienced in the first trimester of pregnancy (heightened symptoms in the third month). As the name suggests, it appears frequently in the morning upon rising, but can be present throughout the day. It is important to realize that women who are pregnant have an extremely keen sense of smell at this time. Perhaps it is a safety feature nature has programmed into the female's system to protect mother and baby. Certainly with all the physiologic changes taking place, in addition to this heightened odor awareness, nausea is not surprising. Adjust the amounts of essential oils recommended in the following recipes if you need to. Morning sickness can possibly be the result of vitamin B-6 deficiency or a low blood sugar level. However, during this trimester is when the placenta becomes seated within the uterus and is probably the most likely cause of the nausea.

For quick relief of morning sickness inhale the essence of peppermint essential oil. It can bring immediate relief. Warning: It must be used with caution during pregnancy because of its stimulating effects on the central nervous system. Therefore do not use it internally or in large amounts, although spearmint herb tea is fine to drink for nausea and digestive complaints.

Lavender essential oil can relieve nausea by inhalation or a warm compress. It can be used alone or in combination with lemon or peppermint essential oils. For inhalation, try 4 parts Lavender essential oil with one part Lemon or Peppermint essential oil. Put a few drops on a tissue, in an aroma lamp, or run through a diffuser. This will help to minimize other unpleasant odors that may be triggering the nausea. The following recipe is for a warm compress for the forehead to combat morning sickness. If you regularly experience nausea upon rising, you may want to ask your spouse to prepare this for you before you get up in the morning. Lavender is soothing to the nervous system, while the lemon (or peppermint) is gently refreshing.

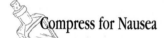

Compress for Nausea

to relieve and prevent morning sickness

warm water

3 drops Lavender essential oil

1 drop Lemon OR Peppermint essential oil

a bowl or sink

washcloth

To a sink or bowl, add about four cups of warm water. Add the essential oils and stir with your hands. Soak the washcloth in the aromatic water. Gently wring the cloth until it is moist, but not too wet. Apply to the forehead. Keep eyes closed. Leave compress on for 10 to 15 minutes or until you have obtained relief.

Essential oils that help to prevent nausea and ease morning sickness are lavender, ginger, lemon, and peppermint. Traditional herbs used to treat this discomfort are chamomile, ginger, orange blossom, fennel, raspberry leaf, and spearmint.

Dietary recommendations include avoiding foods and odors that are unpleasant. These may include rich, highly spiced, and oily foods. Avoid alcohol, tobacco, coffee, and black tea. Small frequent meals may be more appealing than larger, heavy ones. Avoid highly refined foods which contain sugar, salt, and fat.

Can You Help the Swelling of Feet and Hands During Pregnancy?

Most often a symptom in late pregnancy, swelling of the hands and feet is a result of fluid retention and inadequate circulation. The increase of weight of the abdomen interferes with the circulation from the legs due to pressure on the veins in the pelvis. Use of mild diuretics and toning essential oils is helpful, in addition to taking frequent breaks during the day. Elevating the feet several times throughout the day can also help. Regular exercise, including yoga, walking, and swimming promotes good general circulation.

For hand or feet swelling, compresses and foot baths are the methods of choice. I will speak of swelling of the feet primarily, though understand the same recommendations and recipes apply to the hands as well. Use of cool water will provide additional relief to hot, swollen feet as cold water temperatures encourage constriction of blood vessels and aid inflammation. Although local treatment can include massage, many women who are in their last trimester find it difficult to apply oils to their feet due to their enlarging bellies. The easiest method of all to ease swelling and edema of the feet and ankles is the cool compress. A cold wet towel soaked in aromatic water brings welcome relief. Lie down and elevate your feet (at least 8 inches above heart level) on pillows while the compress treatment is done. Alternatively, a footbath can be made using the same amount of essential oils given in the compress recipe, and mixing them in a basin of cool water to soak the feet. This is convenient if you are sitting doing something else; however, it doesn't allow for elevation which is very helpful. This forces you to take a nice relaxing break which is beneficial itself!

Cold Towel Compress

for swollen feet

a towel to wrap feet and ankles
a piece of plastic wrap
sink or tub of cold water
2 drops Lavender essential oil
1 drop Lemon essential oil
1 drop Geranium essential oil

Fill a sink or basin with cool to cold water. See hydrotherapy guidelines in Chapter 11. Add the essential oils and stir with your hands. Soak the towel in the aromatic water. Prepare the place where you will be lying. Place several pillows at the foot of the bed or couch, with a layer of plastic wrap over them to protect from the moist towels. Wring out the towel leaving it moist. Lie down and wrap your feet and ankles loosely with the cool towel compress. Leave on for 15 to 20 minutes, or as long as desired.

Other helpful essential oils to use for swelling and edema of the extremities include mandarin, grapefruit, lime, orange, rose, and rosemary.

Lifestyle recommendations include taking frequent rest breaks and elevating your feet. Wearing supportive hosiery will help, but be careful not to wear tight clothing around the abdomen. Regular exercise, avoiding salt, and eating healthy food will also discourage this ailment. The Wall Butterfly yoga pose described in the next section helps swelling of the feet. Use the adaptation recommendation given there, which suggests leaving the legs in the vertical position as most effective for this ailment.

Relieving Backache Due to Pregnancy

It is not uncommon to experience low backache during your pregnancy, especially in the last trimester, when the baby gains most of his or her weight. This creates pressure on the lower back and pelvis, and changes the center of gravity for the mother. Additionally, at this time hormone levels increase to relax muscles and ligaments in preparation for labor.

This recipe is safe to use during late pregnancy when backache is most common. You can apply the oil yourself by using the palms of your hands and rubbing in circular motions on the low back area. Otherwise, it would be ideal to have someone rub your back for you. Finding a comfortable position to receive a massage when eight or nine months pregnant can be a challenge. You can sit over the back of a chair or use pillows or a bean bag chair on the floor to support your abdomen and allow access to your back.

Massage Oil for Backache

for simple backache due to pregnancy

4 tbls. vegetable oil

5 drops Lavender essential oil

3 drops Rosemary essential oil

3 drops Sandalwood essential oil

1 drop Geranium essential oil

In a 2-ounce amber glass bottle, add the essential oils. Be sure to measure the exact amounts carefully. Add the vegetable or sweet almond oil. Shake well and label contents. To apply this oil simply pour a small amount on the palms of your hands and rub together to warm. Apply by massaging into the sacrum and lower back area for a few minutes. Apply counterpressure with your thumbs, as this can bring additional relief. Take a few deep relaxing breaths.

If your partner or friend is giving you the massage, speak up about any discomfort you may feel, and communicate what works for you and what does not. Review the aromatherapy massage tips in Chapter 12. Sitting over the back side of a chair, with pillows under the abdomen, works particularly well for this treatment.

A very effective yoga exercise called the "Wall Butterfly" can be done daily to prevent backache and also for symptomatic relief of aches already present. It is very helpful for women when they are menstruating and experiencing low backache, and for providing relief for the backache pregnant mothers endure. You can do this exercise two or three times per day, or whenever your body tells you to take a time out! Try using the aromatherapy backache oil blend prior to doing this pose to gain extra benefit.

The Wall Butterfly Pose

Do this exercise with comfortable clothing on and remove your shoes.

Lie on your back on the floor, with your buttocks and legs against the wall. Let your legs drop open and press the soles of your feet together. You can gently press your knees apart and down with your hands to stretch completely. Breathe deeply and slowly through your nose. Close your eyes, concentrate on your breath and relax. Rest in this pose for several minutes or as long as it is comfortable for you.

An adaptation to this pose is to simply leave your legs in the vertical position against the wall, or drop them apart into a "V" formation. Rest your arms out to your sides on the floor, palms open and facing the ceiling. Or you can put your legs up on a chair seat, bending at the knees, if this is more comfortable for you.

Support For Breast Soreness

Breast heaviness and soreness is common for all mothers-to-be. The increasing weight and stretching of the breasts can be uncomfortable. Wearing a good supportive bra, applying cool aromatic compresses on swollen and enlarged breasts, or running cool shower water over the breasts can be very helpful. A massage oil can also be used to diminish soreness and discomfort caused by the additional weight. However, it is important to mention that once you start breastfeeding your baby, do not apply essential oils to your breasts as the baby can ingest them. This section addresses the general discomfort experienced prior to giving birth and breastfeeding.

Occasionally premenstrual breast soreness is experienced. If breast tenderness or pain is present without an apparent reason (you are not pregnant or experiencing PMS), perform a breast self-examination or seek an evaluation from your doctor.

If you experience dry or cracking nipples after childbirth, apply a natural healing ointment made of herbal infused oils, like the ointment recipe given on page 319.

The following compress can easily be made and applied to swollen and sore breasts. Cool water temperature is ideal for conditions that involve swelling.

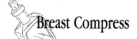 **Breast Compress**

---

to relieve soreness

warm water

2 drops Orange essential oil

1 drop Geranium essential oil

towel, 2 washcloths (or tube socks)

In a bowl or sink, add warm water. Add the essential oils and stir with your hand to mix into the water. Soak the washcloths (or you can use 2 cotton tube socks) in the aromatic water. Wring the cloth until it is moist, but not wet. Wrap the washcloths or socks around each breast. Drape a towel over this and lie down and relax. Leave the compresses on until they become cool or dry, then replace with fresh ones. Leave on for a total of 15 minutes.

To make an aromatic massage oil to apply to sore breasts, the following recipe is very effective. Massage the breasts in a circular motion from the center (midline of chest) outward in a counterclockwise direction. This stroke direction encourages lymphatic drainage away from the congested breasts to the lymph nodes under the arms. This can be applied once per day, or as needed for breast tenderness and feeling of heaviness.

Breast Oil

to relieve soreness (Do not use while breastfeeding)

2 tbls. vegetable oil

4 drops Orange essential oil

2 drops Geranium essential oil

In a 1-ounce amber glass bottle, add the essential oils. Add the vegetable oil and shake well. Label contents with directions for use. Apply daily in an outward circular massage direction.

Aromatherapy Support for Labor and Delivery

More than ever women and their partners are requesting personalized childbirths, including homebirths, birthing rooms in hospitals, and water births. Many of these were unheard of in our mothers' time, but are becoming increasingly popular. It is not uncommon to see women choosing natural supportive therapies, such as aromatherapy, for their childbirth experiences.

I wish I could turn back the clock, and use what I know now when I had my twins. It would have been a much more pleasurable and relaxing experience, I'm sure. Soft lighting, gentle music in the background, and soothing scents would fill the room. After all, this is a special day, a cause for celebration. To many the birth of their offspring is a spiritual experience that will change them forever. Not only does aromatherapy help with pain control, relaxation, and air disinfection, it welcomes the newborn in a very special aromatic way.

Several of the essential oils employed at this time (labor and childbirth) are ones on the cautionary list for pregnancy. These include clary sage, jasmine, nutmeg, and rose essential oils. These essences aid in childbirth by easing labor pain. It is safe to use these oils in labor under the recommendations stated here. Be aware that many women experience periods of disinterest in scents, or possibly episodes of extreme reactions to them, when previously they posed no problems. The mother is priority, and no matter how helpful an essential oil or aromatherapy method may be, if the woman dislikes it at the time, remove it until a later time perhaps. Her comfort is crucial. More often than not, aromatherapy is very well received by mother, partner, and birthing staff. It helps relax everyone and bring the focus to the event at hand. Because most essential oils possess antibacterial properties, disinfection of the room air is an added benefit to using aromatherapy. A room mister, diffuser or aroma lamp is the best option, as fire regulations do not allow burning candles in most hospitals.

Case History: *A 31-year-old first-time mother delivered her baby at home. We had prepared several months in advance for the coming of this baby and had discussed her wishes about the childbirth event. She had experimented with different essential oils beforehand, and knew which essences pleased her. She used a diffuser with lavender and frankincense essential oils to relax her and help with pain control in addition to encouraging her to stay focused and grounded. Massage oils were prepared ahead of time which included lavender and clary sage to aid the labor process. These oils were very effective when massaged into her lower back with counterpressure when she experienced "back labor" and discomfort, and also applied to her lower abdomen to increase and strengthen contractions when needed. One of her favorite aromatherapy treatments was a simple neroli facial mist which she used often over her face and chest for relaxation, uplifting her emotions and to freshen her. It was very pleasant for the birth team members too! She had a birthing tub available, which she used through dilatation to aid in relaxation. She experienced a wonderful birth, and can't wait to have another baby soon. Between the supportive birth team and her partner, the flowers and aromatherapy, the soft lighting and music, and the welcoming of her perfect and precious newborn daughter, the experience was magically memorable.*

The inhalation synergy blend given below is used to help decrease the need for pain medication, promote relaxation, relieve anxiety and help the mother (and birth team) to stay focused and centered during the labor process. The Lavender essential oil is also a mild antiseptic which is helpful in purifying the room air. If a stronger disinfecting blend is needed, as perhaps in a hospital setting, then the *Pure For Sure Blend* found on page 335 would be a good option since it contains more effective essences that are antibacterial. Remember to use aromatherapy inhalation in moderation to provide a subtle ambiance, rather than an overwhelming scent. A room mist can also be made with this blend or with others you create by following the directions on preparation in Chapter 13.

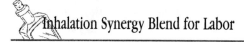

Inhalation Synergy Blend for Labor

to ease pain, promote relaxation and centeredness

8 parts Lavender essential oil

1 part Frankincense essential oil

A very effective labor massage oil blend is welcomed in most births. A combination of lavender, clary sage, and chamomile essential oils is used to massage the lower abdomen to aid contractions to be more effective, help to relax inner tensions in the mother, and aid in pain control. This massage oil can be applied between contractions as discussed above or applied to the lower back and sacrum for "back labor" and pain. Massaging this area of the back with counterpressure from the palm of the hand provides additional relief.

Alternatively, this oil can be massaged into the mother's feet. However, if you are planning to deliver your baby in water, as in a birthing tub, then it is suggested that you wash off the essential oils with a mild soap and water solution to prevent contact of these oils with the newborn. You can make this blend ahead of time so it will be ready when you are.

 Labor Oil

a pain-relieving blend

2 tbls. sweet almond or vegetable oil

2 tbls. St. John's Wort or Arnica infusion oil

8 drops Lavender essential oil

3 drops Clary sage essential oil

1 drop Chamomile essential oil

In an amber glass bottle, mix the essential oils with the carrier oils. Combine well by shaking the bottle and label contents with directions for use. Warm a small amount of oil in your hands before applying to the lower abdomen or lower back area (sacrum).

Essential oils that are frequently used in labor are clary sage, jasmine, lavender, nutmeg, and rose. Those that aid in relaxation, anxiety, and fear are also helpful, and include bergamot, chamomile, frankincense, jasmine, lavender, lemon, mandarin, neroli, orange, rose, and spikenard. Lavender essential oil is key to all your labor oil blends as it is well known in relieving pain and decreasing the need for analgesic drugs. Essential oils which potentially stimulate the production of endorphins, the body's natural painkillers, are useful in pain control and include many of the oils already listed for labor and delivery: clary sage, jasmine, patchouli, and ylang ylang.

If nausea is experienced during labor, placing a drop of peppermint on a tissue and inhaling will help. Also a cool compress of lavender and peppermint is very effective. Use the *Compress for Nausea* recipe on page 277.

For general use, and for refreshing the mother, a facial mist can be made or purchased to use over the face and upper chest. It is very light and cooling for a tired and warm mother in stressful times. It quickly changes both the environment and her outlook. Turn to Chapter 12 for recipes and be sure to include the relaxing and refreshing essences she prefers. This mist can provide a mild deodorant effect which is pleasant to use. Choose neroli, rose, or a citrus essential oil for options.

Healing the Perineum with Soothing Sitz Baths

After the birth of your baby, you can expect to experience discomfort of the perineum area which will vary in degree among women and circumstances. There may be swelling of local tissues, tears, or stitches if an episiotomy was performed. During the first 24 to 48 hours after the delivery cold packs are recommended to diminish inflammation if the symptoms are severe. Otherwise, sitz baths in warm or tepid water with essential oils can increase healing, prevent secondary infection, aid circulation, and decrease swelling. Most hospitals have sitz baths on their post-partum floors. At home you can use the bathtub by filling it only partially, sit in a large basin, or use a baby bathing tub. A low level of water is used to cover the perineum area only. If there is considerable swelling, use the cooler water temperature or cold packs to help. Otherwise a warm water temperature is soothing and relaxing. Witch hazel lotion can be included in the sitz bath treatment for its astringent quality, but is optional.

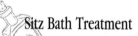 **Sitz Bath Treatment**

following childbirth

2 drops Lavender essential oil

1 drop Patchouli essential oil

1 drop Tea Tree essential oil

1/4 cup Witch Hazel lotion (optional)

1 tbls. honey

Combine the essential oils with the honey. Add the witch hazel to the water, and then the aromatic honey. The honey is used as the carrier and for its anti-inflammatory and antibacterial properties. Stir the water well with your hands to disperse the oils completely. Sit in the water for 15 to 20 minutes. This can be done twice per day to aid healing and to prevent infection.

A peri-wash can be very helpful immediately following the delivery and up to a few days afterwards. Using toilet tissue can cause discomfort to swollen and sore areas, while cleansing with warm aromatic water can be very soothing and aid healing. Keep a plastic bottle at hand in the bathroom for convenience. If you have any itching, try bergamot essential oil instead of the patchouli. If there is any tearing or sutures, substitute tea tree for the patchouli. You may want to use the lavender essential oil all by itself as another option. It doesn't have to be complicated to work well.

Post-Delivery Peri-Wash

to cleanse the perineum

7 ounces warm distilled water

2 tbls. Witch hazel (optional)

1 drop Lavender essential oil

1 drop Patchouli essential oil

In a clean plastic bottle, add the essential oils and witch hazel. Shake well. Add the warm water and shake again to mix well. Before using this peri-wash solution, you must shake it very well as the essential oils float to the top quickly. Alternatively, you can mix the essential oils in a little honey to emulsify them, making them water soluble. After voiding, rinse the perineum with this aromatic solution to be fresh and clean.

Other essential oils that are useful in healing the perineum following childbirth are bergamot, chamomile, and myrrh.

A Guide to Surviving Post-Partum Depression

Post-partum (after childbirth) depression is a common condition for many women several days following delivery up to one year later. Vague feelings of depression, tearfulness, feelings of being overwhelmed, resentment, anger, or deep depression can be experienced in varying degrees. Caused by a fluctuation in hormones, increase in demands put upon the mother, stress, sleepless nights, and the change in family dynamics are all factors in this challenging condition. The primary goal of aromatherapy support for post-partum depression, or the "baby blues," is to relieve stress, encourage relaxation, lift the spirits, and rebalance the physiology. Often, mothers expect perfection from themselves, spouse, and their new baby. It never works that way.

Asking for help, getting nurturing and support (both physically and emotionally), eating healthy foods and getting enough rest are measures that can be taken to support the balancing and recuperation of the new mother. When friends or neighbors offer to help, let them. Or ask for massage gift certificates or baby-sitting "coupons." When I had my twins, I was very overwhelmed and ended up hiring a teenage girl to help clean the house and play with my older child so that I could attend to the newborns more easily and be more relaxed. The fact is, when there is a new addition to the family, some of the other chores must be let go. I'm giving you permission not to do everything!

As you might expect, there are essential oils that can help uplift your mood while being effective for stressful conditions such as post-partum depression. The most frequently used essential oils are bergamot, chamomile, geranium, grapefruit, jasmine, rose, and ylang ylang; I find geranium and bergamot most helpful in regulating the physiology and emotions. Many of the florals, such as neroli, rose, and jasmine, help lift the spirits. Rose, jasmine, clary sage, and grapefruit are euphoric essential oils and can lift mild depression. Ylang ylang essential oil is noted for calming anger, which may not be a conscious feeling you are experiencing, but it is not unrealistic to feel a little resentment towards all the changes taking place around you. Indeed, experts believe some forms of depression may in fact be anger turned inward, instead of outwardly expressed. If this is the case, as I have seen periodically, then ylang ylang is the answer.

This is a synergy blend that can be added to the bath, used in a diffuser or aroma lamp, or applied on the skin in a lotion or oil. Refer to Part Three of this book for different aromatherapy methods that will be convenient and easy for you to use. Refer to the User-Friendly Blending Chart to determine how much essential oils are used in the various aromatherapy methods outlined there. This is a blend well-liked by many; you don't have to be experiencing depression to enjoy it. It is a light, slightly fruity, heavenly scent, sure to lift your spirits and balance the emotions.

Post-Partum Depression Synergy Blend

to balance and uplift the emotions

4 parts Lavender essential oil

2 parts Ylang ylang essential oil

2 parts Clary sage essential oil

1 part Bergamot essential oil

1 part Mandarin essential oil

Mix the above essential oils in an amber glass bottle with screw top. For a large amount, use an eye dropper or teaspoon as the measure. If a smaller amount is needed, simply count them out as drops, using the above ratios.

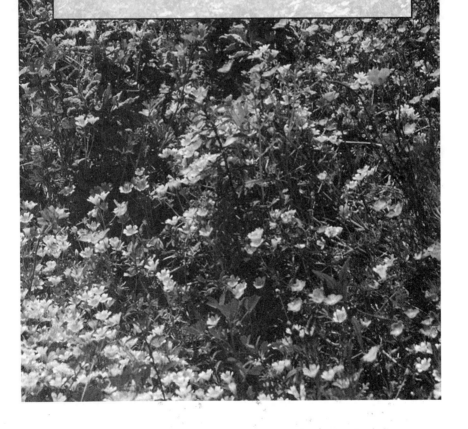

PART THREE

Enjoying
the Aromatic Lifestyle

The most popular and creative methods of enjoying aromatherapy are presented in the following three chapters. Some will be familiar to you, while others may surprise you with their simplicity and effectiveness as new ways to apply essential oils in your bath, on your body, or diffused in the air. Traditional aromatherapy is discussed, as well as new cutting-edge technologies not yet in the mainstream marketplace. You will have fun exploring many new ways of using natural plant essences, and learning which ones will fit easily into your lifestyle. Welcome to the aromatic lifestyle! Be prepared to awaken your senses while you create a more healthful and pleasurable environment for yourself, while healing a multitude of common ailments with these therapeutic essential oils.

CHAPTER 11

The Aromatic Bath —Your Personal Spa

When you hear the word "bathing," what do you think of? A way to get clean, sun bathing, dirty kids, baby baths, bubbles . . . ? This chapter will have you anticipating and planning your next bath after you find out some of the great benefits to bathing with essential oils.

If you can't get away to find rest and relaxation, you can create your own peaceful escape, indulging the senses and nurturing the soul, within the privacy and convenience of your own home. I'll share some of my secrets with you, so you can experience that feeling of "getting away" without ever leaving the tub! Sounds too good to be true, doesn't it? *An hour of aromatherapy can make you feel like you've had the whole day off.* Escape + relax + indulge = Rejuvenation. This formula works every time. And essential oils are involved every single step of the way.

In today's stressful and fast-paced world, we rarely allow ourselves enough time to take a quick shower, let alone a full, relaxing bath. Ironically, those of us who have the least time for this luxury, are the ones who need it the most. But don't despair! Later on in the chapter I'll present quick and easy recipes for the shower, simple foot and hand soaks, and more. I believe once you begin to experience the "aromatic lifestyle" you *will* find the time, even if it's on a weekly basis at first, to enjoy essential oils as part of your daily routine.

Nature's Healing Ritual—The Bath

The bath experience can be totally relaxing and rejuvenating in itself, but once you learn how to incorporate the use of aromatherapy with the basic hydrotherapy techniques described later on in this chapter, you'll be multiplying the bath's effects by many times. Essential oils and baths have synergistic effects.

Humankind has used water in religious rituals since the earliest recordings. However, it was the Greek and Roman cultures that probably contributed the most to this area of combining oils and bathing. You are about to learn how to create your own personal spa or therapeutic bath, free from synthetic fragrances, dyes, etc.

> Hippocrates noted in 500 B.C. that "the way to health is to have an aromatic bath and scented massage every day."

You can use single essential oils or a combination to get a desired effect. It's as highly individual as you are, and comes down to your response to an oil and also your scent preference. Although one can design a purely therapeutic blend for a specific problem, don't use it if you can't stand the smell of a particular essential oil; find an alternative with similar qualities.

Every essential oil has the potential to affect us both physically and emotionally. Essential oils have a tiny molecular structure enabling them to penetrate the skin. Because of the skin's absorption capabilities, essential oils used in the bath can have a multitude of effects on the physical level (See Cross-Section of Skin illustration page 16.). Lavender is a perfect example of this. It has been used traditionally in skin care for acne conditions, oily skin, minor burns, and skin rejuvenation. Essential oils in the bath also affect our moods, because as they evaporate we inhale them. (See psycho-aromatherapy illustration page 14.) Here as well, lavender has a similar effect, soothing the nervous system as well as the psyche. For this reason, it is often found in relaxation blends designed to relieve stress, anxiety and insomnia.

The Carriers—Transporting Essences into the Bath

Decide on what carrier, if any, you want to use for the essential oil blend. Carriers are needed to "disperse" the essential oils in the bath since they are not soluble in water. When using essential oils by themselves (without a carrier) always add them last after the tub has filled, because they evaporate very quickly. It's best to give them a whirl or swish in the water with your hand to insure that they disperse as much as possible.

Some popular oils used as carrier-agents are sweet almond, canola, soy, and safflower. (See Chapter 15 for more information on carriers). These are wonderful for their moisturizing abilities, leaving a thin film of oil on the surface of the water which will envelop your body as you sink in. However, they also tend to leave an oily ring in the bath tub. I personally prefer using carriers like sweet cream, honey, Castile soap, or a bath salt mixture.

You can mix your essential oils in a tablespoon or two of Castile liquid soap (unscented, of course). For a very luxurious bath, I use honey as a base carrier or heavy cream. (It worked for Cleopatra!) The honey is very nourishing to the skin and has anti-inflammatory properties. The cream is a natural emulsifier that is excellent for dry skin, making it a great alternative to oils. Essential oils dissolve easily in both.

Hydrotherapy—Using Water Temperature to Heal

Literally translated, hydrotherapy means "water healing." This form of therapy involves the extended use of baths or showers in the home using hot or cold temperatures. Hydrotherapy is a very powerful tool, with documentation showing this regime alone can relieve muscle soreness, help in relaxation, increase oxygen, nutrients and lymphatic flow. In general, it strengthens and cleans out the body. I have included only the very basics of hydrotherapy here for you to consider when deciding upon an appropriate bath. Please practice safety by confirming the bath water temperature with a thermometer, especially when using the hot and cold bath temperatures. And never allow yourself to get to the point of fatigue or chills.

A *hot bath* (99°-108° F) is good for insomnia, to increase circulation, help relieve pain and eliminate toxins. Heart rate can increase by as much as 4 times the normal rate the first 5 minutes, then will normalize. Recommended time: 20 minutes or less. Follow with cool water.

A *warm bath* (97°-101° F) is the most common temperature for the average bath. Immersion for 20 minutes to an hour is great for relaxation.

A *tepid bath* (92°-97° F) is helpful when you want to rejuvenate or have inflammatory conditions such as hives, itching, or skin rashes. Recommended time: Up to 1 hour.

Cold applications (59°-68° F) are for very short periods of time and are used most often in the shower or in foot and hand baths. Recommended time: A few seconds.

Caution: If you have low blood pressure, are elderly, obese, have heart problems, or caring for young children, do not use the extreme tempera- tures unless directed to do so by your doctor.

I also like to make my own bath salts to add to the bath and carry the essential oils. Although not as popular as in the great days of the "European Spas," bath salts appear to be making a comeback. The recipe for bath salts I've included in the book have great detoxifying and "drawing-out" bene- fits.

For a full soak make sure your shoulders are totally submerged. A good guidcline for an average bath (outside of the hydrotherapy recom- mendations described in the chapter) is about 20 to 30 minutes to get the full benefit, although I've been known to disappear for more than an hour with a good book, an indulgent essential oil blend, and plenty of hot herbal tea. Near the end of this chapter, I have provided some personal favorite base recipes for aromatic bathing, as well as the essential oil blends to add to them.

> To make an aromatic vanilla honey, heat natural honey gently, then pour into a squeaky clean glass jar to which you have added 1 or 2 four- inch pieces of vanilla bean. Let it age for a week or two, if you're able to stay away from it that long!

Stimulating Showers

If you prefer to shower, you can still enjoy the benefits of aromatherapy. Before you even get into the shower, massage yourself with a cloth or mitt sprinkled with 6 to 8 drops of essential oils (according to this chapter's recipes), then shower as usual. The heat from the water will open your pores, allowing some of the oils to be absorbed, and it will diffuse aromatic scents around you. (This massage method, however, is not recommended for sensitive areas, broken or irritated skin. Additionally, do not use peppermint essential oil undiluted on the skin, or other skin-irritant essential oils. (See Chapter 1: Common Sense Safety.)

Another way of using essential oils in the shower is to apply them after you have washed, but before you get out. Put your essential oils on your wet washcloth and rub yourself all over. Breathe deeply as the water gently runs down your cleanly scented body. Towel-dry gently once out of the shower, taking care not to scrub off all the good oils you just put on. (Keep the bathroom door shut to keep in the vapors, as long as the room has adequate ventilation.)

A fun and easy option for the shower without directly applying essential oils is the Short-cut Steambath method. Simply plug the shower floor drain (a rubber sink drain stopper works well) and add a few drops of essential oils to the water collecting in the bottom of your shower. You will be inhaling the beneficial steam as the vapors rise, as well as soaking your feet in the aromatic water below. If you take a really long shower, like my oldest son, keep an eye on the water level!

I recommend avoiding as much as possible harsh deodorant soaps and all toiletries made with synthetic fragrances. They tend to undo the aromatic benefits and strip your skin of its natural moisture, as well as remove the delicate essential oils just applied. Using gentle, pure vegetable-based soaps made with essential oils is the best choice, and there are now many natural alternatives for hair care. By using aromatherapy-based skin and hair care products, you are using aromatherapy in the shower!

> "Water is the most healing of all remedies, and the best of all cosmetics."—Old Arab Proverb

Most essential oils have some deodorizing effect since they help kill bacteria and germs; consequently they help with body odor. Some are more potent in this area than others. (See Chapter 14: *Essential Oil Reference Guide* for individual essential oil characteristics and Chapters 7 and 13—for other references related to this subject.)

Quick 'n' Easy Shortcuts—Foot and Hand Baths

Now, what do you do if you don't even have the time for a quick shower, or just don't feel like totally undressing? What if it's only your feet that need the attention and not your entire body? Foot and hand baths are the answer. These simple yet very effective ways of using aromatics are virtually unknown to the general population. You're going to love how easy they are to use and how great they make you feel.

Maurice Messegué, a famous French herbalist and natural healer, perfected and popularized this form of healing therapy. Although he used mostly fresh and dried herbs that grew along the French countryside for his bath preparations, he demonstrated the positive benefits from using herbal hand and foot baths. I have observed similar results with the use of aromatherapy-adapted foot and hand soaks. If you are an avid runner or your occupation calls for being on your feet all day, you will want to learn about these local treatment baths.

Hand and foot baths are an excellent way to "take your medicine," especially for children. The essential oils are absorbed via this local bath method; however, they benefit the whole body.

M. Messegué favored this way of healing over all other external treatments. We know the beneficial principles of the plants and their essential oils are absorbed through the skin. This form of treatment bypasses the stomach; therefore it does not interfere with digestion, nor do the gastric juices interfere with the medicament.

To prepare a footbath, you need a few basic items: a tub that can fit both feet comfortably, such as a plastic dishpan, a towel, your essential oils, and about 10 to 15 minutes of your time. This can be done easily while reading, writing letters, or watching television. Pick a comfortable place to sit. Fill the tub half full of water, using the hydrotherapy guide on page 294 for the appropriate temperature if you wish, or just warm water for general use. Add the selected essential oils and/or carrier, and jump in! Ten to fifteen minutes is an average amount of time to soak; any longer than that and you'll need to change the water because this small amount gets cold quickly. Towel dry. Apply a massage oil blend to the feet if you wish.

Some Eastern and Western therapies include "Reflexology," which is based on the theory that there are "responsive zones" in the feet and hands corresponding to every part and organ of the body.

Hand baths are basically the same preparation except you may choose to use two separate tubs, one on each side, or you could use the single tub on your lap or on a table top. The hand bath is commonly recommended for arthritis, writer's cramp, swelling, and carpal tunnel syndrome.

With both of these localized bath treatments you will get overall aromatherapy benefits as well. For example, my recipe for tired, aching feet will have an uplifting, stimulating effect on your emotions because of the rosemary and peppermint essential oils, as well as a rejuvenating effect on your feet, making them feel wonderful and ready to dance the night away!

A sitz bath is another local bath treatment useful in healing the perianal region. It means "to sit" literally, and involves using a shallow level of water up to the hips and soaking . It is useful in conditions involving this area, such as cystitis, perineum healing following childbirth, and for local irritations and itching. Use up to 4 drops of essential oil per sitz bath. The use of a carrier is recommended in warm or tepid water. Avoid the essential oils that are known to be skin irritant-prone as the tissues of this area are very delicate. (See Chapter 1 for the listing of such essential oils.)

The A,B,C'S of The Aromatic Bath

A is for *Aromatherapy*—choose the essential oils you want to use to attain a desired effect or because you are drawn to their scent.

B is for *Bath temperature*—if appropriate, choose what temperature will assist you in your goal. Hot, warm, tepid, or cold.

C is for *Carrier*—choose a carrier to mix your essential oils with to disperse them, if desired. Vegetable oil, honey, cream, milk, bath salts, Castile lotion. Or simply sprinkle essential oils directly onto bath mitt or washcloth.

Beauty and the Bath—The Recipes

This is your time . . . so relax and enjoy.

Choose the appropriate essential oils for these basic carrier recipes from the special blends recipes which follow (pages 297 to 305)

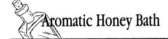

Aromatic Honey Bath

Soothing and anti-inflammatory

Mix 6 to 10 drops essential oil in 1/4 cup of raw honey, then add to bath water.

(can also add 1 or 2 Vitamin E capsules by cutting end off gel cap and squeezing the vitamin E oil into the honey. Mix well.)

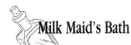

Milk Maid's Bath

Wonderful in winter or when skin is dry

Mix 6 to 10 drops essential oil in 1/4 – 1/2 cup of heavy cream, Buttermilk or Goat's Milk (or can use powdered milk to make a paste)

then add to bath.

Be frivolous! Sprinkle Rose petals in your bath water.

Castile Bath Lotion

Mix 6 to 10 drops essential oil
in 1 to 2 tablespoons unscented Castile liquid soap, then add to bath water.

Botanical Bath

An indulgent bath to replenish and nourish the entire body

1/4 cup aloe vera gel or juice
1/4 cup milk or cream
2 tablespoons honey
2 tablespoons baking soda
1/4 cup sea salt
6 to 10 drops essential oils
1 tablespoon powdered spirulina sea weed
(or whole seaweed frond), optional

Mix in 2-cup measuring cup. Add to bath after it has been drawn.

Bath Oil

Very moisturizing and protective

Mix 6 to 10 drops essential oil in 2 teaspoons of vegetable or seed oil (canola, safflower, soy, or sweet almond oil); add to bath water and swish.

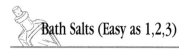

Bath Salts (Easy as 1,2,3)

Useful in detoxifying the body

Add 6 to 10 drops essential oil
to following mixture:

1 teaspoon baking soda
2 teaspoons Epsom salt
3 teaspoons Sea salt

Mix well. Add to bath water.

(Can use up to 1/2 cup of bath salts per bat—but do not exceed the 10 drops total of essential oils per Bath.)

The above bath salts can be made ahead in larger amounts. The typical amount used for one bath is 2 tablespoons. I keep mine in an apothecary jar with a seashell for a scoop. Keep away from moisture as it can cake relatively easily.

The following recipes call for a total of *eight drops of essential oils per bath,* unless otherwise noted. In general, six to ten drops can be used for the average aromatic bath.

For foot and hand baths use a total of *four drops of essential oils* per small local treatment bath, unless otherwise noted.

Do it in the dark. Bathe in complete darkness. Great antidote for sensory overload. Have a flashlight handy.

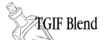

TGIF Blend

For mental exhaustion

Lavender 5 drops

Grapefruit 3 drops

Recommend dim lighting or total darkness for sensory overload. Warm-hot bath.

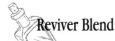

Reviver Blend

(my sister's favorite) Good in morning or to rejuvenate for evening

Bergamot 4 drops
Petitgrain 4 drops
Warm-tepid bath.

Serenity Blend

Relaxing, sleep-inducing

Lavender 5 drops
Bergamot 2 drops
Mandarin 1 drop
Dim lights, candles, quiet or soft music.
Hot-warm bath.

Make a DO NOT DISTURB sign for the bathroom door.

Undress-De-Stress

For nervous tension and anxiety

Lavender 6 drops
Clary Sage 2 drops
Dim lights, one single candle, deep relaxing breaths.

The better the skin's condition, the better the essential oils will be absorbed and utilized.

Tune-Up

Tones the body, good during seasonal changes

Lavender 4 drops
Lemongrass 4 drops
OR
Grapefruit 5 drops
Basil 3 drops

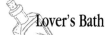

Lover's Bath

an aphrodisiac blend

Ylang-Ylang 4 drops
Clary Sage 2 drops
Bergamot 1 drop
Sandalwood 1 drop
Wait until kids are asleep. Candlelight, soft music.
Warm-hot (be careful it's not too hot.)

Woodstock

An aphrodisiac blend

Patchouli 4 drops
Ylang-Ylang 4 drops
Get out some 60's music.
Burn patchouli incense.

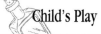

Child's Play

For the young at heart

Lavender 4 drops
Mandarin 4 drops
Use half this amount for children.
Fun bath toys. Warm-tepid bath.

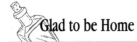

Glad to be Home

Regulating, good for jet lag

Lavender 5 drops

Geranium 3 drops

For hangover, substitute 3 drops of Juniper for Geranium.

Warm bath. Dim lights.

Cool washcloth to forehead.

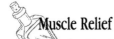

Muscle Relief

For overworked muscles

Great after working in the yard all day, or following a marathon!

Lavender 4 drops

Rosemary 2 drops

Eucalyptus 2 drops

OR

For sore, swollen muscles

juniper helps with excess fluid and toxins

Lavender 4 drops

Juniper 2 drops

Eucalyptus 2 drops

Warm-hot bath.

Dry brushing is a form of stimulating massage. It sloughs off dead skin cells and increases circulation. Always dry brush and massage towards the direction of the heart.

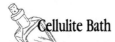

Cellulite Bath

To help with cellulite, rid excess fluid

Cypress 3 drops

Lemon 3 drops
Juniper 1 drop
Lavender 1 drop
Warm bath. Dry brush before bath or use loofah in tub on stubborn areas.
Sip on hot water with lemon juice (daily).

Try growing your own loofah sponges!

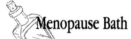

Menopause Bath

Regulates, helps with hot flashes

Geranium 3 drops
Clary Sage 2 drops
Lemon 2 drops
Bergamot 1 drop

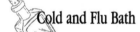

Cold and Flu Bath

Lavender 3 drops
Bergamot 3 drops
Tea Tree 2 drops
Warm to hot bath temperature.
Dry off well. Wrap yourself up in a thick bathrobe.
Go to bed early.

Some specific foot and hand bath recipes.

Footbath for Tired, Aching Feet

Great for joggers and anyone standing feet all day.

Rosemary 3 drops
Peppermint 2 drops

Lavender 1 drop
Tepid-cold bath.

Ask your mate for a foot massage. A test of true love!

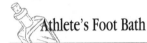

Athlete's Foot Bath

For fungus infection

Tea Tree 2 drops
Cedarwood 1 drop
Cypress 1 drop

Helpful hints for Athlete's Foot: Fungus likes moisture, so wear cotton socks, stay out of sneakers as much as possible, and towel dry completely between toes.

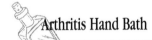

Arthritis Hand Bath

Also helpful with cramping and overuse

Juniper 2 drops
Lavender 1 drop
Cypress 1 drop
Rosemary 1 drop
Warm-tepid bath.

Raynaud's Foot and Hand Bath

To increase blood circulation by dilating capillaries

Geranium 2 drops

Rosemary 2 drops

Lavender 1 drop

Warm-hot bath. Check water temperature carefully, as people with Raynaud's disease often have temperature sensitivity.

CHAPTER 12

All-Over Body Treatments and Special Care for Small Areas

Whole-Body Treatments— Practical Tips to Do It Yourself at Home

In this chapter we will talk about some of the different body treatments where aromatherapy can be applied. This section is divided into two parts. The first part is concerned with whole-body applications, and the second covers small, local and problem areas. One of the major differences between the two is the dilution percentages. Whenever we are applying essential oils to a large area, typically a 2% dilution is recommended. The skin, being our largest organ, can weigh as much as 6.6 pounds and cover more than 2 square yards of area. So it makes sense that we use a smaller amount, since such a large surface area will be utilized to absorb the oils. In contrast, the local treatments cover a much smaller, concentrated area such as a patch of skin, a facial area, or one particular joint or muscle. Therefore a stronger preparation of 4% to 8% can be used safely.

Personalized Body Lotions and Oils

I am about to give you some necessary tools to customize your very own body lotions and oils at home. They will undoubtedly be better for you since you will be adding only what *you* need. You will know exactly what you are putting on your body, and absorbing for that matter, because you are creating your own unique body preparations. *You* will choose what to add and for what reason.

Let's start with the simplest. If you are using a good, unscented body lotion now, all you have to do is add the right amount of essential oils to it to make an easy scented lotion. Most lotions are water-based, emulsified, or blended with vegetable oils. They consist of a solidifier and emulsifier to keep the water and oil from separating.

When purchasing your lotion, be sure to read the ingredients and avoid mineral oil by-products. Mineral oil is produced from tar. It has a large molecular structure which can prevent or block the essential oils from penetrating the skin. Look for aloe vera, herbal extracts, and good nut and seed oils in them to help nourish the skin.

For an all-over *body lotion,* use 40 drops of essential oil for a 4-ounce bottle of neutral lotion, or 80 drops in an 8-ounce bottle. Be sure to mix well by capping the bottle of lotion tightly and shaking. This is a great way to "feed" your body the balancing, calming, or stimulating oils it may need on a regular daily basis. Or you may simply choose an essential oil you are drawn to because of its unique scent, and it brings you pleasure simply because you like it. It's up to you. A helpful hint: when mixing your lotions, start with less than a full bottle, so when you add the essential oils, there will be space in the bottle to allow good mixing to take place when the bottle is shaken well.

There are some fine lotions available in natural health markets these days. Make note of the fluid ounces on the bottle and add the required amount of essential oils. Be sure to label it afterwards. I use an unscented base lotion with a plenitude of herbal extracts, concentrated aloe vera, jojoba oil, etc., and then add my own essential oils. In the summer, when I don't need the richness of this lotion, I opt for a much lighter one with a higher water content.

Much simpler to prepare yourself at home are the body oils. It's amazing how thirsty our skin is for oil. Oils are one of the earliest treatments used for wrinkles, dry skin, and over-all moisturizing protection. They do not call for the emulsifiers and solidifiers needed to prepare lotions. Basically they consist of a base vegetable or nut/seed oil blended with essential oils. I do, however, add vitamin E, wheatgerm, or jojoba oil to them to slow down their oxidizing tendency. See Chapter 15: Blending How-To's for more information on this subject.

Body oils are best utilized when applied to wet skin, so putting them on after a shower or bath is an ideal time. Having the skin pre-moistened ensures an even application of the oils and also "locks" in some of the moisture. When you're finished showering, don't towel dry your body as you normally would. Reach for your body oil instead, and apply it all over your wet skin. Then pat dry with a towel. Oils are very easy to apply this way, and your skin will appreciate the extra moisture!

The amount of essential oils to add to your *body oils* is 50 drops per 4 ounces of base oil. You can cut this amount in half to make a 2-ounce preparation, or double it to make a larger quantity, depending on the need. I recommend making smaller amounts, so you can continually be adjusting the blend, and also it will not be sitting around unused for months. That would be wasteful if it oxidized or the oil was rancid. When mixing your body oils, use clean colored glass bottles. Count out drops slowly and carefully according to the above ratios. Shake well, label, and cap tightly.

Get All Wrapped Up in Aromatic Body Wraps

A Bavarian monk named Father Sebastian Kneipp developed an herbal wrap treatment, along with his widely practiced hydrotherapy and herbal regimens. He used layers of hot, herbal-scented towels to wrap his patients, similar to the aromatic body wraps in use today. In Europe, where this special wrap technique was perfected, often very complex blends of essential oils, seaweed extracts, floral and mineral waters are used. Usually there is an exercise and dietary program encouraged simultaneously to achieve a particular outcome, along with the weekly or bi-weekly aromatic wrap sessions. For example, this form of aromatherapy application is useful with anti-cellulite or weight loss programs, as it facilitates the circulatory and lymphatic systems. When professionally done, clients have lost as much as 6 to 14 inches (total body inches) over an 8- to 10-treatment period, according to reports. Some claim as high as 80 to 90% maintained this inch loss over a one-year period with home maintenance sessions.

You can save hundreds of dollars and enjoy this at home yourself. Few materials are needed for this procedure. A large plastic or vinyl sheet that is waterproof, along with a blanket, large beach towel, and a 12-ounce spray bottle are all that is necessary. A bedroom or open space on the bathroom floor is a good place to do this at home. Lay out the blanket on the floor, put the plastic sheet over that, and the beach towel over the top. Fill the spray bottle with very hot mineral water or distilled water with a total of 10 to 15 drops of your chosen essential oils. Shake well and spray onto the beach towel. Be sure to shake often while spraying; remember that essential oils float on top of water and we want them dispersed as much as possible. Lie down face-up on the beach towel and reach around to grab all the layers, pulling them around the sides and on top of you. You want the blanket on the outermost side to keep the heat in. The plastic wrap keeps the moisture in. You may ask someone to help with wrapping you up. Time is of the essence, because the essential oils are evaporating and the water temperature cools quickly. Consider a hot water bottle or heating pad under the blanket to assist in warming. Close your eyes and relax totally in your "cocoon." You can stay wrapped up as long as you are comfortable and remain warm, about 30 to 60 minutes.

Aromatic wraps encourage your body to detoxify by increasing perspiration, stimulating circulation, and promoting lymphatic drainage. It is a good idea to replenish your body with plenty of water by drinking at least 6 to 8 glasses in the next 24 hours. Of course, a natural vegetable- and fruit-based diet would be helpful if you are trying to detoxify or beginning a healthy weight-reducing program. To customize a *detoxifying* or *anti-cellulite* aromatic wrap use the following combination: Cypress 6 drops, Lemon 5 drops, Juniper 2 drops, and Lavender 2 drops. This makes a total of 15 drops which should be added to 12 ounces of hot mineral water in your spray bottle.

The other major benefit of using aromatic wraps is the relaxing quality of being cocooned. Therefore, a *relaxation* blend of essential oils can be most enjoyable. Try 15 drops of a single oil like lavender, or a blend using Lavender 10 drops, Bergamot 3 drops, and Mandarin 2 drops. For *regulating* and *balancing* the body use Lavender 10 drops, and Geranium 5 drops. I don't recommend stimulating or "wake-me-up" blends for aromatic wraps; those are best utilized for showers and foot baths with cold water applications.

Aromatherapy Massage

An aromatherapy massage combines the relaxing and balancing properties of essential oils with the benefits of touch and therapeutic massage. Several body systems can be involved during an aromatic massage. Lymphatic drainage and muscular relaxation are encouraged with every massage stroke while essential oils are absorbed through the skin's surface. They promote a state of relaxation and initiate the central nervous system as they enter the respiratory tract and olfactory system.

A good massage takes practice and a few developed skills. However, you can incorporate massage at home to help with muscle and joint aches and pain, cellulite control, stress reduction and other discomforts, or simply for the pleasure of it! There are many books written on massage, so if you want more information on this art please refer to those that specialize in this topic. You will need to recruit someone as your massage partner.

Perhaps a close friend or spouse might be willing to trade massages with you.

A full aromatherapy massage may last 1 to 1 1/2 hours. Its main effect is to be relaxing and nurturing. A few basic recommendations are offered to assist you in preparation and hands-on application for this wonderful experience. Massage therapists use special tables in their practice, but a futon or padded floor area will work at home. A bed isn't firm enough and makes it awkward for the masseuse. A large bath or beach towel covered with a cotton bed sheet works well for both the floor or futon method. You will need another large towel or blanket to cover your partner with. Also, a hot water bottle for under the feet and/or heating pad for under the floor towel will be useful. Make sure the room is sufficiently heated, lights are dim, and outside noise is at a minimum. All these things encourage relaxation. Soft background music or nature sounds and candlelight can further enhance a feeling of relaxation. Try to create a special "retreat" for your partner. Following these helpful hints will insure a positive experience:

- Empty your bladder right before the massage.
- Massage strokes should be slow and gentle, light and sensitive, each movement blending into the next.
- Always massage toward the heart, from extremities to body center. This encourages blood flow back to the heart.
- Masseuse must be relaxed and comfortable before "working" on someone else.
- Maintain constant contact with your partner's body.
- Keep extremities and parts not being worked on covered and warm. Heat also increases oil absorption.
- Keep conversation to a minimum to encourage relaxation and slowing the mind.
- Try to prevent distractions ahead of time (TV, telephone, etc.).
- Encourage feedback from partner if discomfort or pain is experienced.
- Avoid applying pressure directly over the spine and joints.
- Avoid stimulants such as caffeine, alcohol. Eat lightly before massage and drink plenty of water afterwards. Full body massage should be avoided if *flu, fever, or any serious condition exists.*

A trained aromatherapist or massage therapist never starts a massage without a thorough consultation. Medical history, allergies, lifestyle and diet, physical conditions, and mental state should be a few of the things considered prior to treatment. According to the individual's needs, a treatment blend is prepared. For at-home use, decide what the goal or aim is for the massage. Are relaxation and nurturing the emphasis for stress-release, or perhaps a big dose of pampering is what you want.

Sweet almond oil, coconut oil, or a blend of several vegetable and seed oils is used for massage. Refer to Chapter 15 for oil choices and their specific properties. Warm oils and hands before the massage. Keep oil in a bowl to dip fingers into, rather than pouring from a bottle. To make a typical oil for full body massage use 25 drops for 2 ounces of carrier oil.

If you or your partner find the full body massage too much to handle at first, you may want to practice back massages. They are much easier to do and don't take as long. Give special attention to the lower back and neck area where we tend to store tension and stress. The skin on our backs is evenly distributed and thick, making it a perfect area for application of essential oils. This part of our bodies is often neglected because it is so difficult to reach ourselves.

Head to Toe in Mud—Body Masks and Scrubs

Who would ever have thought that as grown adults we'd even consider such an idea as covering our bodies with mud? It has become a popular attraction in some European and American spas. The primary ingredients used in "mud" baths and body masks are clay, herbs, aromatics, and water. Clay has the amazing quality of being able to draw and absorb oils, dirt, and bacteria out from the skin's surface. It dries naturally at room temperature and, as it does, waste products adhere and become trapped in the hardening mask.

There are several clays to choose from. Kaolin, Bentonite, Fuller's Earth, and French green clay are some popular types. You can purchase them at natural health food markets in the cosmetics section.

It is best for several reasons never to allow a clay mask to completely dry and crack on the skin. One reason is that it can drain the skin of moisture and oil, robbing the mantel or top layer of the skin of this vital protective coating. As clay dries, it also pulls and tightens underlying skin and muscular structures and can cause unnecessary stretching during movement such as talking or smiling. I do not recommend the use of clay masks for dehydrated or extremely dry skin because replenishment of moisture is needed.

Most clays can absorb as much as 200 times their weight in water.

Aromatic mud or clay body masks are most beneficial for oily, slug-gish, or congested skin that calls for the extra drawing power clay seems to offer. Here is a nice recipe to use at home in the privacy of your own bathroom. Customize the mask by changing the essential oils you pick.

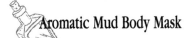 ## Aromatic Mud Body Mask

Honey 2 teaspoons

Yogurt 2 tablespoons

Vegetable oil 1 teaspoon

Mineral or Floral water 1/2 cup

Clay (powdered form) 1/3 cup

Essential Oils 10 drops total

Mix honey, yogurt, and vegetable oil together. Add clay to this mixture, adding small amounts of water at a time until it becomes a smooth, creamy and thick paste. When it is the right consistency, add the essential oils. Mix well.

Start with your hands and arms, then feet and legs, working always toward the body center and heart. Massage lightly as you spread this on, spending 1 to 2 minutes on each body section. Take your time, leaving a thick layer of clay on the skin. You can either lie in an empty bathtub or on a towel for 15 minutes or so, *or* relax in a full bathtub of warm water for 15 to 20 minutes. You will still get the clay benefits even though the water dilutes and washes some of the clay off. Shower with warm water after, forgoing the soap. Pat dry gently and wrap yourself in a thick bathrobe or wool blanket. Rest for a good 15 to 30 minutes to further the treatment's effect. Perspiring means more toxins are being eliminated.

You're probably asking yourself what could possibly be next? We've covered massage, body wraps, and mud masks. But how about exfoliation? An enthusiastic whole body scrub is what's missing. Here's the best all-around *body scrub* I know. Certainly daily use of loofah sponges and cac-tus cloths are great. I wouldn't be without them. But it feels really great when you do a full body scrub with some ingredients from the kitchen pantry and a special blend of essential oils to tingle and enliven your skin and senses. The better the condition of your skin, the more efficient the essential oils will work. Therefore exfoliating the dead skin cells and deep cleansing are very helpful. Do not use this or any other scrub on broken or irritated tissue.

Aromatic Body Scrub

Sea Salt 1/4 cup

Medium-ground cornmeal 1/4 cup

Olive oil 1/3 cup

Essential oils 10 drops total

Mix sea salt and cornmeal together. Combine warm olive oil and essential oils together and mix with dry ingredients. Add additional oil if necessary to form a paste-like consistency.

We lose 1 to 2 pounds of cells per day, both inside the body and out. Externally, our skin is constantly sloughing dead skin cells and generating new ones. On the inside, our body (including blood cells) is under a constant renewal process.

Definitely do this scrub in the shower or standing in the tub; it can be messy. Take small handfuls at a time and lightly rub in a circular motion from the extremities inward, working toward the body center and heart. Do not use on the face; I have a finer facial scrub to suggest later in this chapter. Once your entire body has been scrubbed, sloughed, and stimulated, rinse completely in the shower with warm water. Do not use soap. Gently pat dry. I guarantee your skin will feel smoother and have a healthy glow. Consider this a skin workout, increasing circulation, getting rid of dead skin cells, and an aromatherapy treatment all in one.

You can use any of the essential oil combinations already mentioned previously, as well as the stimulating blends. However, when using peppermint essential oil in the bath or whole body treatment, do not exceed a total of 5 drops since it can cause skin irritation in concentrated amounts. One of my favorite stimulating, pick-me-up blends is:

Good Morning

Ginger 2 drops

Rosemary 3 drops

Peppermint 4 drops

Local Areas With Special Needs—Made Simple

In this second half of the chapter we focus on specific body areas with special needs, from facial massage to first-aid ointments and compresses. We will be covering a wide variety of aromatherapy specialties you can put into practice at home. You don't have to be a nurse or doctor to learn how to apply compresses and poultices. Nor do you have to be an expert in cosmetology or skin care to customize your personal care needs. I'll give you the necessary tools it will take for you to be successful in these areas.

Concentrated Massage Oils for the Face, Hands, Feet, and Other Small Areas

Hand massages and foot massages are another way to use aromatherapy. Both the elderly and children seem especially receptive to hand massages. My school-age children love them. And I never met anyone who passed up a foot massage. Barter, bribe, do what you must for those small indulgences! For an easy foot or hand massage oil use any of the listed oils in Chapter 15. Pure vegetable oils like olive, safflower, or sesame work well. To one tablespoon of carrier oil add 3 to 5 drops of essential oils. Mix well. Remember, warming the oil and your hands prior to the massage helps a lot with relaxation and penetration of the oils.

And let's not forget the *facial massage*. You can do this one yourself. However, do use the finer seed oils like hazelnut, apricot kernel, or avocado. And always moisten the face before applying the oils. Floral waters work well and can be misted over the facial area with the eyes closed. This allows a smaller amount of oils to be used, provides extra moisture, and facilitates an easy "glide" surface when applying oils that may otherwise pull the skin or just sit there and soak in. Avoid the delicate eye area; this tissue is very fragile and has very little muscular structure. Use 3 to 5 drops of essential oils, depending on your skin type, and mix with 3 teaspoons of carrier oil. Adding evening primrose oil, vitamin E, or carrot seed oil will add to the anti-aging benefits of doing this massage regimen. Here is a basic, but excellent, face oil recipe you can make.

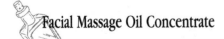 **Facial Massage Oil Concentrate**

Hazelnut, avocado, or other fine oil 2 teaspoons

Sweet almond or Olive oil 1 teaspoon

Vitamin E capsule, or several drops of evening primrose oil

Essential oils 5 drops total—choose on basis of skin type

For example: If you have oily skin, make the above facial massage oil concentrate, and add to it the following essential oils for oily skin types: Lavender 2 drops, Lemon 2 drops, and Juniper 1 drop. For dry skin opt for this blend: Frankincense 2 drops, Geranium 2 drops, and pure Rose oil 1 drop. You always have the choice of using a single essential oil as well; Lavender is wonderful on its own and good for all skin types.

I'm including some simple illustrations on how to give yourself a mini-facial massage using this aromatherapy facial massage oil. Facial massage is very beneficial if done correctly and regularly, since there is a multitude of facial muscles involved in this type of massage. It is well practiced by many Asian cultures for its benefit in preventing wrinkles and age lines. It will bring a healthy glow to your complexion, and with it nutrients and oxygen to the skin's surface. Do not use this technique on broken, irritated, or sunburned facial skin. These are problems that will tend to worsen with added stimulation.

Homemade Facial Steams, Scrubs, Masks, and Sprays

Facial Steams are a well-kept secret for sure. You just don't hear much about them and all their benefits to good skin health. Facial steaming helps open pores, detoxify, and soften the skin. My guess is they aren't popular because they're too simple and easy! You need only four items: a towel, bowl, hot water, and a few drops of essential oil. Heat water to near boiling and pour into a ceramic or glass bowl. Add 2 to 3 drops of essential oil. Drape the towel over your head to make a "tent" over the bowl of steam. Keep your eyes closed as essential oils are volatile. Relax. If the steam is too hot, release it by lifting the towel momentarily. Your face should be about 8 to 10 inches away from the bowl. Do this steam for as long as the heat lasts, about 5 to 10 minutes. Mist face with floral water or mineral water to close pores and balance the pH of the skin.

Floral waters and hydrosols can be purchased from essential oil companies since these are byproducts of distilling the oils from the plants. Refer to illustration of Steam Distillation Chapter One for this process explained. To make a floral water or *facial spray* simply put distilled or mineral water in a spray bottle; one with a fine mister works best. If you have a 4-ounce size spray bottle use a total of 6 to 8 drops of essential oils. *Shake well before each use.* Use the essential oils that correlate with your skin type as charted earlier.

Facial masks are basically moisturizing, toning, or cleansing. Their application will depend on your specific skin care needs at the time. If it's the mid-

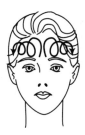 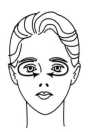 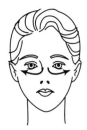

Step 1:
Apply dabs of the product to entire face. Massage your forehead upward. Do this three times, making seven circles each time.

Step 2a:
Draw gentle circles around your eyes. Do this five times.

Step 2b:
Now, press the inner corners of your eyes, draw one stroke outward, then press your temples.

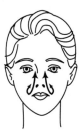 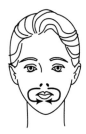 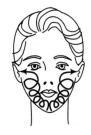

Step 3:
Massage up and down the top of your nose ten times, then five times up and down the sides of your nose. Finally, draw semicircles around your nose five times.

Step 4:
Draw semicircles around your mouth five times, stroking upward.

Step 5:
Draw circles upward from your chin toward your temples using the inside length of your fingers, then press in at the temples. Do this three times, making seven circles each time.

Printed with permission from NOEVIR U.S.A., Inc. 1995

Five-Step Daily Massage

This quick and easy massage was specifically designed for today's fast-paced lifestyles. This invigorating facial massage promotes circulation and keeps your skin looking toned not to mention the relaxation it brings after a long day. Follow these five easy steps, massaging at a hearbeat pace using the entire hand. Do not use this massage if your facial skin is irritated or sunburned.

dle of winter, you may need a deep moisturizing mask as I do! This time of
year is spent mostly indoors, where central heating depletes our skin's moisture reserves. Many of these skin treatments are designed to be used on an
occasional basis or once or twice weekly at most. Don't overdo them.

For oily skin I suggest a facial mask with clay. This will decrease the oil
on the skin, deep cleanse impurities and tighten pores which are often large.

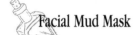

Facial Mud Mask

Powdered Clay 2 tablespoons

Mineral or Floral water—enough to form a paste

Essential oils 3 to 5 drops total

Mix the clay and water to form a smooth consistency. Add the essential oils
and mix well. Apply with fingertips, avoiding the eye area and hairline.
Leave on for 10 to 15 minutes, but do *not* allow to completely dry and
crack. Relax facial muscles and avoid talking or smiling when it's drying. To
remove the mud mask apply a warm wet washcloth over the face and
moisten. Rinse well with warm water. Follow with facial spray.

A moisturizing mask is just the opposite of a clay mask. Instead of
drawing out impurities etc., a moisturizing mask is meant to replace or
replenish moisture. Its aim is to nourish and calm the skin's surface. Good
for both dry skin types and combination skin, there are endless possibili-
ties of what can be added to this type of facial mask such as floral and
herbal waters, seaweed extracts, oils, yogurt, honey, mashed avocado or
papaya, etc. This particular recipe is easy to prepare, very moisturizing, and
has a good consistency.

Moisture-Balanced Facial Mask

Natural Yogurt 1 teaspoon

Honey 2 teaspoons

Vitamin E capsule

Oat flour 1 teaspoon (or can use finely-ground oatmeal)

Essential oils 5 drops total

Combine yogurt and honey. Squeeze vitamin E capsule's contents into this
mixture and stir well.

Add oat flour and mix into a smooth paste. Adjust flour as necessary. When
it looks right, add essential oils and mix. Apply with fingertips. Lie down
and relax. Wait 15 to 20 minutes before removing with warm water.

How about trying an exfoliating scrub that will leave your face feeling softer than you can imagine? And you won't need any blush after this because you will have a *natural* rosy glow! I call it Farm Fresh because of all the ingredients used and because it reminds me of the clean, young-looking skin of a country girl.

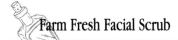

Farm Fresh Facial Scrub

Fine- to medium-ground oatmeal 1 teaspoon

Finely ground cornmeal 1 teaspoon

Honey 1 teaspoon

Natural yogurt 1 teaspoon

Brewer's yeast 1/2 teaspoon (optional)

Mineral or floral water (enough to make a paste)

Lavender essential oil 3 drops

Combine oatmeal, cornmeal, honey, yogurt, and brewer's yeast. Add just enough water to make a paste-like consistency. Add Lavender essential oil and mix well. Apply to face with fingertips, massaging very gently in upward and circular movements. You can follow the facial massage guidelines on page 316 if you'd like. Do not rub hard or near the eyes. Rinse well with warm water.

First Aid to the Rescue—Ointments, Compresses, and Poultices

Ointments are made with various oils or fats and beeswax to form a coating over weakened or soft areas of skin that need extra protection to heal. You can make the ointment soft or firm depending on the ration of oils to beeswax that you use. This preparation is one of the highest concentrations of essential oils used, abut an 8% dilution. However, ointments are designed to be used sparingly and in acute situation as a general rule.

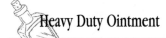

Heavy Duty Ointment

Extra virgin Olive oil 1/4 cup (or homemade Calendula oil see Chapter 15 to make)

Natural Beeswax 1 tablespoon*

Vitamin E capsule 2 or 3 (200IU each)

Essential oils 80 to 100 drops total

*If you desire a softer ointment, use less beeswax.

Combine the above ingredients in the top of a double boiler and melt together. Once melted, remove from heat and allow to cool. If adding essential oils, wait until the oils have cooled somewhat so they don't evaporate away quickly. Stir them in completely and pour into a sterile or very clean colored glass jar. Cap tightly and label contents. You can hasten the cooling by putting the jar in the refrigerator. Use a tongue depressor or small spatula to take out what you need with each use as not to contaminate the contents.

Compresses are moistened pieces of cloth soaked in medicine, in this case, aromatic medicinals—essential oils and water. They are useful in spot treatment of specific areas that need healing such as wounds, muscle injuries, and joint pain. Compresses involve hydrotherapy techniques as well. Refer to Chapter 11 for review of the use of water temperature if you need to. In general, a warm water temperature encourages circulation, where as a cool water temperature decreases circulation, having a "cooling" effect that would be useful for such ailments as headaches or simple burns.

To prepare a compress you will need a piece of flannel, gauze, or soft cloth that will cover the area in question, a towel, bowl, saran wrap, gloves (optional), about 4 to 8 ounces of water or herbal tea, and 8 to 10 drops of essential oils. To apply a compress, you soak the cloth in water and essential oil mixture in a bowl. Wring out the cloth so much of the excess liquid is squeezed out and not dripping. Place on affected area and wrap with saran wrap lightly, then wrap towel around that to keep the heat and aromatics in. When the compress cools or dries, repeat the process. Compress treatments range from 15 minutes to 1 hour.

Poultices are similar to compresses, with one major difference: poultices use the *whole* herb. To make a poultice fresh herbs are best, although dried herbs can be used by adding mineral water or herbal tea to them. Blend herbs and mineral water in a blender until a thick paste-like consistency is made. Additionally, aloe vera gel can be added in place of some of the water. Rub skin with a thin layer of vegetable oil to prevent the herbs from sticking when they dry on the skin. Lay the herbal poultice on the affected area to be treated about 1/2 inch thick or more. Apply gauze over the top of the herbal poultice to hold them in place. Then wrap with saran wrap and tape to secure. Leave this on for 1 to 2 hours. It will naturally cool to body temperature, you do not need to reapply.

CHAPTER 13

Breathe Easy— The In's and Out's of Inhalation

Environmental Air Purification

Have you ever thought about why we are attracted to and feel creative in certain places like pristine evergreen forests, fragrant herb gardens, sun-drenched ocean beaches, and fresh-mown hay fields? Is it because of the visual beauty and quiet calmness these places seem to offer us? Or could their positive attraction also be attributed to the pure fresh air and natural aromatic ambiance these places create? In the old days, doctors would actually "prescribe" a vacation or healing retreat to the mountains, in order for the patient to "take in the fresh air" and get well, much like in the story *Heidi* when the doctor suggested that Heidi's friend go to the mountains to recuperate and heal at the Uncle's cabin. He knew it was health promoting and had incredible regenerating influence over city dwellers' failing health conditions.

This chapter not only involves the air we breathe but also our immediate environment and personal spaces. We can positively influence our surroundings as well as personalize them. The desire is to have healthy and pleasurable home and office environments. It can be likened to bringing part of nature into our "unnatural" and sometimes toxic personal spaces.

We spend at least 1/3 of our lives in bed. Therefore the bedroom is a great location to utilize many of the inhalation methods such as diffusers, aroma lamps, etc.

In this chapter we will explore a variety of methods used for inhalation, the process by which we take air (and aromatic molecules such as essential oils) into our lungs. Inhalation is perhaps one of the oldest ways in which aromatics were used by ancient cultures. For centuries incense and aromatic woods have been burned in religious ceremonies and purification rites, and are prime examples of inhalation methods. Today, the U.S., Europe, and Japan lead the way in using modern applications of inhalation for improving air quality and enhancing workplace and home environments.

The benefits of inhalation of essential oils basically fall into four major areas:

1. environmental air purification,
2. natural fragrancing,
3. healing the respiratory tract, and
4. regulating/balancing moods and emotions.

Since most essential oils are antiseptic to some degree and all possess natural fragrance, the first two areas will inherently be dual benefits whenever essential oils are used with inhalation methods. However, when healing of the respiratory system and regulating the emotions are the goals, the outcome will depend upon the specific essential oils chosen.

Inhalation treatments for ailments related to the respiratory tract, such as sinus problems, chest colds, and other related infections, are covered in greater detail within the chapter that addresses that specific ailment in Part II of this book. However, steaming, vaporization, and diffuser use, discussed here, are very therapeutic inhalation methods still used today.

In general, the inhalation method is best utilized for challenges that involve the respiratory and nervous systems, as well as for affecting the emotions and for mental alertness. It relates directly to the process of respiration and the connection between the olfactory system and the limbic brain. Refer to page 14 for illustration of the Olfactory System (nose-brain link). Ailments of the respiratory system, such as colds, sore throat, sinus problems, and coughs, can be easily rectified through this approach. The cardiovascular, psychological, and immune systems can also be positively influenced by this modality.

"Environmental fragrancing" is a term heard often these days, relating to the process of diffusing essential oils (or synthetic fragrances) into our living and working spaces. We don't even have to be consciously aware of the scent; it can be subliminal. As a matter of fact, it is best utilized when the scent-scape is barely noticeable and merely in the background. Interestingly, Japanese companies have studied particular scents and their effect on brain waves. Those scents that were calming demonstrated a smooth wave pattern (〰〰) versus the stimulating scents that caused dramatic peaks and dips (∿∿∿) in brain wave measurement.

Synthetic chemical environmental fragrancing has been used to influence consumers for the last 10 to 15 years or more, from the used car salesperson who may use a "new vinyl" scent for selling cars, to the shopping malls which pipe in "food" smells to entice hungry shoppers. You'll even find creative and resourceful real estate agents who will encourage their sellers to bake pies, cookies, or bread during an open house to convey a message of " *Welcome, this warm and cozy home is for sale.*" It is very effective or it wouldn't be employed as a sales tool as often as it is.

Virtually everything sold in the marketplace is scented to some degree; even items that boast "unscented" on the packaging are sometimes lightly scented to mask the original or natural smell of the product. (For example, most mineral oil products are scented to cover up its unique odor.) Scents are used most often in the sale of retail consumer products, from the skin and hair care products and facial tissue in your bathroom to the paper towels, dish soap, and cleaning supplies in the kitchen. Even things we normally don't think of as being scented, like women's hosiery, athletic sneakers and even the packaging itself, in fact are, to subconsciously lure potential buyers.

More than 60,000 different synthetic chemicals are presently available on the market, with about a thousand new chemicals being introduced per year. Prior to 1930, nostalgic scents included natural odors like flowers, cut grass, manure, and burning leaves. It is interesting to note that after 1930 up to the present day , synthetic odors prevail as the nostalgic scents. Crayons, Play-doh, chlorine bleach, fabric softener, window cleaner, motor oil, and plastic can evoke childhood memories for those born during this era.

Natural Deodorizing Essences

Essential oils have the potential to kill germs (germicidal), destroy bacteria (bactericidal), and eliminate offensive odors due to their antiseptic qualities. They do *not* merely cover up or mask bad odors, as some might think, but actually alter the physical and chemical molecular structure. Some are very powerful in this area. Numerous studies have established the efficacy of essential oils in disinfecting room air. Since it has been determined that some essential oils are rich in terpenes, phenols, alcohols, and aldehydes, their germ-killing ability is now confirmed.

Hippocrates was one of the earliest physicians to document using aromatic essences for their antiseptic qualities, such as when he ordered the city of Athens to be "fumigated" during the plague epidemics. Although we have only recently been able to confirm the reason *why* essences are powerful disinfectants, they have been used for this purpose for thousands of years.

A few of the microorganisms tested that were drastically inhibited by the diffusion of essential oils were: E. Coli, Neisseria gonorrhea, Streptococcus faecalis, Staphylococcus aureus, and Pneumococcus. Some essential oils work directly on neutralizing these harmful organisms.

> Dr. Jean Valnet demonstrated the bactericidal properties of Eucalyptus essential oil. A 2% dilution in spray form killed 70% of the airborne staphylococcal bacteria.

It is no accident that we equate lemon and pine smells with cleanliness. Just count the number of cleaning solutions and room deodorizers that include these particular scents. Unfortunately, virtually all are of synthetic origin. But don't despair! Scent your own natural Castille or Castor oil-based organic cleansers with essential oils like Citrus, Pine, and Peppermint. They will be gentler and safer alternatives to what you may be currently using and will have great deodorizing and germ-killing benefits.

> Put a few drops of Lemon, Orange, or Grapefruit essential oil on the vacuum cleaner bag or filter for extra cleaning power and for an added uplifting scent to a not-so-uplifting chore!

In the workplace, gyms, and schools, we often have large numbers of people (and their germs), higher levels of stress, etc., all of which contribute to health problems, increase in infectious diseases, and job-related stress. Prevention is the key: proper maintenance of heat and ventilation systems, including regular and thorough consistent cleaning, replacement of filters, and use of bactericidal, deodorizing, and disinfecting essences only.

Some essential oils shown to have high *antiseptic* and *antibacterial* properties include the following:

Bergamot	Orange
Citronella	Peppermint
Eucalyptus	Petigrain
Juniper	Pine
Lavender	Rosemary
Lemon	Sandalwood
Lemongrass	Tea Tree

The *antifungal* properties of essential oils are gaining more notice as there seems to be a rise in Candida albicans and other yeast and fungal infections in the general population. The essential oils known to have an antifungal effect include the following:

Roman Chamomile
Fennel
Geranium
Lavender
Tea Tree

In Australia, Tea Tree is commonly used in ventilation systems to control bacteria and mold growth.

Nature's #1 Air Filtering System—The Clean Air Plants

There is a solution for indoor air pollution and poor air quality. Not only do plants produce life-sustaining oxygen, they are living air filters, taking in "dirty" air and *consuming* or *digesting* the multitude of chemical pollutants that can cause various health problems and even cancers. They help clean the air, making it safer for us to breathe. Refer to page 95 for the illustration of our lungs and trees, and the similarities between the two.

Currently, there are a number of biochemists and other scientists who are studying correlations between certain plant species and the toxins they are capable of digesting, making a specialized list of toxin-specific plant categories. For example, Boston Ferns digest formaldehyde, while English Ivy seems to be especially effective in consuming benzene. A few of the NASA plant experiments in the 1980's involved placing plants in highly polluted enclosed rooms containing chemical toxins. Within a 24-hour period many of the toxins had been digested by the plants and previous toxin levels were greatly reduced.

The Clean Air Plants

Some plants, such as the following, are especially good for filtering air pollution and cleaning the air. Keep plants clean and dusted, as this increases their effectiveness. Excellent air-filtering plants include:

Areca Palm

Arrowhead Vine

Boston Fern

Chrysanthemums

Dwarf Date Palm

English Ivy

Golden Pothos

Peace Lily

Spider Plant

Striped Dracaenea

Modern Devices—Diffusers and Ventilation Systems

Becoming increasingly popular both commercially and for personal use are the natural aromatic environmental fragrancing machines and devices. There are electric-powered machines that emit airborne essential oils into the atmosphere of a room, portion of a house, or an entire office building. The chief goal is to purify and positively enhance the indoor air quality of work spaces and homes. The essential oils employed in this form of inhalation can also be chosen for their beneficial effects on the emotional and mental states. For example, Japan undertook an extensive study involving the use of different scents, and found that Lemon essential oil increased the acuity of typists and computer programmers when piped in through the air conditioning system. Eucalyptus oil was found to be very effective for keeping the night-shift employees awake and more alert, with fewer mistakes and accidents.

The basics of these modern electric diffusers include an air pump, essential oil chamber, and glass nebulizer. The air is used to propel the essential oil (liquid state) into the nebulizer part which is often a complex union of convoluted glass chambers. When the essential oils are "pushed" through these glass bubble-like structures, the oils break apart into smaller fragments that become airborne, thereby "diffusing" essential oils into the air in a fine mist. The aromatic molecules stay suspended in the air, doing their work for several hours. They change the environment and how we "perceive" it by purifying and refreshing the air, and by revitalizing, relaxing, or stimulating us through the nose-brain link.

We have several in our home including one in the main kitchen and family room area. In the main part of the house, I have an electronic timer attached to the diffuser and programmed to turn on several times during the day for 5 to 10 minutes. Ideally, it goes on before the family comes down to eat breakfast, once during the day, again before the children return home from school, and one more time before dinner or late evening. If colds are going around at school, I use a cold/respiratory blend. But most often I like to use a nice relaxation blend that also promotes a sense of well-being and has anti-bacterial and purifying qualities (see recipes). It should be one that is liked by everyone in the family.

In the office, I am particularly fond of a blend I put together called Mint Conditioning. It has quite a few stimulating oils, as well as mental and memory invigorating ones. This blend helps to keep me awake and alert, my mind clear, and enhances my level of concentration. You will want this recipe if you do a lot of writing, paper work, office-type work, or just need a little extra help when you sit down to pay the bills!

With 6 million smell receptor cells, we can distinguish approximately 10,000 different odors.

In Japan they are using a delivery system with computerized scent attached to very large ventilation systems. The air conditioning system filters the air, then adds scent and recirculates it. Improving alertness, increasing productivity, and relaxation can be some of the desired outcomes of this type of mass ventilation. The scent that is emitted from these systems can be changed according to the time of day or shift. For example, a fresh pleasant lemon scent may be piped in during early morning to help wake up and gently stimulate. In early afternoon a more stimulating scent may be used, then perhaps a relaxing blend ventilated in right before the work day is over to aid in relaxation and preparation for evening. The United States is also implementing some of these ideas but on a much smaller and limited scale in comparison to Japan where it is more widely accepted.

Large commercial systems are now being developed and implemented for the workplace. Customized "signature" scents are becoming popular and are being developed by aroma experts for large and exclusive hotels, as well as for commercial malls and movie theaters.

> **Many fragrances used today are 90% synthetic in origin. These include room deodorizers, perfumes, cleaning supplies, etc.**

The actual amount of essential oils needed to induce a positive effect on us and the surrounding environment is quite small. Even if we do not consciously perceive the scent, our central nervous system continues to respond. The goal is to perceive a background scent, not one that is overwhelming.

However, aromatic fragrancing can be abused. Consider those individuals who may have allergies, asthma, or related sensitivities. There may be a thin line between what is considered *adding to* the quality of our environment and what may be *interfering* with it. Personal sensitivities, allergies, and public awareness need to be considered.

Nevertheless I think the use of essential oils for purifying the air, for naturally deodorizing and killing potentially harmful germs, and for creating an uplifting aroma is an example of essences taking a giant step toward a positive influence on our environment and assisting humankind in staying connected to nature.

Some places that can easily adapt aromatic fragrancing to benefit their surroundings are listed below.

Schools and Study rooms—to increase mental alertness and memory stimulation.

Psychotherapy and Hypnotherapy—for deeper relaxation and hypnosis. Or to help recover childhood memories, etc.

Hospitals, Medical and Dental offices, nursing homes, MRI and CAT scanning rooms where long tests are performed—use purifying, anti-bacterial blends that relax and soothe the nervous system.

Labor and Delivery Rooms, Home births—blends that help with pain control, focusing, and relaxing.

Home—kitchen, living areas, bedrooms—depending on the goal, relaxation, colds & flu blends, mental stimulants, etc.

Hotel Lobbies—ambient, inviting "background" scents customized.

Workplace—increase air quality, purify and clean air, help with stress; anti-bacterial to help decrease spread of colds.

Health clubs, Gyms and Locker rooms—combat body odors and related bacterial and fungal growth that is often prevalent in these places.

The following is a case history of aromatic diffuser use in our family's dental office. In the waiting room a calming blend is used to aid in relaxation and to purify the air. As a result, the patients are exposed to fewer germs, they feel more relaxed as they wait for their appointments, and there is a pleasant ambiance to the office environment. Lavender and Lime blossom essential oils are used to help with pain control and relaxation in other dental treatment areas.

Healing Treatments for the Respiratory Tract

Steaming or *vaporization* combines heat, vapor (steam) and essential oils providing direct inhalation of moist heat and aromatics. Used for many years, this method is particularly effective for upper respiratory infections and catarrh. It is considered an intensive inhalation aromatherapy treatment, and is commonly prescribed and practiced by aromatherapists, naturopaths, nurses, and grandmothers, even today!

It is almost exactly like the facial steam except that you are using different oils specific for the respiratory tract, and you are inhaling deeply through the nose and mouth to either help clear mucus and/or kill bacteria in those areas. To do this at home you need a glass or ceramic bowl, towel, hot water, and your oils. Pour hot water (not quite boiling) into the bowl, and add your essential oils. About 2 to 3 drops is all you need. Quickly cover your head with a towel, forming a tent over the bowl. Keep eyes closed, and breathe slowly and deeply. You may want to set a timer for 5 to 10 minutes, so you can get the full benefit of this type of inhalation treatment.

You can also heat water in a pan on the *stove* and add several drops of your favorite essential oil. The heat from the hot water will encourage evaporation of the essential oils. Similarly, you can keep a kettle of water on the *radiator* and add the oils there. This has the benefit of adding moisture to the air, similar to a humidifier. My mother always did this in the winter months. We had those old iron radiators that made banging and clinking noises as the steam built up. We also had an old wood stove in the kitchen (just like the Walton's), and a parlor stove where open kettles of water were kept.

If you own a *humidifier*, you probably can add essential oils to the water or to the compartment made for the addition of medicinals. Read the directions specific to your unit, as metal and rubber parts can be affected by the oils over time. We own a small cool water humidifier and use it frequently during the winter months in the kids' room. It helps prevent dry nasal passages, colds, and nosebleeds due to the heated air.

Inhaling essential oils right from the bottle is often overlooked as a way of utilizing aromatherapy. (Due to their potency, they should never be in reach of young children.) This method is especially helpful and simple to carry in your purse. For nausea, motion sickness, car sickness or menopausal hot flashes I recommend carrying a tiny bottle of Peppermint essential oil. Some airlines and hotels, particularly in Great Britain and Australia, are offering essential oils to sniff from tiny bottles to help travelers counteract jet lag. For jet lag use Lavender and Lemon. You just open the top and take a good whiff or two. It really works!

Tissue, handkerchief, blotting paper, cotton balls are all examples of putting essential oils onto something that is easily carried on your person, or in a pocket. An effective way to prolong the scent short-term is to put a few drops of essential oils on the absorbent material, then slip them into a plastic baggie.

Ancient and Modern Methods for Natural Fragrancing

Before the invention of diffusers and complicated air systems, some very simple, yet effective, inhalation methods were utilized. Probably the first known to us was the burning of aromatic herbs and woods, called fumigation. *Incense* was derived shortly after, combining sometimes very complex mixtures of thirty or more various plants, resins, gums, powdered roots, grasses, and mosses. Incense was also known as perfume. From the Latin derivation "per" meaning *through,* and "fume" meaning *smoke,* it was used by many ancient civilizations, particularly in religious practices.

The role aromatics played and their importance to people and their environments is clearly seen in history, especially in spirituality. Aromatic plants were pulverized and blended into the mortar used to build some of the ancient churches. Sometimes the entry doors, floors, and altars were carved from aromatic woods such as Sandalwood, Cypress, or Cedarwood. Incense and candles were often used as early forms of inhalation as part of various ceremonies, while anointment oils contained plant essences as well.

Potpourri, which translated from French literally means "*rotten pot,*" is a medley of moist or dry ingredients derived from flower petals, herbs, woods, and spices. We are most familiar with its dry version. Many of the classic recipes include rose petals, wood shavings, spices and herbs, and a fixative, such as orris root. Depending on its country of origin, potpourri can differ greatly. In France, it often consists of the common plants native to that region. They may include roses, violets, bay, lavender, jasmine, rosemary, and various spices. From England you might expect roses, juniper, lavender, thyme, geranium, and sweet fern. In India, sandalwood, patchouli, citrus, and spices are the dominant scents.

I have a huge three-foot tall urn in the foyer, about half full with potpourri. A collection of past summers' flowers, herbs, and dried fruit. When I go through the pantry cupboards, instead of throwing out the old spices, herb teas etc., I happily toss them in the urn and give them a stir! An old-ashioned way of fragrancing that still has a welcomed place in our home.

Potpourri, comprised of mostly dried plant parts, does contain a minute amount of essential oil content imparting its gentle aromatic fragrance. However, you can easily add pure essential oils to your old potpourri to refresh it, or simply add the essences to a newly-made batch. Using a fixative, such as orris root, can help "hold" or "fix" the scent so it will last longer.

Candles are another fairly simple form of environmental fragrancing. They provide a much milder background scent; however, the soft scent coupled with the gentle glow of candlelight provides a most romantic atmosphere. Candles usually are made of a paraffin base, or a combination of bees wax. Instead of buying synthetic candles, make your own. I made some really wonderful candles for Christmas gifts this past year. I custom blended particular scents for each individual, depending on what I perceived them needing or preferring. You can make sand candles and forgo the mold altogether. Or pour your candles into wide-mouth sturdy spice jars, sea shells, or regular candle molds. I made votive candles. You simply add essential oils to them making them aromatherapy candles.

For a short cut method, you can add one to two drops of essential oils into the melted wax of a burning candle. Be extremely careful not to put them directly on the flame; they are flammable! Similarly, do not burn candles unattended or in a child's room. Most aromatherapy candles only need to be lit for 15 to 20 minutes to emit their soft fragrance into the room.

Light bulb rings are used for room fragrancing as well. However, some are made of asbestos-absorbent material, which I wouldn't recommend using. I don't particularly like them for two reasons. One, it's difficult to vary scents, because you're using the same ring over and over. Secondly, I find they can get extremely hot on some higher watt bulbs and I can detect a burnt odor. You can find some made of different materials like ceramic and lightweight metals, that are used to hold the oils rather than absorb them.

One particularly nice way of incorporating aromatherapy into fragrancing a room is by way of the *aroma lamp* or *potpourri burner.* A votive candle or tea light is used as the heat source under a small cup-shaped saucer that holds the heated water. You place 3 to 5 drops of your essential oil selection in the hot water so it will slowly evaporate and do its thing. Aroma lamps come in a wide variety of shapes, sizes, and colors. Most are made of ceramics and are relatively inexpensive. A few new designs I'm beginning to see in the marketplace are of intricate and artistic form with details of glass, stone, and metal. All aroma lamps and potpourri burners are ideal to use when the more expensive and rare essential oils are desired, or when the viscous oils that can't be run through a diffuser are warranted. A helpful hint when using the aroma lamp: make sure you begin with hot water in your burner; otherwise the candle has to heat it and that can be a slow process.

Other old fashioned ways of using aromatherapy are pomanders, sachets, herbal pillows, and homemade lavender wands for linen closets, drawers, and bedrooms.

My family, especially my youngest twin boys, love the *sleep pillows* I have made for them. Any sleep-inducing, relaxing herbs and flowers will suffice. I researched this idea several years ago and cross referenced many herbal medicine books and aromatherapy literature to come up with my own special blend. I got fancy one year and made little pillow cases with eyelet lace and ribbon for the little 4x6-inch muslin pillows. To refresh them simply put a few drops of Lavender and Chamomile on the pillow. Fluff in the dryer for a few minutes along with a damp washcloth.

Sweet Dreams

Valerie's Sleep Pillow Recipe

Sweet Woodruff 4 parts *(smells like fresh mown hay)*

Lemon Balm 2 parts

Lavender 2 parts

1 part *each of the following herbs and spices:*

Hops, Rosebuds, Chamomile, Marjoram, Thyme,

Sage, Rosemary (grind the leaves so they don't poke through the pillow),

Southernwood, Mugwort, and Cinnamon

Powdered or finely grated orris root 1 part

Lavender, Chamomile, and Marjoram Essential oils

Mix the above combination of sleep-inducing herbs, flowers, and spices in a large bowl. If you are making one pillow, the portions can be 1 table-spoon = 1 part. If you are making enough for gifts, use 1 cup = 1 part. However, when it comes time to add the essential oils, add about 3 to 5 drops per pillow. To do this, simply count out the drops onto the orris root and mix well with a spoon or mortar and pestle. Then add this to the pre-mixed herbs in the bowl. Put about 1 to 1 1/2 cups of herbs into each pil-low, depending on the size. Sew up the opening. Now tuck your sleep pil-low inside your bed pillow. Sweet Dreams . . .

Have you ever seen *eye pillows?* They are rectangular shaped pillows filled with lentils, rice, oats, or other grains. You use them by laying them across your face and over your eyes. The pillows have a nice gentle pres-sure or weight to them, and often smell nice. I'll give you my recipe. I keep mine on my night stand and would not be without it. It is one of those lit-tle necessities that comes in handy when you suffer from eye strain, ten-sion headaches, or mental fatigue. The pillow should fit sideways across your face covering your eyes and a little beyond to each side. An average size is about 3 1/2 x 8 1/2 inches. I use a soft fabric like satin or silk to make mine and fill with flax seeds and lavender flowers.

Eye Pillows

great for tension headaches and eye strain

Flaxseed 1 cup

Lavender 1 cup

Lavender essential oil 3 to 5 drops

Mix the flax seed and lavender together in a bowl. Sprinkle the essential oils in the mixture and blend well with a spoon or spatula. Put into eye pillow and sew opening. Keep by the bedside; if you don't see it, or if you can't find it, you won't be able to enjoy the benefits of using it.

Aromatic Room Mists are an easy way to change the milieu of any room in a hurry, without the use of electrical hookups, danger of candle flames, etc. You can make your own by simply adding 10 to 20 drops of essential oils to a 4-ounce spray bottle of distilled water. You must shake well before each use because the oils do not mix with water naturally. Mist over head and about the room. The fine misters are best.

I've made room misters for friends to use in their workplaces. One friend is a psychotherapist and likes to spray the chairs and couches with a floral and purifying blend to help with body odors between client sessions. Another friend uses it in the bathroom for a natural room deodorizer. Be sure to label and direct use when it's left out on a counter for general use. Before some of my public lectures, when a diffuser is not practical, I use a room mister. My favorite blend for this setting is Lavender 20 drops and Peppermint 10 drops in a 6-ounce spray bottle. Lavender helps soothe the nervous system, while peppermint stimulates alertness, and both are well received by most people.

Aromatic jewelry is not a new concept, though it is gaining popularity among those who enjoy the benefits of aromatherapy, or who just like having their personal favorite perfume scents handy to reapply during the day. Perhaps the most common is the pendant necklace that can hold a few drops of essence in its small compartment. Some are quite elegantly made of hand-blown colored glass, sterling silver, or hollowed-out hard woods. Aromatic jewelry can also come in the form of pins and earrings.

Clay potteries and aromatic pots are often small pots or jars made of clay or of natural unfinished woods that hold and absorb the essential oils, then slowly allow them to evaporate from their surfaces. These are handy for the car, drawers, and small places like bathrooms. Small carved pieces of cedar work nicely. They have a scent of their own, but you can easily add a few drops of oil to them. Cedar shavings were known to keep moths away from linen and hope chests in our grandmothers' time. I like bringing a few aromatic pots with us on camping trips. Citronella or Geranium essential oils help keep the bugs and mosquitoes away, while peppermint deters the picnic ants!

Direct From the Source—The Scented Plants

These are the plants that are highly scented and are natural environmental scent-enhancers. Most are seasonal, offering their scented gifts at certain times of the year. My favorite scented plants are *Lavender* and *Rosemary*.

Oh, and I love *Basil.* Although these are best grown outdoors in the heat of summer, they can be brought indoors for enjoyment but are a bit of a challenge. I adore all the scented *Roses, Lilacs, Peonies,* and *Phlox* that grow in our yard in the spring and summer months. One of my favorite places is in my herb and vegetable garden, especially in the summer, when it is blooming full of the sweet, spicy, and fruity scents. I even purchased some fragrant *Alpine strawberry* plants from France last year to grow at the foot of my gliding settee in the garden. *Scented geraniums, Heliotrope, Sweet peas,* and *Mints* of every variety surround me all summer long.

The deck off the master bedroom is a perfect setting for the evening blooming flowers. Sweet-scented *Nicotiana, Moonflowers,* and *Marvel of Peru* are a few of my favorite annuals that are easy to grow. They perfume the night air with their sensual aromas all summer long.

In the winter months, when the Seattle weather threatens months of dreary drizzle and cool damp temperatures, I concede reluctantly to move indoors where I create an entirely different setting of scented pleasures. I take great care and joy in creating a softly fragrant world in my home with nature's living things. At my side, close to where I sit to dine, is *Neroli,* a *Calamondin orange* tree I picked out for my Christmas present last year. Its blooms are so intensely fragrant they're difficult to describe in words. They bloom in December and January and make winter bearable after all.

Bearr's Lime is another citrus that has wonderfully scented blossoms. I also force bulbs of *White Narcissus* and *Hyacinth* in the slower months of October and November. Winter blooming *Jasmines, Sweet Violets,* and *Scented Geraniums* have their places in sunny corners and windowsills of the house. Another highlight, that ranks right up there with my Calamondin Orange, is *Stephany,* my *Stephanotis* plant that I've had for three years. Its unforgettably fragrant little trumpet-like flowers open around January and early February.

Gardenias, Camellias, Lemon verbena, and *Lily of the Valley* are more options for fragrant indoor growing.

Psycho-Aromatherapy Recipes

Here are a few of my favorite recipes for inhalation and natural room fragrancing tht I use most often for the home and office settings. They can be used in any of the forms discussed in this chapter for inhalation and room fragrancing, unless other wise noted. Recipes are given in "parts", allowing different amounts to be mixed according to need. If you are making a blend for diffuser use, a larger amount of at least 1/4 ounce or more may be necessary. If an aroma lamp is to be used, only 3 to 5 drops is needed. Therefore, one part can equal on drop, one teaspoon *or* one ounce, depending on the amount you wish to make. Be consistent throughout that particular recipe with the same measures.

Pure for Sure

for general antiseptic use

Lavender 5 parts
Eucalyptus 3 parts
Pine 3 parts

Cold and Flu Relief

antibacterial, ant-flu, and respiratory enhancing blend

Hyssop 4 parts
Rosemary 3 parts
Peppermint 3 parts
Eucalyptus 3 parts
Lemon 3 parts

Slow Down and Relax

a very special calming blend

Lavender 6 parts
Ylang Ylang 5 parts
Sandalwood 3 parts
Marjoram 3 parts

I Love My Job

an uplifting, puifying, and anti-stress office blend

Lavender 9 parts
Lemon 3 parts
Geranium 2 parts
Bergamot 2 parts

Mint Conditionaing for the Mind and Memory

Valerie's office blend for mental and memory stimulation

Lemon 5 parts
Spearmint 2 parts

Peppermint 2 parts
Black Pepper 2 parts
Rosemary 2 parts

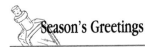 ## Season's Greetings

a warm and inviting holiday blend

Pine 8 parts (or 4 parts Pine, 4 part Spruce)
Lavender 3 parts
Sandalwood 3 parts
Frankincense 2 parts
Nutmeg 1 part
Mandarin 1 part

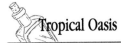 ## Tropical Oasis

a citrus fresh reminder of summer for the mid-winter doldrums

Lemon 3 parts
Mandarin 3 parts
Lemongrass 2 parts
Grapefruit 2 parts
Bergamot 2 parts

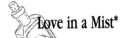 ## Love in a Mist*

an aphrodisiac and euphoric blend for special occasions (to be used sparinly and for short durations, not drop measurent)

Ylang Ylang 10 drops
Patchouli 2 drops
Black Pepper 2 drops
Clary Sage 3 drops
Neroli 2 drops
Rose 1 drop
Jasmine 1 drop

*Not intended for diffuser use. Use an aroma lamp or potpourri burner. Put 3 to5 drops in lamp.

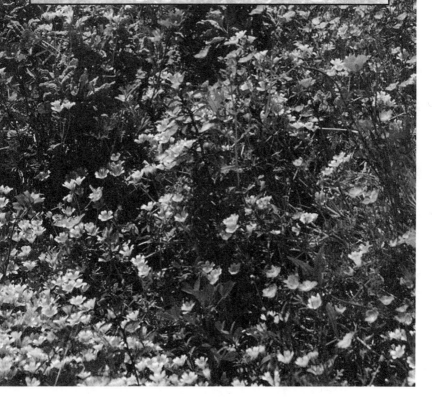

PART FOUR

The Pure Essentials

CHAPTER 14

Essential Oil
Reference Guide

The essential oils discussed in the following pages are referenced according to common English names. The Botanical (Latin) names are included to insure that the correct plant essential oil is discussed. You will find other information of interest such as Plant Origin, the part of the plant used to obtain the essential oil, along with the Extraction Method listed as well. A simple description of that particular Aroma essence by is also given.

For the purpose of blending, Evaporation Rates have been included and are listed according to the following ratings:

Top Notes   = High Evaporation number
                  (1 – 14 evaporation rate)

Middle Notes   = Mid-range evaporation number
                  (15 – 60 evaporation rate)

Base Notes   = Low evaporation number
                  (61 – 100 evaporation rate)

Refer to Chapter 15 *Blending How-To's and Helpful Hints* for a detailed explanation of the meaning and use of these.

Odor Intensity is also included for each essential oil to aid in satisfactory blending. The ratings are referenced accordingly:

Low	= rating of 4 or below
Medium	= rating of 5
High	= rating of 6
Very High	= rating of 7
Extremely High	= rating of 8 or 9

For more information on the meaning and application of these ratings refer to Chapter 15 *Blending How-To's and Helpful Hints*.

The Medicinal properties are the most important actions demonstrated by that specific essential oil. Because every person is unique, it is impossible to promise outcomes when using specific essential oils. However, knowing the traditional and medicinal uses of each will be of great assistance in guiding your choice of the correct oil! Caution: Do not attempt to self-diagnose or treat a serious condition.

Safety Precautions are given whenever there are contraindications to the use of a specific essential oil. However, if you are pregnant, elderly or caring for small children, extra care is warranted. For example, lower dilutions (of 1% or less) are recommended, as well as checking for skin sensitivities to new oils, and adhering to the guidelines in Chapter One: Common Sense Safety. The thirty essential oils introduced in this section were chosen both for their wide variety of applications and for their safety. Responsible use of all medicine, both herbal and prescription, is in the hands of the caregiver. Therefore, use this information as a resource, as it was intended—an Essential Oil Reference Guide.

Common ailments and possible benefits are included in the following pages as they relate to each essential oil. I have divided them into two basic categories: Physical Benefits and Psycho-Emotional Benefits. Most often essential oils work on several body systems at once, so there will be overlay or dual-action between both categories.

As you might imagine, I could not possibly include every known use of every essential oil produced. As I said earlier, these oils were chosen for their wide range of benefits, safety, and well documented therapeutic applications. They will create a strong foundation from which to work in using aromatherapy for prevention and treating everyday health challenges.

Oral administration of essential oils are not the topic of this book. With ailments related to the gastrointestinal tract (i.e., indigestion, stomach ache, acid stomach), the fresh or dried herb can be used. The following methods are recommended to take herbs by mouth:

Fresh herb—in salads, cooking, condiments, tea

Dried herb—dressings, cooking, seasoning, tea

Spice—cooking, seasoning, condiments, tea

Herbal Honey—herb gently heated in raw honey and strained. Used in hot tea.

Herb capsules (medicinal)—ground herbs in capsule form; take according to directions on label.

Herbal tincture (medicinal)—herbs extracted in alcohol; take according to directions on label.

Basil
THE HERB OF ROYALTY

Botanical Name	Ocimum basilicum
Plant Origin	Herb
Extraction Method	Distillation
Aroma	Fresh, light, slightly spicy
Odor Intensity	Very High
Evaporation Rate	Top note

Medicinal Properties: Antiseptic, antispasmodic, carminative, digestive, emmenagogue, expectorant, febrifuge, stomachic, tonic, antidepressant, cephalic, nervine, diaphoretic, adrenal stimulant, estrogen-like hormone qualities, decreases uric acid in blood.

Safety Precautions: Avoid in pregnancy. Possible irritant to sensitive skin. Avoid long term use with history of estrogen-dependent cancer.

Physical Benefits	*Psycho-Emotional Benefits*
Headaches	Encourages concentration
Stress-related allergies	Calms nervous system
Sinus congestion	Mild depression
Loss of smell from chronic sinusitis	Anxiety
Asthma	Insomnia
Bronchitis	Mental fatigue
Colds, Flu	PMS mood swings
Coughs	Hysteria
Mouth ulcers/Herpes	
Skin toner	
Hair loss	
Muscle aches and pain	
Painful and scanty menstruation	

Gout
Insect bites
Colitis
Hiccups
Gastric spasms

Herb: Take orally for gastric upset and pain, nausea, and hiccups.

Bergamot
NATURE'S WAY TO BALANCE

Botanical Name	Citrus bergamia
Plant Origin	Fruit
Extraction Method	Expression or steam distillation
Aroma	Spicy, citrus
Odor Intensity	Low
Evaporation Rate	Top note

Medicinal Properties: Analgesic, anti-infectious, antibacterial, anti-toxic, antiseptic, anti-depressant, antispasmodic, diuretic, digestive, deodorant, expectorant, febrifuge, anti-parasitic, tonic.

Safety Precautions: Will increase a sunburn, phototoxic. Possible irritant for sensitive skin or in strong dilution. Do not confuse with Beebalm, the herb Bergamot. A rectified (terpeneless) oil is available, and is considered safer to use.

Physical Benefits	*Psycho-Emotional Benefits*
Eczema	Depression
Acne, blemishes	Anxiety
Varicose veins, hemorrhoids	Stress-related disorders
Bad breath	Nervous tension
Mouth infections, Herpes Simplex	PMS
Colds, flu, bronchitis, tonsillitis	Insomnia
Deodorant	Regulates appetite due to anxiety
Insect repellant	Anger
Helps scar tissue form	Frustration
Cystitis	
Intestinal parasites	
Intestinal colic	
Colitis	

Cedarwood
A Wood That Cleanses

Botanical Name	Cedrus atlantica (Atlas Cedarwood)
Plant Origin	Wood
Extraction Method	Distillation
Aroma	Warm, balsamic, woody
Odor Intensity	Low
Evaporation Rate	Base note

Medicinal Properties: Antiseptic, astringent, diuretic, expectorant, fungicidal, sedative, insecticide, tonic.

Safety Precautions: Avoid in pregnancy. Possible irritant to sensitive skin or in strong dilution. Do not confuse with other Cedars or cedar leaf (thuja).

Physical Benefits	*Psycho-Emotional Benefits*
Skin infections	Nervous tension
Acne, blemishes	Anxiety
Oily skin	Meditation—focusing
Dandruff	Stress
Hair loss	Fear
Bronchitis	Anger
Coughs	
Catarrh (increase in mucous discharge)	
Cystitis	
Insect repellant	
Cellulite	
Air purifier	
Arthritis	
Immune stimulant	
Fungus	

Chamomile
Relief for Inflammations

Botanical Name	Anthemis nobilis
Plant Origin	Flowers
Extraction Method	Distillation
Aroma	Slightly fruity, herbal
Odor Intensity	Extremely high
Evaporation Rate	Middle note

Medicinal Properties:	Analgesic, anti-convulsive, antidepressant, anti-inflammatory, anti-neuralgic, antiphlogistic,antiseptic, antispasmodic, anti-allergic, carminative, digestive, diuretic, emmenagogue, febrifuge, sedative, tonic, antiparasitic.
Safety Precautions:	Avoid in first trimester of pregnancy. Avoid long term use with estrogen-dependent cancer.

Physical Benefits	*Psycho-Emotional Benefits*
Asthma	Stress
Allergies	Nervous Tension
Headache, migraine	Insomnia
Acne, boils	Anxiety
Dermatitis	Anger
Inflammations	Irritability
Arthritis, bursitis, sprains, neuralgia, teething	Fear, worries
Burns, blisters, wounds, ulcers	
Broken capillaries	
Herpes	
Psoriasis	
Gastritis	
Colitis	
Toothache	
Menopause and PMS symptoms	
Possibly neutralizes bacteria toxins	
Chronic infections	

Herb: Take orally for abdominal cramping, gas and pain, colitis, stomach ulcers, diarrhea.

Chamomile floral water or herb tea: Use for eye inflammations and infection.

Clary Sage
A WOMAN'S HELPER

Botanical Name	Salvia sclarea
Plant Origin	Herb
Extraction Method	Distillation
Aroma	Sweet,warm, nutty-herbal
Odor Intensity	Medium
Evaporation Rate	Middle note

Medicinal Properties: Anticonvulsive, antidepressant, antiseptic, antispasmodic, aphrodisiac, astringent, deodorant, digestive, emmenagogue, hypotensive, nervine, sedative, tonic.

Safety Precautions: Use with caution in pregnancy. Do not use while drinking alcoholic beverages (may increase narcotic effect). Do not over-use as it can cause headaches. Do not confuse with common garden sage. Do not use if history of low blood pressure. Avoid with history of estrogen-dependent cancer.

Physical Benefits	*Psycho-Emotional Benefits*
Physical debility	Depression
Inflamed skin	Nervous tension
Tones the skin	Panic states
Deodorant, profuse sweating	Sedative
Scanty, painful menstruation	Encourages feeling of well-being (euphoria)
Stimulates menstrual flow	Aphrodisiac
Uterine tonic	Migraine
Encourages labor	Fatigue
PMS symptoms	Stress
Menopause, hot flashes	Fear
Muscle spasms, cramps	
Hypertension	
Acne, boils	
Dandruff	
Hair loss	
Aged skin	
Varicose veins	
Constipation	

Cypress
ALL-TIME SKIN TONER

Botanical Name	Cupressus sempervirens
Plant Origin	Wood, branches
Extraction Method	Distillation
Aroma	Fresh, spicy-wood
Odor Intensity	Low
Evaporation Rate	Mid to base note

Medicinal Properties:	Antirheumatic, antiseptic, antispasmodic, astringent, deodorant, diuretic, febrifuge, insecticide, restorative, sedative, tonic, vaso-constrictive, anti-infectious, decongestant.
Safety Precautions:	Avoid in pregnancy. Avoid with hypertension. Avoid with history of estrogen-dependant cancer.

Physical Benefits	*Psycho-Emotional Benefits*
Asthma	Irritability, PMS
Spasmodic coughs, bronchitis	Stress-related conditions
Varicose veins, hemorrhoids	Nervous tension
Bruises	Restlessness
Puffy, watery skin	Debility
Cellulite	Anger
Broken capillaries	
Nose bleeds, sinusitis	
Excessive perspiration	
Hot flashes, menopause	
Painful, heavy menstruation	
Insect repellant	
Poor circulation	
Sore throat, hoarseness	
Arthritis	
Muscle cramps	
Bleeding gums	

Eucalyptus
AN OLD FAVORITE FOR COLDS

Botanical Name	Eucalyptus globulus, Eucalyptus radiata, Eucalyptus smithii
Plant Origin	Tree, leaves
Extraction Method	Distillation
Aroma	Medicinal, pungent, fresh
Odor Intensity	Extremely high
Evaporation Rate	Top note
Medicinal Properties:	Analgesic, antiseptic, antispasmodic, deodorant, decongestant, diuretic, expectorant, febrifuge, stimulant, anti-neuralgic, antiviral, increases circulation, antifungal, antibacterial, anti-infectious.

Safety Precautions: Avoid if taking homeopathic remedies. Do not use in strong dilutions on the skin. Avoid if history of epilepsy or hypertension.

Physical Benefits	*Psycho-Emotional Benefits*
Asthma	Lack of concentration
Colds, flu	Increase alertness, stay awake
Chest and throat infections	Clears the mind
Catarrh	
Viral infections including herpes	
Cystitis	
Arthritis, bursitis	
Abscesses, boils	
Cuts, wounds, burns	
Blisters, ulcers	
Headache, migraine	
Neuralgia	
Muscle stiffness, bruises, sprains	
Stings, insect bites	
Fever	
Insect repellant	
Air purifier	
Immune stimulant	
Swollen glands	

Frankincense
THE ESSENCE OF ANTIQUITY

Botanical Name	Boswellia carteri
Plant Origin	Tree, resin
Extraction Method	Distillation
Aroma	Balsamic, spicy
Odor Intensity	Very high
Evaporation Rate	Mid to Base note

Medicinal Properties: Antiseptic, astringent, diuretic, expectorant, sedative, uterine tonic, anti-inflammatory, antidepressant, immune stimulant.

Safety Precautions: Avoid in pregnancy.

Physical Benefits

Dermatitis

Aging skin, wrinkles

Wounds, ulcers

Shortness of breath

Asthma

Sinus congestion

Bronchitis

Laryngitis

Uterine tonic

Cystitis

Acne, pimples

Scars

Diarrhea

Psycho-Emotional Benefits

Anxiety

Nervous tension

Stress

Obsessive thinking

Helpful during labor

Post-partum depression

Meditation, focusing

Depression

Fear, nightmares

Geranium
THE HORMONE REGULATOR

Botanical Name	Pelargonium graveolens
Plant Origin	Herb
Extraction Method	Distillation
Aroma	Rose-like, green
Odor Intensity	High
Evaporation Rate	Middle note

Medicinal Properties: Analgesic, anti-inflammatory, anticoagulant, antidepressant, antiseptic, astringent, diuretic, deodorant, insecticide, tonic, vasoconstrictor, immune stimulant, antibacterial.

Safety Precautions: Avoid in early pregnancy. Possible irritant to sensitive skin. Can cause insomnia and restlessness if overused. Avoid long term use with history of estrogen-dependent cancer.

Physical Benefits

Menopause

Heavy menstruation

Breast tenderness and swelling

Tonic to liver and kidneys

Cystitis

Excess fluids, especially lower limbs

Throat infections, tonsilitis

Psycho-Emotional Benefits

Nervous tension

Anxiety

Depression

Uplifting and balancing emotions

PMS

Stress

Facial neuralgia
Excess mucus
Eczema
Oily or dry skin extremes
Burns
Herpes, shingles
Ringworm, fungus
Insect repellant
Acne
Bruises, broken capillaries
Mature skin
Asthma
Poor circulation
Hemmorhoids, ulcers

Ginger
A WARMING SPICE

Botanical Name	Zingiber officinalis
Plant Origin	Root
Extraction Method	Distillation
Aroma	Warm, balsamic, woody
Odor Intensity	Medium
Evaporation Rate	Middle note

Medicinal Properties: Antiseptic, antispasmodic, aphrodisiac, carminative, diaphoretic, expectorant, febrifuge, laxative, stimulant, stomachic, analgesic, anti-inflammatory, tonic.

Safety Precautions: Possible irritant to sensitive skin. Do not use in strong dilution on skin.

Physical Benefits	*Psycho-Emotional Benefits*
Congestion	Aphrodisiac
Colds, coughs, bronchitis	Mental fatigue
Excess fluids, swelling	Nervous exhaustion
Spasms, diarrhea	Debility
Throat infections	Aids memory
Fever	
Headaches	
Arthritis	
Sprains	

Bruises, soreness
Poor circulation
Varicose veins
Raised body temperature
Toothache
Nausea

Use the *spice or fresh ginger root* for: Loss of appetite, gas, abdominal cramps, painful digestion, laxative.

Grapefruit
THE BEST BODY TONIC

Botanical Name	Citrus paradisii
Plant Origin	Fruit
Extraction Method	Expression
Aroma	Fresh, citrus, bright
Odor Intensity	Very high
Evaporation Rate	Top note

Medicinal Properties: **Antidepressant, antiseptic, astringent, diuretic, stimulant, tonic.**

Safety Precautions: **Phototoxic. Shorter shelf life.**

Physical Benefits	*Psycho-Emotional Benefits*
Obesity	Stress
Cellulite	Euphoric, uplifting
Cleansing effect on: Circulation, Kidneys, Lymphatic system	Tiredness
	Depression
PMS	Nervous exhaustion
Headache	Jet lag
Acne	Drug/alcohol withdrawal
Congested skin	
Oily skin	
Skin toner	
Muscular fatigue, stiffness	
Hair loss	

Fresh juice: Take for digestive aid, cleansing and detoxifying the body.

Hyssop
AN INCREDIBLE LUNG TONIC

Botanical Name	Hyssopus officinalis
Plant Origin	Herb, flowers
Extraction Method	Distillation
Aroma	Fresh, herbal, spice-like
Odor Intensity	High
Evaporation Rate	Mid-base note

Medicinal Properties: Antiseptic, antibacterial, antispasmodic, antiviral, diuretic, decongestant, expectorant, emmenagogue, febrifuge, sedative, circulatory and respiratory tonic, astringent, pulmonary anti-inflammatory, hypertensive.

Safety Precautions: Use in moderation. Avoid during pregnancy. Do not use with history of epilepsy or hypertension.

Physical Benefits	*Psycho-Emotional Benefits*
Asthma	Anxiety
Bronchitis	Fatigue
Colds, flu, swollen glands	Nervous tension
Coughs	Stress-related conditions
Chest congestion	Grief
Sore throat	Aids concentration
Tonsillitis	
Colic, indigestion	
Bruises, cuts, wounds	
Dermatitis	
Eczema	
Acne	
Cystitis	
Water retention	

Jasmine
THE KING OF FLOWERS

Botanical Name	Jasminum grandiflorum, Jasminum officinale
Plant Origin	Flowers
Extraction Method	Solvent extraction

Aroma	Warm, exotic, floral
Odor Intensity	Very high
Evaporation Rate	Base note

Medicinal Properties: Antidepressant, antiseptic, antispasmodic, aphrodisiac, emollient, sedative, uterine tonic, mild analgesic, anti-inflammatory.

Safety Precautions: Use with caution during pregnancy. Use in low dilution. Do not overuse. Narcotic-like properties.

Physical Benefits	*Psycho-Emotional Benefits*
Helpful during labor	Depression
Strengthens contractions, relieves pain	Nervous tension
Uterine spasms	Emotional imbalance, suffering
Promotes milk production	Post-partum depression
Menstrual cramps, pain	PMS
Bronchial spasms	Eurphoric
Spasmodic coughs, hoarseness	Aphrodisiac
Dry, sensitive skin	Fear, paranoia
Skin softener	Pessimism
Strengthens sexual organs	
Catarrh	

Juniper
AID IN DETOXIFYING THE BODY

Botanical Name	Juniper communis
Plant Origin	Tree, berries
Extraction Method	Distillation
Aroma	Fresh, woody
Odor Intensity	Medium
Evaporation Rate	Middle note

Medicinal Properties: Antirheumatic, antiseptic, antispasmodic, astringent, diuretic, anti-toxic, tonic, nervine, anti-infectious, anti-arthritic, circulatory stimulant.

Safety Precautions: Avoid in pregnancy. Avoid if history of kidney disease. Do not use in strong dilution or for prolonged use. Use with caution on sensitive or damaged skin.

Physical Benefits	Psycho-Emotional Benefits
Acne	Aphrodisiac
Boils	General debility
Oily skin, blocked pores	Nervous disorders
Arthritis, gout	Mental exhaustion
Cellulite	Anxiety
Detoxification, overindulgence	Stress-related conditions
Cystitis	Clears the mind, strengthens nervous system
Poor urinary flow	Jet lag
Hair loss	Poor memory
Varicose veins, hemorrhoids	
Water retention	
Colds, flu, infections	
Possibly helps in diabetic conditions.	
Ulcers	

Lavender
GRANDMOTHER'S INCREDIBLE REMEDY

Botanical Name	Lavendula officinalis, Lavendula angustifolia
Plant Origin	Flowers
Extraction Method	Distillation
Aroma	Floral, slightly herbal
Odor Intensity	Low
Evaporation Rate	Middle note
Medicinal Properties:	Analgesic, anticonvulsive, antidepressant, antiphlogistic, hypotensive, antirheumatic, antiseptic, antispasmodic, antiviral, decongestant, anticoagulant, deodorant, anti-toxic, diuretic, restorative, sedative, nervine.
Safety Precautions:	Avoid in first trimester of pregnancy. Avoid if blood pressure is extremely low.

Physical Benefits	Psycho-Emotional Benefits
All inflammations of the skin	Nervous tension
Palpitations	Balances emotions
Hypertension	Irritability
Convulsions	Helpful during labor
Muscle spasms	Insomnia
Pain related to: arthritis, sprains, strains	Stress
	Hysteria

Headache

Acute stages of respiratory ailments

Scanty and painful menstruation

Loss of hair

Nausea, vomiting

Burns, sunburn

Acne

Eczema

Psoriasis

All wounds, cuts, bites, scarring

Hiccups

Scars

Anxiety

Soothes nervous system

Exhaustion

Manic depression

Anger

Lemon
A SUNNY DISPOSITION

Botanical Name	Citrus limonum
Plant Origin	Fruit peel
Extraction Method	Expression
Aroma	Fresh, citrus, bright
Odor Intensity	Very high
Evaporation Rate	Top note

Medicinal Properties: **Antirheumatic, antiseptic, antispasmodic, anti-toxic, astringent, bactericidal, diaphoretic, diuretic, febrifuge, hypotensive, antifungal, insecticide, tonic, immune stimulant, antiviral.**

Safety Precautions: **Shorter shelf life. Phototoxic. Possible irritant to sensitive skin. Use with caution on sensitive or damaged skin.**

Physical Benefits

Acne, boils

Exfoliant

Oily skin

Corns, warts

Cellulite

Obesity

Fever

Inflamed and painful joints

Arthritis, gout

Hypertension

PMS

Psycho-Emotional Benefits

Depression

Confusion

Lethargy

General debility

Brain stimulant

Aids Concentration

Jet lag
Throat and upper respiratory ailments
Mouth ulcers, herpes
Hair loss
Lightens skin pigmentations
Poor circulation
Asthma
Nosebleeds

Use *fresh lemon juice* for: Detoxification, high acid system, obesity.

Lemongrass
SUPPORT FOR SAGGING SKIN

Botanical Name	Cymbopogon citratus
Plant Origin	Grass
Extraction Method	Distillation
Aroma	Fresh, lemon-like
Odor Intensity	Medium
Evaporation Rate	Top note

Medicinal Properties: Antiseptic, analgesic, antidepressant, astringent, diuretic, deodorant, febrifuge, insecticide, nervine, tonic, anti-inflamatory, astringent, fungicidal, parasiticide.

Safety Precautions: Possible irritant to sensitive skin or when used in strong dilution. Do not use on damaged skin. Avoid in pregnancy.

Physical Benefits	*Psycho-Emotional Benefits*
Vertigo	Lack of concentration
Palpitations	Mental fatigue
Increases milk production	Stress-related conditions
Deodorant	Headaches
Athlete's foot, skin parasites	Nervous exhaustion
Enlarged pores	Irritability
Loose skin	
Fever	
Recovery from illness	
Jet lag	
Excessive perspiration	
Bruises, sprains	

Oily skin, hair
Cellulite
Arthritis
Muscle soreness
Colitis
Indigestion

Use *fresh or dried herb* for: indigestion, colitis, difficult digestion, abdominal spasms.

Mandarin
PROMISING FAVORITE OF CHILDREN

Botanical Name	Citrus reticulata
Plant Origin	Fruit
Extraction Method	Expression
Aroma	Sweet, orange-like
Odor Intensity	High
Evaporation Rate	Top note

Medicinal Properties: **Antiseptic, antispasmodic, digestive, diuretic, sedative, tonic.**

Safety Precautions: **Phototoxic. Shorter shelf life.**

Physical Benefits	*Psycho-Emotional Benefits*
Acne	Stress
Oily skin	Insomnia
Skin toner	Irritability
Obesity	Mental fatigue
Excess fluid	Favored by children
Scars, stretchmarks	Overactivity
Muscle spasms	Nervous tension
Hiccups	Restlessness
Cellulite	
Obesity	
PMS	

Use *fresh juice* for: gas, abdominal cramping, burping, stimulate appetite.

Marjoram
#1 SEDATIVE

Botanical Name	Origanum marjorana
Plant Origin	Herb

Extraction Method	Distillation
Aroma	Warm, slightly spicy, herb-like
Odor Intensity	Medium
Evaporation Rate	Middle note

Medicinal Properties: Analgesic, antiseptic, antispasmodic, digestive, expectorant, hypotensive, laxative, nervine, sedative, tonic, anaphrodisiac.

Safety Precautions: Avoid if history of very low blood pressure. Avoid during pregnancy. Do not use on young children, or the elderly without advice from a health professional.

Physical Benefits	*Psycho-Emotional Benefits*
Asthma	General debility
Colds, spasmodic coughs	Mental exhaustion
Bronchitis, sinusitis	Mental/emotional instability
Headache, migraine	Anxiety
Palpitations	Insomnia
Arthritis	Nervous tension
Hypertension	Agitation, hyperactivity
Muscular spasms, stiffness	Grief, heartache, sorrow
Painful menstruation	Anaphrodisiac
Bruises	PMS
Flu	Hysteria
Mouth ulcers	Stress
	Obsession

Herb: Take orally for abdominal cramping, colic, gas and constipation.

Myrrh
MIRACULOUS MOUTH CARE

Botanical Name	Commiphora myrrha
Plant Origin	Tree, resin
Extraction Method	Distillation
Aroma	Warm, smoky, balsamic
Odor Intensity	Very high
Evaporation Rate	Base note

Medicinal Properties: Anti-inflammatory, antifungal, antimicrobial, antiphlogistic, anticatarrhal, antiseptic, astringent, emmenagogue, expectorant, sedative, uterine tonic.

Safety Precautions: Avoid during pregnancy. Use in moderation.

Physical Benefits	*Psycho-Emotional Benefits*
Cuts, ulcers	Extreme emotional states
Wounds	Confusion
Dry, cracked skin	Hysteria
Aging, mature skin	Fear, panic
Athlete's foot, ringworm	Emotional coldness
Asthma	Apathy
Bronchitis	
Sinusitis	
Mouth ulcers	
Gum infections, gingivitis	
Oral thrush	
Loose teeth/weak gums	
Inflamed skin	
Sore throat	
Loss of voice	
Hemorrhoids	

Neroli
A PERFECT CHOICE FOR SENSITIVE SKIN

Botanical Name	Citrus aurantium
Plant Origin	Flowers
Extraction Method	Distillation/Solvent extraction
Aroma	Sweet, floral, slightly citrus
Odor Intensity	Medium
Evaporation Rate	Middle note

Medicinal Properties: **Antiseptic, anti-depressant, antispasmodic, deodorant, sedative, tonic, hypnotic.**

Safety Precautions: **Use in moderation.**

Physical Benefits	*Psycho-Emotional Benefits*
Dry, mature, sensitive skin	Insomnia
Deodorant	Aphrodisiac
Headache	Depression
Neuralgia	Chronic anxiety
Scarring	Stress
Stretchmarks	Post shock
Radiated or extremely sunburned skin	PMS

Poor circulation

Palpitations

Varicose veins

Hemorrhoids

Aids labor

Irritability

Menopause

Sadness

Floral water: Useful for sensitive, mature skin.

Patchouli

THE RENEWAL ESSENTIAL OIL

Botanical Name	Pogostemon patchouli, Pogostemon cablin
Plant Origin	Shrub
Extraction Method	Distillation
Aroma	Pungent, earthy
Odor Intensity	Medium
Evaporation Rate	Base note

Medicinal Properties: Anti-inflammatory, antiseptic, fungicide, insecticide, cell regenerator, antidepressant, deodorant, diuretic, sedative, tonic, antiphlogistic, aphrodisiac, astringent, decongestant.

Safety Precautions: Use in moderation.

Physical Benefits

Acne

Dermatitis

Dry, cracked skin

Eczema

Hemorrhoids

Fungal infections

Athlete's foot

Dandruff

Wounds, sores

Insect repellant

Possible appetite suppressant

Loose skin

Enlarged pores

Scars

Aging skin

Varicose veins

Psycho-Emotional Benefits

Depression

Aphrodisiac

Anxiety

Nervous exhaustion

Stress-related conditions

Emotional coldness

Confusion

Menopause

Lethargy

Peppermint
Cooling Relief in a Bottle

Botanical Name	Mentha piperita
Plant Origin	Herb
Extraction Method	Distillation
Aroma	Strong, sharp, minty
Odor Intensity	Very high
Evaporation Rate	Top note

Medicinal Properties: Analgesic, antiphlogistic, antiseptic, antispasmodic, astringent, carminative, expectorant, febrifuge, nervine, stomachic, vasoconstrictor, decongestant, ant-inflammatory, anti-infectious, antifungal, digestive.

Safety Precautions: Possible irritant to skin. Do not use in strong dilution. Avoid in pregnancy and lactation. May antidote homeopathic remedies. Do not use on sensitive or damaged skin.

Physical Benefits	*Psycho-Emotional Benefits*
Constricts capillaries	General debility
Palpitations	Lethargy
Headache	Hysteria
Painful menstruation	Mental fatigue
Fever	Depression
Asthma	Nervous stress
Colds, sinusitis	Shock
Chronic bronchitis	
Nausea, dizziness, fainting	
Neuralgia	
Muscular spasms, aches	
Ringworm	
Toothache	
Bad breath	
Laryngitis	
Arthritis	
Hypotension	
Decreases lactation	

Herb: Take orally for indigestion, abdominal cramping, gas, high-acid stomach, intestinal parasites and/or worms, bad breath.

Petitgrain
A NATURAL SKIN TONER

Botanical Name	Citrus bigardia
Plant Origin	Tree, leaves
Extraction Method	Distillation
Aroma	Fresh, green, slightly floral
Odor Intensity	Medium
Evaporation Rate	Middle to Top Note

Medicinal Properties: Antiseptic, antidepressant, antispasmodic, deodorant, nervine, stimulant, tonic.

Safety Precautions: Shorter shelf life. Possible irritant to sensitive skin.

Physical Benefits	*Psycho-Emotional Benefits*
Acne	Insomnia
Skin toner	Anxiety
Oily skin	Sedative
Enlarged pores	Mental fatigue
Excessive perspiration	Nervous tension, exhaustion
Deodorant	Stress-related conditions
Muscular spasms	Calms anger, panic
Encourages relaxed breathing	Mild depression
Recovery from illness	
Respiratory infections	
Asthma	
Arthritis	
Palpitations	

Pine
THE TRUE DIS-INFECTANT

Botanical Name	Pinus sylvestris
Plant Origin	Tree
Extraction Method	Distillation
Aroma	Fresh, forest-like
Odor Intensity	High
Evaporation Rate	Middle note

Medicinal Properties: Antiphlogistic, antirheumatic, antiseptic, antineuralgic, antiviral, antiscorbutic, deodorant, decongestant, diuretic, disinfectant, expectorant, stimulant, tonic, antifungal.

Safety Precautions: Possible irritant to sensitive skin. Do not confuse with other pines. Avoid with history of prostate cancer. Do not use on sensitive or damaged skin.

Physical Benefits	*Psycho-Emotional Benefits*
Asthma	Fatigue
Bronchitis, laryngitis	Nervous exhaustion
Colds, flu	Stress-related conditions
Sinusitis	Debility
Cystitis	
Prostatitis	
Arthritis, gout	
Sciatica, neuralgia	
Muscular stiffness, soreness	
Psoriasis	
Insect repellant, lice	
Excessive perspiration	
Eczema	
Ringworm	
Sore throat	
Fever	

Rose
THE QUEEN OF FLOWERS

Botanical Name	Rosa damascena
Plant Origin	Flower
Extraction Method	Distillation/solvent extraction
Aroma	Intense, floral, honey-like
Odor Intensity	Very high
Evaporation Rate	Middle note

Medicinal Properties: Antidepressant, antiphlogistic, antiseptic, antispasmodic, aphrodisiac, astringent, emmenagogue, hemostatic, sedative, tonic.

Safety Precautions: Use with caution during pregnancy.

Physical Benefits	*Psycho-Emotional Benefits*
Nausea	Depression
Headache	Emotional coldness
Irregular menstruation	Impotence
Broken capillaries	Aphrodisiac

Aging, mature skin

Balancing and rejuvenating to skin

Uterine tonic

Possible hormone balancing

Eczema

Palpitations

Mouth infections

Insomnia

Nervous tension

Post-partum depression

Encourages feeling of well-being

Grief, sadness

Stress-related conditions

Poor memory

Rose floral water or rose petal tea: Use for inflammation of the eye, puffiness, conjunctivitis.

Rosemary
THE OIL-FREE ESSENCE

Botanical Name	Rosmarinus officinalis
Plant Origin	Herb
Extraction Method	Distillation
Aroma	Fresh, woody, herbal
Odor Intensity	High
Evaporation Rate	Middle note

Medicinal Properties: Analgesic, antirheumatic, antiseptic, astringent, antispasmodic, aphrodisiac, carminative, cytophylactic, diaphoretic, digestive, decongestant, diuretic, emmenagogue, hypertensive, nervine, parasitic, restorative, stimulant, tonic.

Safety Precautions: Avoid during pregnancy. Avoid if history of high blood pressure. Avoid if history of epilepsy. Do not use on sensitive or damaged skin.

Physical Benefits

Hypotension

Physical fatigue

Asthma

Bronchitis

Painful menstruation

Arthritis, gout

Headache

Muscular soreness, bruising, cramps

Weakness of limbs

Skin toner

Oily hair, dandruff

Hair loss

Psycho-Emotional Benefits

General debility

Mental fatigue

Nervous tension

Amnesia

Stress-related conditions

Hysteria

Depression

PMS

Grief, apathy

Lethargy

Acne, blemishes
Insect repellant
Varicose veins
Tonsillitis
Sinusitis
Colds, flu
Swelling

Herb: Take orally for high cholesterol in the blood, mild constipation, and upset stomach.

Sandalwood
AID IN INFECTION CONTROL

Botanical Name	Santalum album
Plant Origin	Tree, wood
Extraction Method	Distillation
Aroma	Exotic, woody
Odor Intensity	Medium
Evaporation Rate	Base note

Medicinal Properties: **Antiphlogistic, antiseptic, antispasmodic, aphrodisiac, astringent, diuretic, emollient, expectorant, sedative, tonic, decongestant, insecticide, antifungal.**

Safety Precautions: **Use in moderation.**

Physical Benefits
Urinary tract infections
Chronic asthma, bronchitis
Acne
Dry, cracked skin
Aging, mature skin
Dehydrated skin
Dry cough
Immune stimulant
Cleansing action on sexual organs
Laryngitis, sore throat
Muscle spasms
Varicose veins, hemorrhoids
Neuralgia
Respiratory infections

Psycho-Emotional Benefits
Insomnia
Nervous tension
Aphrodisiac
Aggression
Meditation, focuses
Depression
Stress-related conditions
Obsession
Grief

Tea Tree
NATURE'S FIRST AID

Botanical Name	Melaleuca alternifolia
Plant Origin	Tree, leaves
Extraction Method	Distillation
Aroma	Sharp, medicinal
Odor Intensity	Very high
Evaporation Rate	Top note

Medicinal Properties: Antibiotic, antibacterial, antifungal, anti-inflammatory, antiviral, diaphoretic, expectorant, immune stimulant, anti-parasitic, anti-infectious, decongestant.

Safety Precautions: Possible irritant to sensitive skin.

Physical Benefits
Cuts, abrasions, insect bites
Burns
Mouth ulcers, cold sores
Air purifier
Herpes, chicken pox
Boils, warts
Nail infections
Jock itch
Asthma
Bronchitis
Chest colds, catarrh
Sinusitis
Acne, blemishes
Immune stimulant
Athlete's foot
Dandruff
Ringworm
Tonsillitis
Upper respiratory infections
Varicose veins, hemorrhoids
Parasites

Psycho-Emotional Benefits
General debility
Post-shock
Nervous exhaustion

Ylang Ylang
THE FLOWER OF FLOWERS

Botanical Name	Canaga odorata
Plant Origin	Flowers
Extraction Method	Distillation
Aroma	Sweet, heavy, exotic
Odor Intensity	High
Evaporation Rate	Middle to base note

Medicinal Properties: Antiseptic, aphrodisiac, antidepressant, hypotensive, sedative, euphoric, tonic, nervine.

Safety Precautions: Avoid if history of low blood pressure or apnea. Use in moderation. Avoid use on damaged or very sensitive skin.

Physical Benefits	*Psycho-Emotional Benefits*
Hypertension	Aphrodisiac
Palpitations	Insomnia
Rapid breathing	Emotional coldness
Scalp tonic	Depression
Hair loss	Nervous tension
Uterine tonic	Anxiety
Insect bites	Panic
Acne	Fear, anger
Fever	Shock
	Encourages feeling of well-being, euphoria
	PMS

CHAPTER 15

Blending How-To's and Helpful Hints

In this section we will walk through the blending basics that will assist you in creating your own personal aromatherapy favorites. The chosen essential oils, the method of application, coupled with which type of carrier used, all play a significant role in the end result. However, more important are the correct preparation ratios and dilutions. This chapter covers carrier oil choices, blending instructions, and quick reference charts.

Keys to Successful Blending—"Less is More": An Aromatherapy Paradigm

"Blending" is a word frequently heard within the aromatherapy field. According to Webster's dictionary it means "to mix thoroughly; to prepare by mixing different varieties; to combine into an integrated whole; to harmonize, merge or mingle." All the above are accurate descriptions of this artful process. Blending aromatherapy oils is a creative and highly personal art, rather than a science. However, there are a few "keys" to this subjective process that will assist you in preparing satisfying and well-balanced aromatherapy blends.

When a therapeutic blend is needed to remedy a particular ailment, the main focus is to choose essential oils for their specific characteristics.

For example, Lemon and Pine may be chosen for their antiseptic properties, Lavender or Chamomile for their anti-inflammatory qualities, or Geranium and Tea Tree because they are anti-fungal. However, even therapeutic blends such as these should be somewhat agreeable and pleasant for you to use, and by adding two or more essences together you increase their effect considerably.

Alternately, when you wish to make a purely pleasurable concoction (e.g., an aphrodisiac oil, a personal perfume oil, a very pampering bath salt mix, or a luxurious body lotion), these blending tips will be most useful for referencing.

Evaporation rates are given in terms of Top, Middle, and Base Notes for use in blending. The Top notes are noticed first in a blend, as they evaporate most quickly. In contrast, the Base notes are the slowest to evaporate and help in making the blend's scent longer-lasting. The Middle notes help "hold together" the entire range of scents.

Odor Intensity is rated Low, Medium, High, Very High and Extremely High. These describe how powerful an essential oil is on an odor or scent intensity scale. The highest rating refers to the most dominating essential oils. These will overpower a blend if not used sparingly. Conversely, the low rating reflects a softer, more mellow, and gentler scent that will be lost if not adjusted and taken into account when used with higher or more intense essential oils.

For example, Chamomile is referenced as an extremely high scent, while Lavender is rated low as listed in the *Essential Oil Reference Guide*. This means that twice as much Lavender or more will need to be added to the blend if its lighter fragrance is to be noticed when combined with Chamomile.

There are no hard and fast rules to blending. Absolute exactness does not exist when deciding which essential oils "should" be used and how much. Some like to incorporate less scientific methods such as intuition, or simply following their nose in finding the right combination or blend. I personally use essential oils for their therapeutic effects, as well as for their psycho-aromatherapy benefits. However, the final choice is made among scents I find to be most desirable and favored for personal use. If you are drawn to a certain oil, it may be because you need that particular oil at that time.

> Essential oils are *holistic* healing agents whereby they are capable of sometimes influencing several body systems.

Over the past 70 years, some general and traditional guidelines and theories have proven successful over time and with consistent use. We note differences among countries, their cultures, and healing philosophies. For example, in France where they specialize in the medical applications of aromatherapy and phytotherapy, doctors often employ much stronger dosages than in the United Kingdom and the United States. The English focus their aromatherapy applications on massage. The Japanese seem to be primarily working in areas of mental/mood and performance aromatherapy adaptation. I look to the United States and see how we are embracing all these and more, adopting aromatherapy into our lifestyle.

All in all, there appears to be agreement among many aromatherapists regarding treatment of young children, the very old and frail, as well as pregnant women. Considering these populations, we find they generally will be more sensitive and responsive to most treatments. Also, since body weight and size can vary dramatically compared to that of the average adult person, we advise you, when caring for such a family member, to always divide the normal adult essential oil dose by half or more. See Chapter One: *Common Sense Safety* for hazardous essential oils related to this subject.

What does it mean "Less is More"? When it comes to aromatherapy, you must forget the "more is better" philosophy. Although many cultures and health philosophies agree with this, consider Homeopathy and Bach Flower Remedies. They constitute a form of medicine that is based on treatments with minute (almost undetectable) amounts of "remedy" to stimulate or support the body in healing. In Ayurveda, the ancient system of healing from India, very small amounts of specific herbs and spices, including aromatherapy oils, are commonly prescribed to promote health and balance.

It is also interesting to learn that the "whole" essential oil, as it appears naturally, is found to be more effective than its single isolated constituents. Laboratory tests have shown that the original complete and naturally occurring oil was far more effective than its constituents (e.g., increase in spasmolytic action, increase in sedative effect, increase in expectoration, etc.). Aromatic plants as seen in nature consist of a range of essential oil content from .01% to 10%, with an average of 1% to 2%—exactly the amount most often used in skin application. Indeed, various studies have proven that increasing the essential oil dose actually *diminished* the desired outcome or response!

Unlike antibiotics (which literally means "against life") essential oils work holistically with the natural forces of the body to encourage balance and healing, enhancing life.

Hence, *balance* and *moderation* are key in using essential oils for positive, health-promoting aromatherapy. Be sure to use the guidelines given in this chapter and direct yourself to the helpful charts designed for easy reference that appear in the following pages.

Synergy is a common term often applied to aromatherapy. If we take apart the word we can easily find its meaning: "syn" means *together* while "ergon" means *work*. Taking it one step further, synergy also relates to the theory that the whole is greater than the sum of the individual parts. When we combine 2, 3, or 4 different essences, they make up a whole new compound. The individual effects of each essential oil based on its chemical "parts" or components do not equal the sum of the effects when added together. They will most often become much more powerful and treatment-specific since the combination is now "working together" for a focused outcome.

By mixing 3 or 4 single essential oils together within the same (therapeutic) group, we can create a blend that works synergistically. The individual oils will often complement one another and potentiate the blend. For example, if a respiratory blend was needed, a combination of Eucalyptus, Cedarwood, Pine, and Peppermint would be more effective and "respiratory-enhancing" than a single oil such as Cedarwood or Eucalyptus.

It has been noted that a blend of 5 essential oils or more can become too complex and difficult to blend for the inexperienced. So I recommend simpler blends that consist of 4 or fewer different essential oils; I also recommend trying the variety of recipes given in this book to help increase your success rate early in your aromatherapy experiences.

Lavender essential oil can be added to most aromatherapy blends to complement the mixture. It can almost be called a "potentiator" in that it virtually always "adds to" the blend it is part of; it soothes the nervous system and has a healing, balancing, and anti-inflammatory effect on the skin.

Let's look at how synergy can work on the treatment level, in the aromatic bath, for example. The bath involves several factors, or treatment parts such as (1) hydrotherapy, (2) essential oils (amount, quality, combinations), (3) the carrier chosen, and (4) the length of time or duration of the bath (treatment). All the above parts added together create a whole new powerful and specialized treatment.

So Many Choices—Vegetable, Nut and Seed Oils as Carriers

Carriers are necessary to "carry" or transport other substances, such as essential oils or infusion oils, that cannot be directly applied to the skin by themselves. Those most frequently used are oils such as sweet almond, sunflower, and olive. You can use a neutral unscented body lotion as well for your essential oils as discussed in Chapter 12. The benefit of using lotions as a carrier medium is that they are water-soluble and will not leave a heavy or oily feeling on the skin. They are much lighter in consistency and water-based. Although carrier oils are most often used for their ease and simplicity, they benefit the skin in several ways. Various vegetable and seed oils contain natural vitamins, minerals, and protein. Some of them are high in antioxidants and can help slow the aging of skin. Oils have been traditionally used in massage, skin care, and aromatherapy applications because of their inherent "glide" feel and adaptability to massage. Therefore, we could say that the natural "tools of the trade" are the essential oils themselves, and the carrier vegetable oils.

Essential Oils + Carrier Oils = Aromatherapy Basics for Body Application

Most vegetable, nut, and seed oils you typically find in grocery markets are highly refined and contain solvent and petroleum residues. These are most often processed under high heat to produce a lighter and odorless oil. They contain preservatives such as BHA and BHT to prolong their shelf life indefinitely. For this reason, they are less expensive than their natural chemical-free counterparts.

Unprocessed oils are the best for skin care preparations. Similarly, *organic* and *cold-pressed* oils are the most sought-after for aromatherapy application. As the name suggests, they are pressed from the nut, seed, or fruit; little or no heat is used, nor any chemical solvents to extract them. These oils are inherently rich in vitamins, minerals, and proteins which nourish the skin. Expect to pay more for these oils, and store them safely after opening.

I recommend keeping all your vegetable carrier oils under refrigeration and stored in colored glass bottles. You may even want to date the bottles to insure you use the older oils first. It is a good idea to add an antioxidant to your oils before storing them, or add them at the time when you prepare your aromatherapy mixtures. Doing this will naturally prolong their shelf life considerably. Excellent choices include Vitamin E oil or capsules, Wheatgerm oil, Jojoba oil, or Evening Primrose Oil. Only a small amount, about 2% of Vitamin E or 10% of Wheatgerm or Jojoba, is needed to preserve your oils. Remember, even though some essential oils are good for a few years, once they are mixed in with a carrier oil, the shelf life of the mixture will equal that of the vegetable oil. Most oils have a shelf life of approximately 6 months if kept under refrigeration and tightly capped.

The Carrier Oils (*appearing in alphabetical order*):

Almond, or *Sweet almond* as it is sometimes referred to, is considered a nut oil of light to medium weight. It is used frequently in massage oils for its protein-rich, lubricating, penetrating, and odorless qualities. It is expeller-pressed and good for all skin types. Commonly used in body oils and lotions.

Apricot kernel oil is an extremely fine, light seed oil high in Vitamin A and B, which helps with healing and rejuvenating skin cells. It is used frequently in facial preparations and for delicate, prematurely aging, inflamed, and sensitive skin. Good for all skin types.

Arnica oil is an *infusion* oil made from the *Arnica montana* plant. An "infusion" means it was made by soaking or infusing portions of a plant in a base oil like olive or sunflower oil to extract its medicinal properties. This oil is excellent for bruises and inflammation. Do not use on broken skin.

Avocado oil is made from the large seeds of the fruit's center. It contains a multitude of vitamins and skin-loving nutrients, making it ideal for undernourished, aging, or dry skin types. It has a very rich and heavy quality that spreads easily and has a slight sunscreen effect. Definitely keep this oil refrigerated and buy in small quantities as it has a short shelf life. Good for all skin types.

Borage oil is obtained from the seeds of the *Borago officinalis* plant. This oil is high (about 20%) in GLA (gamma linoleic acid), which is responsible for important metabolic functions, healthy hair, nails, and skin. An excellent choice to add in facial and special blends for problem areas in 10% dilution to stimulate and regenerate skin cells. Used as an alternative to Evening Primrose oil.

Calendula oil is an *infusion* oil made from the flowers of the *Calendula officinalis* plant. It excels in healing and moisturizing and has been traditionally used in first aid ointments, lip salves and lotions for dry, damaged skin. I use it in most of my body oils, as a portion of the entire blend of carrier. I couldn't be without it in the dry winter months when a "healing" oil is called for. If you have trouble finding it, here's my recipe you can use to make your own.

Calendula Oil Recipe. You can use fresh or dried flower heads. However, if you choose to make it with fresh flowers, be sure all the moisture is removed. Fill a slow cooker or crock pot with the clean, dry flower tops. Pour in enough olive oil to cover them completely and heat very slowly on the lowest setting for 24 hours. Alternatively, you can place them in a large glass jar in the sun for a few days. Strain well into squeaky-clean amber glass bottles and label. Add several Vitamin E capsules or oil to prolong the shelf life. Keep refrigerated.

Canola oil is made from the *Canadian rapeseed*. It is very light in texture and is odorless. It is high in linoleic acid, which aids in its longer shelf life. Used frequently in massage blends for easy absorption.

Carrot seed is in fact an *essential* oil of *Daucus carota* but it is most often used as part of a carrier. It has an orange color because it is rich in beta-carotene (antioxidant), vitamins, and minerals. Use in 10% dilution for its anti-aging and skin rejuvenating characteristic. It is used for preventing scar formation before and after surgical procedures and trauma. *Do not* use undiluted on the skin as this is an essential oil!

Castor oil is an expeller-pressed and filtered oil made from the seed of the Castor plant *Ricinus communis*. It is a heavy protective oil useful for sealing in moisture, as in bath oils and lipsticks. Soothing for all skin types.

Coconut oil is expeller-pressed and filtered from the coconut kernel. It is a solid at room temperature and has a melting point of about 76° F, so it melts easily at our body temperature. You must melt it to liquid form prior to adding essential oils. In the past, massage therapists used it extensively; however, as other oils become more readily available and less expensive, coconut oil use has declined. It can cause allergic reactions in some people.

Cocoa butter is a *wax* obtained from the roasted cocoa bean *Theobroma cacao* by expeller-pressing. You must melt this butter down before adding essential oils since it also is a solid at room temperature. It has emollient qualities and absorbs quickly into the skin's surface. It has a light creamy consistency and is used in cream-type moisturizers. Good for all skin types but avoid it if prone to skin allergic reactions.

Corn oil is a medium-weight oil obtained as a by-product of milling corn. It contains vitamins and minerals and is good for all skin types. It has a faint characteristic scent and will thicken upon exposure to air over time.

Evening Primrose oil is very high in GLA; this makes it an ideal antioxidant oil to add to other oil blends to slow down their tendency to become rancid. It is a relatively expensive oil to purchase, but is highly recommended to make preparations for aging skin, psoriasis, and eczema, since it counteracts free-radical damage and rejuvenates skin cells. Use in 10% dilution within another carrier oil. I always include it in my facial blends because it is good for all skin types.

Grapeseed, as its name suggests, is produced from the grape seed. It has a very fine texture and quickly penetrates the skin. It possesses no odor and is used in massage oil blends and facial oils. However, it is solvent-extracted, and if you are prone to acne or blackheads, some aestheticians recommend against its use on problem areas.

Hazelnut is made from the kernel's oil. It is rich in vitamins, minerals, and protein. Useful in facial preparations for its skin nourishing and softening qualities. It is easily absorbed and good for all skin types. One of the more expensive oils.

Hypericum or St. John's Wort oil is an *infusion* oil made from the fresh flowering tops of the *Hypericum perforatum* plant. It imparts a beautiful red color to the base oil and is used for muscle and joint inflammations, nerve-related pain as in neuralgia, and in many first-aid preparations.

Jojoba oil is pressed and filtered from the jojoba plant's bean-like seeds of this desert shrub. It is actually a liquid *wax,* not an oil. It is very similar to the moisturizer our own body produces called sebum. Use it in other carrier oils in 10% dilution to prevent them from going rancid. Good for all skin types, but especially for regulating overly dry or oily skin types.

Kukui Nut is a light, fine-textured and non-greasy oil becoming increasingly popular in some specialized facial blends. It is easily absorbed and high in Vitamins A, E, and F. Good for all skin types.

Lanolin is considered a *wax* and is obtained from the wool of sheep. It has a heavy, thick consistency and provides a protective moisturizing barrier. Used in ointments and lip salves. Not recommended for oily or acne-prone skin types.

Mineral oil is a refined synthetic by-product of petroleum. Because it is inexpensive and has an indefinite shelf life, it is found in many "commercial" cosmetics. Due to its large molecular structure, it prevents nutrients and essential oils from entering the skin surface and blocks moisture or waste from exiting. It is drying to the skin for this reason and is not recommended for personal body care preparations.

Mullein oil is an *infusion* oil made from the fresh yellow flowers of the *Verbascum thapsus* plant. Useful in first-aid oil preparations for painful and inflamed conditions like earache, wounds, and hemorrhoids.

Olive oil is expeller-pressed from olive fruit. You can purchase different grades of this oil. The first pressing is dark green, has the highest amount of vitamins and minerals and is called "extra virgin." The second pressing is referred to as "classico" or "virgin" olive oil and is golden in color. All varieties of this oil will have some distinct fragrance; therefore 50% dilution or less is recommended for its use as a carrier.

Peanut oil is prepared from the shelled and skinned seeds of the peanut plant. It is rich in vitamins and proteins and is an alternative to using olive and almond oil in skin care preparations. Has a slight fragrance; use as part of the carrier oil base. Good for all skin types.

Peach kernel oil is similar to apricot kernel oil. It is very emollient and helps with cell rejuvenation. Good for all skin types.

Pecan Nut oil is expeller-pressed and of medium weight. It is nutritive for the skin and good for all skin types.

Rosehip Seed oil is expeller-pressed from the fruit of *Rosa mosqueta* (or Rosa rubiginosa). It is high in vitamin C and is very rejuvenating and healing. Useful in scar tissue repair, treating age lines and damaged tissue cells. 10% dilution recommended.

Safflower oil is obtained from the pressed seed of the traditional herb *Carthamus tinctorius*. It softens the skin, is relatively odorless, and has a light-to-medium consistency. Good for all skin types. When left exposed to the air it will thicken.

Sesame oil is made from pressing the seeds. It is a lightweight oil rich in Vitamin E, minerals, protein, and lecithin. It can speed healing, prevent drying, soften the skin, and has a sunscreen effect of SPF4. In Ayurvedic medicine, daily sesame massage is practiced for its skin-aging prevention and balancing of the "doshas." Traditionally used to deter body lice.

Shea Butter is actually a *wax* in semi-solid form. It is made from the nuts of the Shea nut tree in South Africa. High in Vitamin E, it softens the skin and has a slight sunscreen effect. Useful in healing and protecting the skin. Use in 10% dilutions and must be melted before adding essential oils.

Soy oil is made from the soya bean. It has very little odor and is high in Vitamin E and lecithin. Good for all skin types. Is now increasingly popular among massage therapists as an alternative to sweet almond oil.

Squalene is an oil that was traditionally obtained from the liver of sharks. Today, however, it can be produced in smaller amounts from olive oil, wheatgerm oil, and rice bran oil. It is very expensive to purchase for this reason. Used in burn treatments and in specialty skin care products for its emollient, healing, and moisture protection.. Use in 2% to 10% dilutions. Good for all skin types.

Sunflower oil is pressed from the sunflower seeds which are rich in lecithin and Vitamin E. It is medium weight and has a slight detectable scent. Good for all skin types. Very common in massage, body lotions, and oils.

Vitamin E oil is produced by vacuum distillation of various vegetable oils. 100% pure Vitamin E (alpha-tocopherol) is very thick in consistency and is well-known as an antioxidant. It is added to carrier oils to prevent them from oxidizing in 2% dilution. Helps heal scar tissue, prevent aging by rejuvenating skin cellular activity. Can use Vitamin E oil capsules by cutting one end of capsule and squeezing into preparation. As a general guideline, I use 400IU for every ounce of carrier oil, to prevent it from oxidizing and to benefit the skin.

Walnut oil is made from the nut through expeller pressing. It is of medium weight and absorbs relatively easily. It is known to help balance the nervous system. Good for all skin types.

Wheatgerm oil is made from pressing the golden germ of the wheat grain. It is high in Vitamins A, D, and E, and is a natural antioxidant. Wheatgerm strengthens weakened capillaries, healing agent for scars, burns, and stretch marks. It regenerates skin cells and aids in keeping skin soft and supple. Good for all skin types. Use as 10% dilution and keep refrigerated.

Simplified Weight and Measure Equivalents

The following *estimated* equivalents have been provided for your use. The adjusted amounts are simplified in measuring quantity and dilution ratios, making a once complicated and time-consuming task easy and straightforward.

cc = ml

1 cc = 20 drops

5 cc = 1 teaspoon = 100 drops

10 cc = 2 teaspoons = 200 drops

15 cc = 1 tablespoon = 300 drops

30 cc = 1 ounce = 2 tablespoons = 600 drops

1/2 eyedropper holds approximately 10 drops

1 full eyedropper holds approximately 20 drops

1-ounce bottle = 30 cc = 2 tablespoons = 600 drops
2-ounce bottle = 60 cc = 4 tablespoons = 1200 drops
4-ounce bottle = 120 cc = 1/2 cup = 8 tablespoons = 2400 drops
8-ounce bottle = 240 cc = 1 cup = 16 tablespoons = 3600 drops

Carrier Volume   Essential Oil Dilution

	1%	2%	4%
1/2 oz. (1 TBS) [1/4 tsp antioxidant]	3 drops	6 drops	12 drops
1 oz. (2 TBS) [1/2 tsp antioxidant]	6 drops	12 drops	24 drops
2 oz. (4 TBS) [1 tsp antioxidant]	12 drops	24 drops	48 drops or 1/2 tsp
4 oz. (1/2 cup) [2 tsp antioxidant]	24 drops	48 drops or 1/2 tsp	96 drops or 1 tsp
8 oz. (1 cup) [4 tsp antioxidant]	48 drops or 1/2 tsp	96 drops or 1 tsp	192 drops or 2 tsp
16 oz. (2 cups) [8 tsp antioxidant]	96 drops or 1 tsp	192 drops or 2 tsp	384 drops or 4 tsp

Quick 'n' Easy Dilution Table

1% dilution: For children, the elderly, and expenctant mother's preparations

2% dilution: For typical whole body lotions and oils

4% dilution: For concentrated massage oil (local areas)

[ ] = Antioxidant which is the equivalent of 10% of the total carrier volume. This is the recommended amount of antioxidant to add to vegetable oils to prevent them from oxidizing. Optional.

A User-Friendly Blending Chart—How Much?

Method:	Carrier/Amount	Essential Oil/Drops
Whole Body Treatments:		
Aromatic Mud Body Mask	about 1 cup	8 to 10
Aromatic Body Scrub	about 1/2 cup	8 to 10
Aromatic Body Wrap	12 ounces	10 to 15
Aromatic Body Lotion*	8 ounce	80
Aromatic Body Oil*	4 ounces	50
Aromatic Bath*	full tub	6 to 10
Aromatic Shower	wet washcloth	6 to 8
Aromatic Sauna	3 cups water	3
Aromatic Jacuzzi	full tub	5 drops per person/ (not to exceed 15 total)
Inhalation:		
Steam/Vapor	4 to 6 cups	2 to 3
Humidifier	full	3 to 5
Aromatic Room Mist	4 ounce	10 to 20
Aroma Lamp	3/4 full	3 to 5
Light Bulb Ring	–	1 to 2
Tissue/Handkerchief	–	1 or 2
Local Treatments for Small Areas:		
Facial Mist	4 ounce	6 to 8
Facial Scrub	3 to 4 teaspoons	2 to 3
Facial Masks	3 to 4 teaspoons	3 to 5
Facial Steam	4 to 6 cups	2 to 3
Facial Oil	3 teaspoons	5
Concentrated Massage Oil*	2 ounces	50
Chest Rub*	2 ounces	30 to 50
Ointment	2 ounces	80 to 100
Compress	4 to 8 ounces	8 to 10
Poultice	1/4 to 1/2 cup	2 to 4
Foot/Hand Bath*	small tub	4 to 6
Hair Oil	1 ounce	20
Shampoo/Conditioner	8 ounce	80 to 100
Miscellaneous:		
Vacuum Machine	bag or filter	2 or 3 drops
Organic Household Cleaner	8 ounces	80 to 100 drops

Caution: Children, elderly, and pregnant women should divide Essential Oil amounts by at least 1/2.

Shall we go over an example? If you want to make a body oil you will need to make a 2% dilution of essential oil in a vegetable carrier. Let's assume you have a 4-ounce amber bottle in which to store your aromatherapy blend. The Dilution Table on the previous page shows you to add as part of the 4 ounces of vegetable oil, 2 teaspoons of antioxidant (optional), and 48 drops of essential oil to make the desired 2% dilution equivalent. If you want the blend to last longer than a month, I recommend you add jojoba, wheatgerm, or other antioxidant to prevent your fine creation from turning rancid.

To do this, count out the 48 drops of essential oil into the 4-ounce bottle. Then add 2 teaspoons of wheatgerm or jojoba oil as the antioxidant. Now all you have to do is fill up the remainder of the bottle with your chosen carrier vegetable oil. Note: if you know the size of the bottle, you don't have to measure the carrier. However, if you are not certain of how much the bottle holds in volume, measure it out. Refer to the *Simplified Weight and Measure Equivalents* for easy and fast measuring amounts.

Recycle your herbal extract and tincture amber bottles. These are useful for your aromatherapy blends. Make sure they are squeaky-clean or sterilize them.

Some bottles have a plastic stopper inside the bottle's neck. To count out drops using this built-in dropper, simply turn bottle upside down, (not on an angle) to count out single drops. However, when the bottle becomes half empty, I find it has a tendency to pour rather than drip its contents. If this is the case, it is best to remove the plastic stopper completely and use an eyedropper.

Practical Tips for Preparing Aromatherapy Blends

This can also be used as a checklist!

[ ] Work in an area that is well-lighted, well-ventilated, and without interruption.

[ ] Have exact dose or dilution rate, essential oil, carrier oil, charts, etc. handy to refer to.

[ ] Double-check the essential oils to be used as well as the dilution amount.

[ ] Do not use any essential oils that may be hazardous. Refer to Common Sense Safety, Chapter One.

[ ] Measure or count essential oils into clean amber bottle. If adding an antioxidant, add it next. Then add additional carrier oil to equal what is needed. For example, if you're using a 2-ounce bottle, just fill it to the top; there is no need to measure if you are certain it holds 2 fluid ounces. *When in doubt, measure it out.*

[ ] Measure drops by using an eyedropper. Use rubbing alcohol to clean and rinse the droppers between use, avoiding cross-contamination of different essential oils.

[ ] Label contents.

[ ] Keep a journal of aromatherapy blends you have made, with the corresponding results. When you make an effective blend or one you particularly like, you will want to be able to make the exact mixture again.

[ ] Wipe up any spills as essential oils can affect varnished wood surfaces and sometimes stain.

[ ] Wash hands thoroughly after measuring and mixing your preparations. Essential oils can be irritating to eyes and skin.

[ ] Keep screw tops securely closed when not in use; essential oils evaporate quickly.

[ ] Store essential oils out of reach of children, and away from light and heat sources.

The Resource Place

All of the essential oils discussed in this book are available through mail order from the following company as 100% pure botanical, genuine, and authentic, chemical-additive-free essential oils. Please write or send a facsimile request for a current price list.

Samara Botane
300 Queen Avenue, N., Suite 378
Seattle, WA 98109
1-800-782-4532
FAX 206-284-3592

Associations:

American Alliance of Aromatherapy
P.O. Box 750428
Petaluma, CA 94975-0428

National Association of Holistic Aromatherapy
P.O. Box 17622
Boulder, CO 80308

American Holistic Nurse's Association
P.O. Box 2130
Flagstaff, AZ 86003-2130

American Botanical Council
P.O. Box 201660
Austin, TX 78720-1660

The Herb Research Foundation
1007 Pearl Street, Ste. 200
Boulder, CO 80302

Education:

Atlantic Institute of Aromatherapy
1601 Saddlestring Drive, Dept. VC
Tampa, FL 33612

Pacific Institute of Aromatherapy
P.O. Box 6723
San Rafael, CA 94903

Journals:

The International Journal of Aromatherapy
P.O. Box 750428
Petaluma, CA 94975-0428

The Aromatherapy Quarterly Magazine
P.O. Box 421
Inverness, CA 94937-0421

Scentsitivity Newsletter
NAHA Administation Office
836 Hanley Industrial Court
St. Louis, MO 63144

The Aromatic Thymes
75 Lakeview Parkway
Barrington, IL 60010

Books of Interest:

*Creative Healing, An Introduction to Joseph B. Stephenson's "Hands-On"
Healing*, Patricia B. Bradley, Editor, Copyright 1993, The Joseph B. Stephenson
Foundation, Inc., P.O. Box 8446, Santa Rosa, CA 95407-1446.

Bibliography and Suggested Readings

Balacs, Tony, Hormones and Health, *International Journal of Aromatherapy*, Vol. 5, No. 1, Spring 1993, Aromatherapy Publications, USA.

Balacs, Tony, Safety in Pregnancy, *International Journal of Aromatherapy*, Vol. 4, No. 1, Spring 1992, Aromatherapy Publications, USA.

Bradley, Patricia B., *Creative Healing*, Joseph B. Stephenson Foundation, Inc.

Breecher, Maury, MPH, *Healthy Homes in a Toxic World*, John Wiley and Sons, 1992.

Burns, Ethel and Susanne Fischer-Rizzi, Inge Stadelmann, Karen Cutter, Dedicated to Better Birth, *International Journal of Aromatherapy*, Vol. 4, No. 1, Spring 1992, Aromatherapy Publications, USA.

Burns, Ethel and Caroline Blamey, Soothing Scents in Childbirth, *International Journal of Aromatherapy*, Vol. 6, No. 1, 1994, Aromatherapy Publications, USA.

Chopra, Deepak, MD, *Perfect Health—The Complete Mind/Body Guide*, Harmony Books, NY.

Colbin, Annemarie, *Food and Healing*, Ballantine Books, NY.

Colino, Stacey, Body/Mind News, *Self*, December 1994.

Coltrera, Francesca, Stress Busters, *Longevity*, November 1994.

Cox, Paul Alan and Michael J. Balick, The Ethnobotanical Approach to Drug Discovery, *Scientific American*, June 1994.

Diamond, Harvey and Marilyn, *Fit For Life*, Warner Books, NY.

Diamond, Harvey and Marilyn, *Living Health*, Warner Books, NY.

Ericksen, Marlene, Aromatherapy for Childbearing, *Mothering*, No. 71, Summer 1994.

Fawcett, Margaret, RGN, RM, LLSA, *Aromatherapy for Pregnancy and Childbirth*, Element Books Limited, Great Britain, 1993.

Facetti, Aldo, *Natural Beauty*, Simon and Schuster, NY, 1990.

Fettner, Ann Tucker, *Potpourri, Incense and Other Fragrant Concoctions*, Workman Publishing Co., NY, 1977.

Gattefosse, Rene-Maurice, *Gattefosse's Aromatherapy*, C.W. Daniel Co. Ltd., 1993.

Green, Mindy, Sex and Smell—Do Women Really Need Men?, *American Alliance of Aromatherapy News Quarterly*, Spring 1994.

Griggs, Barbara, *Green Pharmacy—The History and Evolution of Western Herbal Medicine*, Healing Arts Press, Vermont, 1981.

Grunwald, Jorg, Ph.D., The European Phytomedicines Market—Figures, Trends, Analyses, *HerbalGram* No. 34, The Journal of the American Botanical Council and The Herb Research Foundation, USA.

Guenier, Juliette, Essential Obstetrics, *International Journal of Aromatherapy*, Vol. 4, No. 1, Spring 1992, Aromatherapy Publications, USA.

Gumbel, Dr. Dietrich, Herbal Essence Therapy, *International Journal of Aromatherapy*, 1995, Vol. 6, No. 3, Aromatherapy Publications, USA.

Heinerman, John, *First Aid With Herbs*, Keats Publishing, Inc., USA.

Hirsch, Alan R., Scentsation, *International Journal of Aromatherapy*, Vol. 4, No. 1, Spring 1992, Aromatherapy Publications, USA.

Hirsch, Dr. Alan, Underrated Senses...Taste and Smell, Laura Lee Productions, Tape #191, WA.

Johnson, Kirk, The Herbal Love Potions, *East West*, February 1990.

Lad, Dr. Vasant, *Ayurveda—The Science of Self Healing*, Lotus Press, New Mexico.

Lawless, Julia, *The Encyclopedia of Essential Oils*, Element, USA.

Liddell, Dr. Keith, Smell as a Key to Diagnosis, International Journal of Aromatherapy, Vol. 3, No. 1, Aromatherapy Publications, England.

Maury, Marguerite, *Marguerite Maury's Guide to Aromatherapy—The Secret of Life and Youth: a Modern Alchemy*, C.W. Daniel Company Limited, England, 1989.

Mills, Simon Y., *Out of the Earth—The Essential Book of Herbal Medicine*, Viking, 1991.

Monte, Tom, *World Medicine—The East West Guide to Healing Your Body*, Putnam Publishing, 1993.

Murray, Linda, A Guide to Your Sexual Health, *Longevity*, January 1995.

Murray, Michael, ND., and Joseph Pizzorno, ND., *Encyclopedia of Natural Medicine*, Prima Publishing, 1991.

Ody, Penelope, *The Complete Medicinal Herbal*, Dorling Kindersley, NY.

Pugliese, Peter T., MD., *Advanced Professional Skin Care*, APSC Publishing, USA.

Richardson, Sarah, The Brain-Boosting Sex Hormone, *Discover,* April 1994.

Schnaubelt, Kurt, Pacific Institute of Aromatherapy Course, 1985.

Scholes, Michael, Recent Innovations in Environmental Fragrancing Technology, *Beyond Scents,* Spring 1993, Aromatherapy Seminars, USA.

Sheppard-Hanger, Sylla, *The Aromatherapy Practitioner Reference Manual,* Atlantic Institute of Aromatherapy, Tampa, Florida, U.S.A., 1995.

Stanway, Dr. Andrew, MD., MRCP., *The Natural Family Doctor,* Simon and Schuster, Inc., NY.

Steele, John, Environmental Fragrancing, *International Journal of Aromatherapy,* Vol. 4, No. 2, Summer 1992, Aromatherapy Publications, USA.

Sutcliffe, Dr. Jenny and Nancy Duin, *A History of Medicine,* Barnes and Noble Books, 1992.

Tisserand, Robert B., *The Art of Aromatherapy,* Healing Arts Press, Vermont, 1977.

Tisserand, Robert, Medicine For Sick Buildings, *International Journal of Aromatherapy,* Vol. 3, No. 3, Autumn 1991.

Tucker, Arthur O., Herbs vs. Bugs, *Herb Companion,* June/July 1994.

Upton, M. D., and Graber, M. S., *Staying Healthy in a Risky Environment—The New York University Medical Center Family Guide,* Simon and Schuster, 1993.

Watt, Martin, *Plant Aromatics—A Data and Reference Manual on Essential Oils and Aromatic Plant Extracts,* Atlantic Institute of Aromatherapy, Tampa, Florida, U.S.A.

Watt, Martin, *Plant Aromatics—Effects on the Skin of Aromatic Extracts*, Atlantic Institute of Aromatherapy, Tampa, Florida, U.S.A.

Woodward, Alexander, *How To Improve Brain Capacity Naturally*, Special Report IV, William L. Fischer, Publisher.

Woodward, Alexander, *The Truth About a More Exciting Sex Life*, Special Report I, William L. Fischer, Publisher.

Woodward, Alexander, *Nutritional Secrets to More Youthful Skin*, Special Report, William L. Fischer, Publisher.

Worwood, Valerie Ann, *The Complete Book of Essential Oils and Aromatherapy*, New World Library, USA.

Valnet, Jean, MD., *The Practice of Aromatherapy*, Healing Arts Press, 1982.

_____, Aromatherapy on the Wards, *International Journal of Aromatherapy*, May 1988 Vol.1, No. 2, Aromatherapy Publications, E. Sussex, England.

_____, Frequent Causes of Stress, July 1994 Gallup Poll, *Health*, October 1994.

_____, Snooze News, Healthfront, *Prevention*, Rodale Press, Inc., May 1994.

Personal notes taken Spring 1995, The Psychobiology of Mental Control, Dr. John Madden, Ph.D.., Institute for CorText Research and Development.

_____, Menopause, Women's Survey, *Prevention*, August 1994.

_____, *The Lippincott Manual of Nursing Practice*, Second Edition, J.B. Lippincott Co., 1978.

_____, *University of California, Berkeley Wellness Letter*, Vol. 5 Issue 10, July 1989.

_____, Cancer Facts and Figures—1995, American Cancer Society, Atlanta, Georgia, USA.

Index

A

Abdominal cramping/flatulence:
  anti-gas lozenge, 46
  anti-spasm massage blend, 46
  herb tea for, 47
  symptoms of, 45
Absolutes, 10
Acetylcholine, 222
Acne:
  antiseptic toner for, 176-77
  causes of, 174
  facial steams for, 175-76
  lifestyle/dietary recommendations, 178
  light moisturizing oil for, 177-78
Acute rhinitis, 70-72
Aging skin, See Skin
Agrimony, and sore throat, 36
Allergies:
  Allergy Relief Formula, 106-7
  Allergy Relief Synergy Blend, 105
  causes of, 102-3
  Clear Head Blend, 105-6
  defined, 102-3
  and essential oils, 10
  footbath for, 106-7
  lifestyle/dietary recommendations, 107
  pollen, 103-4
  skin reactions, allergic-type, 106
  and synthetic fragrances, 104
  treatment of, 103
All-over body treatments, See Whole body
    treatments
Almond, 372
  and sensitive skin, 173
Aloe vera:
  and hemorrhoids, 59
  and infection, 190
  and minor cuts/wounds/abrasions, 213
Alveoli, 94
Angelica, 256
Anise, 29
  and colitis, 53
  and digestive problems, 36, 41, 43, 47, 53
Anosmia, 72-75
  causes of, 72-73
  conditions/ailments affecting, 73
  Sense-able Nasal Oil, 75
  stimulating sense of smell, 74
Anti-Anxiety Massage Oil, 235
Anti-Fungal Bath, 210
Anti-Gas Lozenge, 46
Antiseptic Ointment, 213

Antiseptic Toner for Acne, 176-77
Antiseptic Vinegar, 212-13
Anti-Spasm Massage Blend, 46
Anti-stress essences, 53
Anti-Stress Synergy, 227
Anxiety, 234-35
  aromatic bath for, 234-35
  causes of, 234
Aphrodisiacs, 253-58
  angelica, 256
  definition of, 253
  jasmine absolute, 256
  lifestyle/dietary recommendations, 258
  Love Oil, 257
  and olfactory system, 255
  Tea for Two, 257
Apple cider vinegar, and sore throat, 36, 85
Apricot kernel, 314, 372
  and oily skin, 172
  and sensitive skin, 173
Arnica oil, 372
Aroma lamp, 331
Aromatherapy, 198
  and children, 17
  defined, 3-4
  fundamentals of, 3-20
  and pregnancy, 17, 19-20
  treatments:
    for children, 197-20
    for circulatory system, 113-39
    for digestive system, 25-59
    for emotions/moods/memory, 221-58
    for eye, ear, nose, and throat problems, 60-91
    for the musculo-skeletal system, 140-58
    for respiratory system, 92-112
    for skin and hair, 159-96
  See also Essential oils; Psycho-aromatherapy
Aromatherapy massage, 309-11
Aromatic Bath, 183
Aromatic baths, 53, 256, 291-305
  abcs of, 297
  for anxiety, 234-35
  Aromatic Honey Bath, 298
  for arthritis, 145
  Arthritis Hand Bath, 305
  Athlete's Foot Bath, 304
  Bath Oil, 299
  Bath Salts, 299
  and body odor, 183
  Botanical Bath, 298-99
  carriers, 293-95